Advances in
EXTRACTION AND APPLICATIONS OF BIOACTIVE PHYTOCHEMICALS

Advances in EXTRACTION AND APPLICATIONS OF BIOACTIVE PHYTOCHEMICALS

MIHIR KUMAR PURKAIT
Department of Chemical Engineering,
Indian Institute of Technology Guwahati, Guwahati,
Assam, India
Chair Professor, National Jal Jeevan Mission (NJJM),
Government of India, New Delhi, India

DIBYAJYOTI HALDAR
Department of Biotechnology, Karunya Institute of
Technology and Sciences, Coimbatore, Tamil Nadu

PRANGAN DUARAH
Center for the Environment, Indian Institute of
Technology Guwahati, Guwahati, Assam, India

ELSEVIER

ACADEMIC PRESS
An imprint of Elsevier

Academic Press is an imprint of Elsevier
125 London Wall, London EC2Y 5AS, United Kingdom
525 B Street, Suite 1650, San Diego, CA 92101, United States
50 Hampshire Street, 5th Floor, Cambridge, MA 02139, United States
The Boulevard, Langford Lane, Kidlington, Oxford OX5 1GB, United Kingdom

ISBN: 978-0-443-18535-9

For information on all Academic Press publications visit our website at https://www.elsevier.com/books-and-journals

Publisher: Mica Haley
Acquisitions Editor: Andre G. Wolff
Editorial Project Manager: Tracy Tufaga
Production Project Manager: Swapna Srinivasan
Cover Designer: Greg Harris

Typeset by TNQ Technologies

Contents

Author biography *ix*
Preface *xi*
Acknowledgment *xiii*

1. Pharmaceutical prospects of plant-based bioactive molecules **1**
1.1 Introduction 1
1.2 Overview and structural compositions of naturally occurring bioactive phytochemical compounds 3
1.3 Analytical approaches for determining bioavailability and bioaccessibility of bioactive compounds 19
1.4 Commercialization of naturally occurring bioactive compounds 21
1.5 Conclusions and future perspectives 22
References 23

2. Utilization of various parts of the plant for the extraction of phytochemicals and high-throughput screening techniques **29**
2.1 Introduction 29
2.2 Different parts of plants used to produce the pharmaceutically active compound 31
2.3 High-throughput screening techniques for bioactive phytochemicals 44
2.4 Summary 50
References 51

3. Conventional approaches for the extraction of bioactive compounds for pharmaceutical applications **55**
3.1 Introduction 55
3.2 Conventional approaches for the extraction of bioactive compounds 56
3.3 Limitations associated with the conventional techniques 69
3.4 Summary 71
References 71

4. Advancement in bioactive compound extraction from natural products for pharmaceutical applications **75**
4.1 Introduction 75
4.2 Different extraction approaches 76
4.3 Future perspectives 95

4.4 Summary 96

References 96

5. Neoteric solvents for extraction of bioactive phytochemicals 101

5.1 Introduction 101

5.2 Classification of different synthetic solvents 103

5.3 The emergence of solvent-free reactions in pharmaceutical industries 114

5.4 Summary 115

References 116

6. Application and effectiveness of computational methods in improving the production of bioactive phytochemicals 119

6.1 Introduction 119

6.2 Insight into the progress of different computational tools 122

6.3 Insight into the advancement of molecular docking 127

6.4 Insight on molecular dynamics simulation for diseases and drug design 132

6.5 Summary 136

References 137

7. Advances in encapsulation strategies for bioactive phytochemicals 141

7.1 Introduction 141

7.2 Different encapsulation processes for bioactive compounds 142

7.3 Future perspectives 161

7.4 Summary 162

References 163

8. Applications of herb-derived bioactive phytochemicals 167

8.1 Introduction 167

8.2 Treatment of orthopedic diseases using herbal extracts 168

8.3 Influence of herbal plants as immunity boosters in the treatment of COVID-19 and other diseases 177

8.4 Effect of herbal nanoformulation in the applications of tropical delivery 188

8.5 Summary 190

References 191

9. Pharmacologic and therapeutic aspects of various medicinal plants 197

9.1 Introduction 197

9.2 Medicinal effect of *Nigella sativa* in different fields 198

9.3 Selective plants in the treatment of different diseases 203
9.4 Medicinal efficacy of phytochemicals 209
9.5 Summary 213
References 214

10. Applications of plant-derived metal nanoparticles in pharmaceuticals 219

10.1 Introduction 219
10.2 Biosynthesis of metallic nanoparticles for pharmaceutical application 220
10.3 Factors influencing the production of metallic nanoparticles from plant extract 226
10.4 Application of metallic nanoparticles in pharmaceuticals 229
10.5 Limitations and future perspectives 235
10.6 Summary 237
References 238

11. Patents on naturally derived pharmaceuticals 243

11.1 Introduction 243
11.2 Patents on naturally derived pharmaceuticals 245
11.3 Summary 263
References 264

Index *265*

Author biography

Dr. Mihir Kumar Purkait is a Professor in the Department of Chemical Engineering, Chair Professor of National Jal Jeevan Mission, Dean of Alumni and External Affairs, and former Head of Centre for the Environment at Indian Institute of Technology Guwahati (IITG). Prior to joining as faculty at IITG (2004), he received his Ph.D. and M.Tech in Chemical Engineering from the Indian Institute of Technology, Kharagpur (IITKGP) after completing his B.Tech and B.Sc. (Hons) in Chemistry from the University of Calcutta. He has received several awards, e.g., Dr. A.V. Rama Rao Foundation's Best Ph.D. Thesis and Research Award in Chemical Engineering from IIChE (2007), BOYSCAST Fellow award (2009–10) from the DST, Young Engineers Award in the field of Chemical Engineering from the Institute of Engineers (India, 2009), and Young Scientist Medal award from the Indian National Science Academy (INSA, 2009). Prof. Purkait is a Fellow of several academic and professional body/societies. His current research activities are focused in four distinct areas, viz., (1) advanced separation technologies, (2) waste to energy, (3) smart materials for various applications, and (4) process intensification. In each of the areas, his goal is to synthesize stimuli-responsive materials and to develop a more fundamental understanding of the factors governing the performance of the chemical and biochemical processes. He has around 20 years of experience in academics and research and has published more than 250 papers in different reputed journals (citation >12,000, h-index = 64, 10 index = 152). He has 10 patents and has completed 35 sponsored and consultancy projects from various funding agencies. Prof. Purkait has guided 20 Ph.D. students. He is the author of 10 books and several book chapters published in reputed internal journals.

Dr. Dibyajyoti Haldar is an Assistant Professor in the Department of Biotechnology at Karunya Institute of Technology and Sciences (Deemed to be University), Coimbatore, India. He is a former Post-Doctoral Fellow at the Centre for the Environment, Indian Institute of Technology Guwahati (IITG), India. He obtained his Ph.D. in Chemical Engineering from the National Institute of Technology Agartala (NITA), India, and his M.Tech in Environmental Science and Technology from the National Institute of Technology Durgapur (NITDGP), India. His research work includes conversion of lignocellulosic biomass into fermentable sugars, enzymatic hydrolysis, biofuels, formation of value-added products derived from agricultural wastes, and processes kinetics and modeling. He has published more than 25 scientific research and review papers in various reputed international journals. He is the author of several book chapters and two books (ISBN: 9780128188019 and ISBN: 9780128235348) published by Elsevier. Dr. Haldar is the Review Editor for Frontiers in Chemistry journal (SCI indexed) in the Green and Sustainable Chemistry Section. He is the recipient of Most Cited Review Paper Award for his review article, "A review on the production of fermentable sugars from lignocellulosic biomass through conventional and enzymatic route—A comparison" published and downloaded for the period 2016—20 in International Journal of Green Energy organized by 13th International Green Energy Conference on July 18th, 2021, in Beijing, China. He also received International Teaching Excellence Award in Biochemical Engineering in Global Annual Education & Research Excellence Awards 2021 by Centre for Professional Advancement (CPACE, AP) on December 18th, 2021. During his Ph.D., he received the Best Oral Presentation Award in a 1-day workshop on "Current Trends in Scientific Research" at Research Scholars' Day 2018 organized by the National Institute of Technology Agartala, India. He is a potential reviewer of various SCI-indexed international journals. He has attended several conferences of national and international repute.

Prangan Duarah is a doctoral research fellow at the Centre for the Environment in the Indian Institute of Technology, Guwahati. He worked on a research project at the Indian Institute of Technology, Bombay, before joining IIT Guwahati as a research fellow. He graduated from North-Eastern Hill University in Shillong, India, with a B.Tech in Energy Engineering. His current field of study focuses on naturally derived pharmaceutical compounds and green nanomaterial synthesis for various applications. He is a recipient of the prestigious Prime Minister's Research Fellowship (PMRF), which is given to the country's most outstanding research scholars as a token of encouragement to pursue their research. He has published more than five journal papers and several book chapters in peer-reviewed international publications.

Preface

In the realm of naturally derived pharmaceuticals, tremendous advancements have emerged during the last several decades. However, these pharmaceutical lead compounds confront a number of challenges, including the need to separate the various compounds from the original extract and the risk of investing time and money in an activity that may not produce a unique compound. The book explains the fundamental and advanced topics involved with the technologies for extracting and utilizing plant-derived pharmaceutically active compounds. The uniqueness of this book lies in the fact that it covers every aspect related to the topic, including extraction method, high-throughput screening techniques, computational advancements, utilization for critical illness treatment, encapsulation techniques, and patent-related details. A primary goal of this study is to address the recent contributions and advancements of natural products in pharmaceuticals. The first introductory chapter of the book is more prominent exactly for beginners or new readers of pharmaceutical and chemical backgrounds. This chapter will highlight the importance of various naturally derived bioactive components and their commercial aspect. Chapter 2 is based on the extraction and high-throughput techniques for screening pharmaceutically active compounds from various plants and their different portions. Chapter 3 will give an insight into the basics of various conventional extraction methods to separate bioactive elements from the source material. Chapter 4 features the advanced bioactive element extraction from natural products for pharmaceutical applications. Chapter 5 discusses the influence of neoteric solvents on the extraction process. Chapter 6 is for the readers to develop a fundamental knowledge of and highlight the development in computational techniques such as artificial intelligence for simulation, drug design, and molecular docking. Chapter 7 focuses on the advancement in the encapsulation techniques for bioactive elements. Thereafter, chapter 8 highlights the treatment of orthopedic diseases using herbal extracts as well as the influence of herbal plants as immunity boosters in the treatment of COVID-19. Chapter 9 explores selective plants for the treatment of some acute diseases such as asthma, diabetes, cancer, etc. Thereafter, chapter ten is based on the synthesis of metal nanoparticles using plant extract for pharmaceutical applications. Finally, chapter eleven features some of the patented processes related to the extraction and use of the bioactive compound. According to the authors, this is the first time that the readers will be provided with a book in which fundamental and advanced concepts of extraction of plant-based pharmaceutically active compounds are presented. There is something for everyone in the book. The readers will find the book and its content exciting and will be able to grasp the topics very easily.

Acknowledgment

The successful completion of this book has been a long scholastic journey embedded with love, trust, and support from some of the most valuable people and communities of our lives. Today, at the acme of our publication, we greatly remember our parents, family, friends, and well-wishers. Without their enthusiastic support and active participation, this book would not have taken shape. The honor is elevated manifold because of the very opportunity bestowed upon us by our esteemed institutions: the Indian Institute of Technology, Guwahati, and Karunya Institute of Technology and Sciences, Coimbatore. We will be forever grateful for that. We would also like to express our gratitude to Indian National Academy of Engineering, Gurgaon, India, for the support.

CHAPTER 1

Pharmaceutical prospects of plant-based bioactive molecules

1.1 Introduction

Nature has been exploited by people in the hunt for food and bioactive substances to use as poisons and to cure various illnesses from the dawn of time. Photosynthetic organisms on land and at sea have the ability to collect carbon dioxide and use their numerous sophisticated mechanisms to make bioactive compounds when combined with natural light and water. Plants have historically been the most important source of such compounds [1,2].

We have grown more vulnerable to a wide range of life-threatening illnesses due to our shifting diets and lifestyles. In this scenario, various plant-based products such as vegetables, fruits, and seeds, in particular, may help avoid chronic diseases such as malaria, hypertension, inflammatory bowel illnesses, cancer, coronary heart disease, diabetes, and other diseases caused by pathogens, to name a few. Macronutrients (comprising calcium, magnesium, phosphorus, sulfur), micronutrients (such as iron, copper, manganese, zinc, sodium, molybdenum, and boron), a protein with essential amino acids, dietary fiber, and vitamins are all found in plants, and their presence aids the human body's defenses against pathogens like bacteria, viruses, and parasites. Furthermore, compounds found in plants have significant antioxidant activity, which helps to boost immunity and reduce age-related health problems [3,4]. Various studies have been conducted throughout the years to better understand the advantages of such compounds. Additionally, the separation, purification, and structural identification of single compounds from plant extracts have become possible due to the advancement of analytical methods, such as gas chromatography, nuclear magnetic resonance spectrometry, mass spectrometry, and high-performance liquid chromatography. These cutting-edge methods aid in identifying a broad spectrum of physiologically active molecules known as

Advances in Extraction and Applications of Bioactive Phytochemicals
ISBN 978-0-443-18535-9
https://doi.org/10.1016/B978-0-443-18535-9.00013-2

"phytochemicals." These phytochemicals are nonnutrient bioactive molecules produced by secondary metabolism in plants that operate as a defense system, protecting them from pest and disease infections, environmental pressures such as drought and salt stress, ultraviolet (UV) exposures, and other harmful situations [5]. They vary from primary metabolic substances in that they are exclusively formed in particular cells and are not produced by either catabolic or anabolic metabolism [6].

Many studies show that phytochemicals can reduce the risk of major noncommunicable chronic illnesses if taken daily. Many live cells interact with bioactive phytochemicals that prevent DNA damage while slowing the formation of aberrant or damaged ones, such as cancerous cells, by reducing their ability to divide and multiply. There are several ways phytochemicals work against tumors, including destroying rapidly proliferating cells, decreasing oxidative stress, altering the function of growth hormones in cells, inducing apoptosis, and blocking the formation of new blood vessels in malignant tissues. Due to their pharmacologic effects and the fact that they are nontoxic to human cells, they might serve as essential sources for producing drugs to treat a variety of malignancies and other disorders.

To prevent oxidative stress in cell, components including proteins, nucleic acids, and lipids, antioxidants must be present. Antioxidants work by inhibiting the generation of reactive oxygen species or free radicals during various metabolic processes. As a result, a diet rich in plant-based foods provides a wide range of phytochemicals, which are well-known to protect against disease. A wide variety of phytonutrients, including polyphenols, organosulfur compounds, terpenes, steroids, etc., may be found in vegetables and other plant-based meals. The advent of high-sensitivity analytical tools has made it feasible to detect and extract these phytonutrients, as well. It is possible to extract phytochemicals, compounds found in plants, from a wide variety of plant parts and then conduct in-depth analyses to see whether they may be used to treat or prevent certain health conditions [7].

Some of the most important phytochemicals and the biologic roles they play are covered in this chapter. Additionally, various physical and chemical properties of phytochemical groups are highlighted. The chapter also emphasizes analytical methodologies for assessing the bioavailability and bioaccessibility of bioactive substances.

1.2 Overview and structural compositions of naturally occurring bioactive phytochemical compounds

1.2.1 Polyphenols

For treating metabolic syndrome in vitro and in vivo, polyphenols, which are found in many plants, are the most active ingredients. The biologic efficiency of these compounds has been the subject of several studies and reviews. In general, polyphenols are naturally occurring chemicals that share phenolic structural characteristics chemically. As a collective name, "polyphenols" encompasses a variety of chemicals, although the term has been misused, and its inferred chemical structures have proved ambiguous to researchers. In the scientific community, the word "polyphenols" is used to describe plant polyphenols, whereas "plant phenols" is also used to describe the same by some researchers. The term "polyphenols" is still favored for corporate communication, according to Quideau et al. [8]. According to this definition, the term "phenols" encompasses the arene ring and its hydroxy substituents, and the term "polyphenol" should be limited to structures with at least two phenolic moieties, regardless of the number of hydroxy groups they each contain [8].

One of the most abundant and widely dispersed families of secondary metabolites in plants is phenolic compounds. Polyphenols include compounds not only with a polyphenol structure but also molecules with only one phenol ring, such as phenolic acids and phenolic alcohols, as previously discussed. Although polyphenols are technically defined as compounds having phenolic structural properties, they are a varied collection of natural products that include various subgroups of phenolic compounds. Biogenetically, phenolic compounds are generated by two metabolic pathways: the shikimic acid pathway, which produces phenylpropanoids primarily, and the acetic acid pathway, which produces simple phenols primarily. Carbon from photosynthesis is believed to be used to produce between 100,000 and 200,000 secondary metabolites. The phenylpropanoid pathway, which is used to make most phenolic compounds in plants, accounts for approximately 20% of all carbon used in photosynthesis [9]. Flavonoids, the most abundant category of phenolic chemicals in nature, are formed when both processes are combined. Condensed tannins or nonhydrolyzable tannins are created along the biosynthetic routes to flavonoids production, among the not well-understood condensation and polymerization stages. Gallic acid or hexahydroxydiphenic acid derivatives are examples of hydrolyzable tannins. Polyphenols may be connected with numerous organic acids or with one another, in addition to their chemical variety.

More than 1000 different polyphenolic compounds with a diverse range of structures have been discovered (including over 8150 flavonoids). Phenolic phytochemicals are classified into three groups based on their dispersion in nature: those that are broadly dispersed, those that are widely distributed, and those that are polymeric. Similarly, based on the chemical structure, polyphenols can be divided into three distinct categories (phenolic acids, flavonoids, and nonflavonoids), as shown in Fig. 1.1 [10,11].

Aglycone-based categorization is the most used method of categorizing polyphenols. However, polyphenolic substances can be categorized in a variety of ways following this approach. Harborne [12] classified phenolic chemicals into 16 primary classes based on their carbon chain, as shown in Table 1.1.

Apart from the chemical categorization, researchers classify polyphenols according to the amount of phenol rings they possess and the structural features that connect the rings (Fig. 1.2). Moreover, the list of polyphenolic categories is nonetheless consistent. Of all the phenolic chemicals found in plants, flavonoids are by far the most prevalent and well researched. Anthocyanidins, flavones, isoflavones, flavonols, flavanols, flavones, and flavanones are among the most significant flavonoid groups, which are further classified by the degree of hydroxylation and the existence of a $C_2{-}C_3$ double bond in heterocyclic pyrone rings. There are considerable structural changes in the three-ring structures of these compounds depending on the degree of hydrogenation and hydroxylation that has occurred in these groups [14]. About 8000 compounds of flavonoids have been identified so far, many of which are sulfate or methylated, conjugated with mono- and disaccharides, lipids, amino acids, carboxylic acids, and organic acids [15].

Phenolic acid is another popular type that belongs to the group polyphenols. One or more of the following groups can be found in the molecular structure of phenolic acid: carboxylic group, benzenic ring, hydroxyl, and/or methoxyl groups. Phenolic acid can be broadly categorized into two types, i.e., benzoic acids and cinnamic acids. Benzoic acid is one of the simplest phenolic acids found in nature, with seven carbon atoms ($C_6{-}C_1$). Cinnamic acids ($C_6{-}C_3$), which have nine carbon atoms, are seldom seen in plants in their free form.

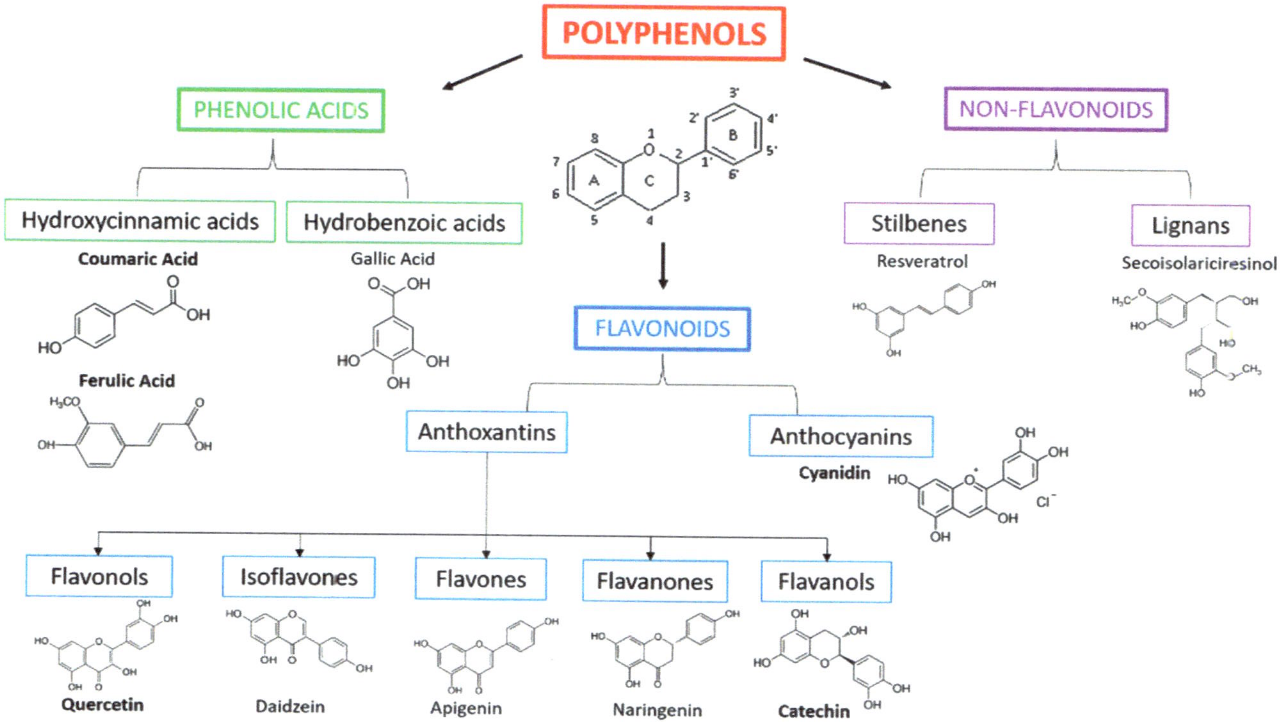

Figure 1.1 Classification of polyphenols based on their chemical structure [10].

Table 1.1 Classification of phenolic chemicals based on their carbon chain.

Phenolic class	Carbon chain skeleton
Simple phenols	C_6
Benzoquinones	C_6
Phenolic acids	$C_6{-}C_1$
Acetophenones	$C_6{-}C_2$
Phenylacetic acids	$C_6{-}C_2$
Hydroxycinnamic acids	$C_6{-}C_3$
Phenylpropenes	$C_6{-}C_3$
Coumarins and isocoumarins	$C_6{-}C_3$
Chromones	$C_6{-}C_3$
Naphthoquinones	$C_6{-}C_4$
Xanthones	$C_6{-}C_1{-}C_6$
Stilbenes	$C_6C_2C_6$
Anthraquinones	$C_6{-}C_2{-}C_6$
Flavonoids	$C_6{-}C_3{-}C_6$
Lignins	$C_6{-}(C_3)_n$
Lignans and neolignans	$C_6{-}(C_3)_2$

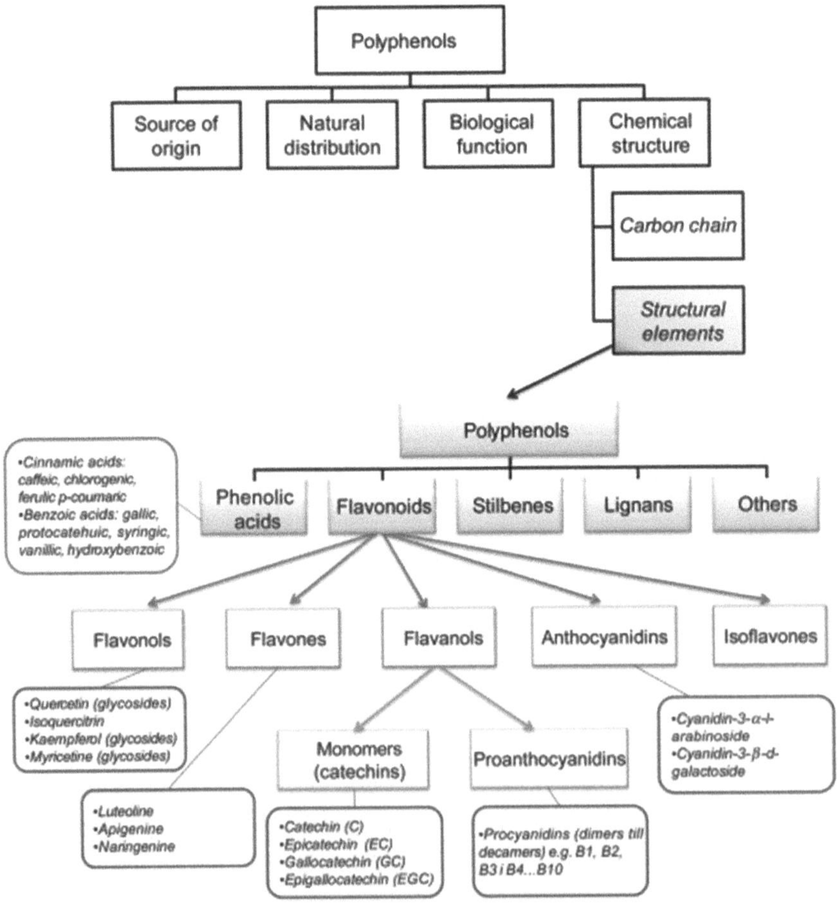

Figure 1.2 Plant polyphenols and polyphenolic groups classified by number of phenol rings and structural components. *(Reproduced with permission from Cvitanović et al. [13].)*

A cyclic alcohol acid is usually seen in combination with the ester form of these compounds. Caffeoyl ester is the most important combination of neochlorogenic acid, isochlorogenic acid, chlorogenic acid, and crypto-chlorogenic acid, all of which are esters that include cyclic alcohol-acids like quinic acid and cinnamic acid [16]. Phenolic acids, in fact, constitute one-third of all phenolic compounds found in the human diet, according to Yang et al. [17]. The quantity of hydroxyl groups in phenolic acids and their esters influences their antioxidant activity. Among the two types, cinnamic acids that have been hydroxylated are more efficient than benzoic acids in general.

Other forms of polyphenols found in dietary sources include lignans and stilbenes. Two phenylpropane units make up lignans. Linseed, which provides secoisolariciresinol (up to 3.7 g/kg dry wt.) and modest amounts of matairesinol, is the most abundant dietary source. Linseed has up to 1000 times more lignans than dairy products as well as other cereals, grains, fruits, and vegetables [18]. Stilbenes are found in tiny levels in the human diet, yet they are beneficial. Wine contains many antioxidants, one of which, resveratrol, is found in modest concentrations (15 mg glycosides/L in red wine and 0.3 to 7 mg aglycones/L in white wine) and has been extensively studied for its anticarcinogenic qualities [19].

1.2.1.1 Properties of polyphenols

Polyphenols have a diverse variety of qualities depending on their specific structural configurations. Based on the vast amount of research available on plant polyphenols and their capabilities, the most important attributes of polyphenols may be grouped into many categories.

For polyphenols, solubility is a critical factor. When the plant phenolics have been entirely esterified, etherified, or glycosylated, polar organic solvents tend to dissolve them. The corresponding aglycones of most phenolic glycosides are water-soluble; however, this is not always the case. Water solubility generally rises with the amount of hydroxyl groups present, with a few notable exceptions.

UV absorption is intense for all phenolic compounds; colorful phenolic compounds also absorb heavily in the visible range [20]. Phenolic chemicals are classified according to their different classes based on their absorption properties. In the 250–290 nm range, phenols and phenolic acids exhibit their spectral peak; similarly, at wavelengths of 250 and 350 nm, cinnamic acid derivatives exhibit absorption bands of approximately equal strength; flavones and flavonols have absorption bands at around 250 and 350 nm that are roughly comparable in strength; chalcones and aurones have a strong absorption peak at 350 nm and a weaker band at 250 nm. When measured at wavelengths between 475 and 560 nm and between 535 and 545 nm, anthocyanins and betacyanins show a similar absorption peak, respectively, whereas their secondary absorption peak is 270–275 nm. These compounds are secondary metabolites generated by plants, and they are employed to safeguard them against the harmful effects of UV radiation and disease.

1.2.2 Alkaloids

W. Meissner created the term "alkaloids" in 1818 to describe all organic substances derived from plants that have a basic structure. Later research revealed that alkaloids include a heterocyclic ring system that contains the nitrogen atom. Primary, secondary, tertiary, and quaternary amines are all included in this definition [21]. There have been various scientific breakthroughs since then that have helped shape the characteristics that define this class of substances, which has resulted in numerous chemical structures being introduced into this class. Alkaloids have been found in plants, animals, and microbes, including humans, marine creatures, fungi, and other bacteria. Compounds possessing side chain–bearing nitrogen, nitrogen-containing functional groups, or any combination of these were also categorized as alkaloids because of their neutral nature [22].

It is possible to categorize alkaloids based on their chemical structure, biologic activity, biosynthesis mechanism, and occurrence into heterocyclic and nonheterocyclic alkaloids, as shown in Fig. 1.3.

1.2.2.1 Heterocyclic alkaloids

Fig. 1.4 depicts the basic structure of the naturally occurring alkaloids. Heterocyclic alkaloids have a nitrogen atom in their structure. They are made biosynthetically from the amino acids they are named after, and they are frequently generated after a decarboxylation procedure. Based on the amino acid of origin, six primary categories of alkaloids have been identified so far. L-ornithine, L-tyrosine/L-phenylalanine, L-lysine, L-tryptophan, L-histidine, and glycine/aspartic acid are all derivatives of these amino acids [23]. Derivatives of these primary groups also play a significant role. For example, isoquinoline alkaloids, a derivative of L-tyrosine/L-phenylalanine, are a class of compounds that are among the most diversified natural compound in the world. In their skeleton, they have an isoquinoline or tetrahydroisoquinoline ring that is biogenically produced from

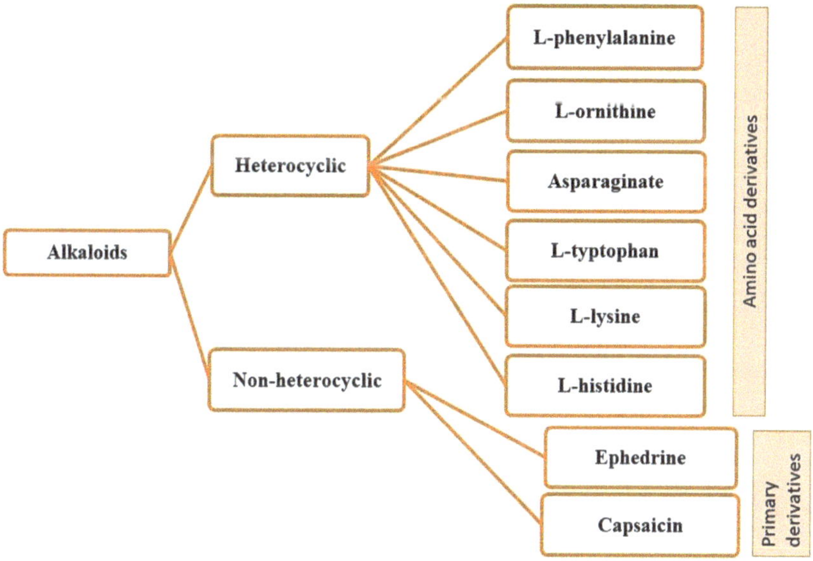

Figure 1.3 Classification of alkaloids.

phenylalanine and tyrosine [24]. The isoquinoline alkaloids are a diverse category of compounds that are not structurally homogenous. There are eight subgroups within this group (i.e., benzylisoquinoline, aporphine, protoberberine, protopine, benzo[c]phenanthridine, morphinan, phthalideisoquinoline, and emetine alkaloids), each with a distinct degree of oxygenation and intramolecular rearrangement, as well as a varied pattern of distribution and the occurrence of additional rings linked to the main system.

When it comes to alkaloids, protoberberines represent about a quarter of all structures revealed so far, making them the most common nitrogen-containing secondary metabolites found in nature. Isoquinoline alkaloids may be found in Berberidaceae, Papaveraceae, Fumariaceae, Ranunculaceae, Menispermaceae, Rutaceae, and Annonaceae, as well as in a variety of other plant groups (in the dehydro forms). Plants of the Magnoliaceae and Convolvulaceae families are also rich in these alkaloids [25,26].

Proline and L-ornithine, two amino acids, are shown to be precursors of the alkaloids nicotine, tropane, stachydrine, necine, and pyrrolizidine. Tropane (L-ornithine derivatives), another major alkaloid, is one of the world's oldest plant medicines, with ethnopharmacologic uses including analgesia, hallucinogens, and poisons. Esters (mono-, di-, and tri), tropanes

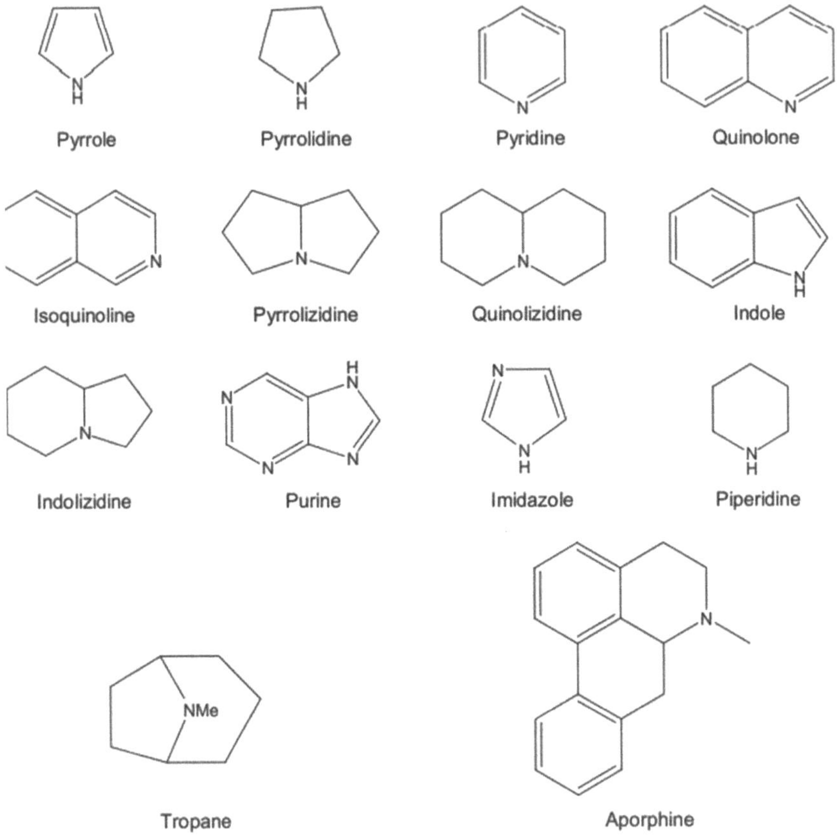

Figure 1.4 Basic structure of naturally occurring alkaloids.

(carboxylated and benzoylated), and ornithine-derived compounds are prevalent in the Solanaceae (family of flowering plants), Convolvulaceae (bindweed or morning glory family), Brassicaceae (a large and commercially significant flowering plant family), Erythroxylaceae (a family of flowering trees and shrubs), and Euphorbiaceae (the spurge family) [27]. Due to a tropic acid residue connected to the ecgonine nucleus as an ester, some of these alkaloids have chiral structures. Racemic mixtures can arise during alkaline extraction, especially when the former exists naturally in its R form (for example, the synthesis of (+)-atropine from (−)-hyoscyamine). Tropanic, benzoic, acetic, tiglic, isobutyric, isovaleric, and anisic acids were all found in the tropane alkaloids, as were a number of other acids. Drugs like scopolamine (a tropane alkaloid) are routinely used to treat digestive and urinary system spasms. Ophthalmologic eyedrops usually contain atropine to increase pupil size, paralyze the accommodation reflex and facilitate ophthalmic examinations. To enhance their appearance, ladies have been using *Atropa belladonna* juice to make their pupils larger since at least the Renaissance period. However, tropane alkaloids have a long list of adverse effects and contraindications. Cardiac abnormalities, particularly irregular heartbeat, as well as euphoric and disorienting moods, depressed tendencies toward the central nervous system, and dryness of the mucous membranes are all documented side effects. Glaucoma, prostatic hyperplasia, urinary tract illness, and pregnancy should all be avoided [28,29]. The central nervous system action of tropane alkaloids makes them a popular drug of abuse. Cocaine is one of the most well-known of these substances. Cocaine can cause cardiac death at large dosages by blocking sodium channels. In the long run, chronic use might lead to depression, suicide attempts, sleeplessness, or psychomotor retardation. More than 4000 people died as a result of its misuse in 2013. Cocaine's medicinal uses are confined to anesthetic purposes in nasal and lacrimal procedures [30]. The alkaloid's ligand impact on the central nervous system's opioid receptors accounts for its dependence-inducing properties.

Similar to the tropane alkaloids, another derivative of L-ornithine is pyrrolizidine alkaloid (PA), which originate from L-ornithine or L-arginine. With a bridgehead nitrogen atom, it has two five-membered rings linked together. These compounds are commonly found in the Boraginaceae, Asteraceae, and Fabaceae group of plants and may be found in the seeds and flowers of all three of those groups. The hepatotoxicity of these alkaloids is determined by a double bond at C-1 and C-2. PAs are the eaters of necic acid and necines. Necic acids are mono- or dicarboxylic acids with branching carbon chains containing 5−10 carbon atoms. However, double esterification can sometimes occur, resulting in macrocyclic diesters with 11−14 ring systems (for instance, senkirkine) [31]. PA is found in many plant species and is estimated to be present in 3% of the world's flowering plants. These plants are commonly harmful to animals, wildlife, and people. PAs have caused significant human illness and mortality through accidental intake of PA-contaminated food sources or purposeful use of PA-containing alternative therapies. To avoid adverse effects, oral consumption of unsaturated PAs is limited to 0.35 g/day for adults for up to 14 days and 0.007 g PA/kg body weight for members of sensitive groups, such as children. The toxicity of these chemicals in animals is also substantial, prompting a careful investigation of their impact on animal grazing. Animals may develop severe liver disease, cirrhosis, or tumors as a result of a single treatment of PA-containing plants. Toxicities caused by PAs are far more poisonous to animals such as pigs and poultry than to sheep and goats [32].

Purine alkaloids are the derivatives of asparaginate and glutamate. Caffeine, theobromine, and theophylline are the three most widespread alkaloids belonging to this group. Indole alkaloids, β-carboline alkaloids, manzamines, ergot alkaloids, and quinolone are examples of L-tryptophan derivatives. Quinoline alkaloids are generally anthranilic acid derivatives (excluding the cinchona alkaloids and camptothecin, both of which are generated from tryptophan). Their occurrence was discovered in extracts from various Rutaceae, Rubiaceae, Asteraceae species, and fungal (Penicillium species) and bacterial (Pseudomonas species) species.

The extracts of Rutaceae species include furoquinoline alkaloids, which are anthranilic acid derivatives with spasmolytic and photosensitizing effects. It is the mutagenic, antiviral, antiplasmodial, and antibacterial characteristics of plant extracts that are due to dictamnine, skimmianine, or fagarine; these compounds also have anticholinesterase capabilities [33]. Another important anthranilic acid derivative is acridone alkaloid. There are just a few acridone alkaloids, but acronycine, isolated from the Australian plant *Sarcomelicope simplicifolia*, is the most critical example. This class of alkaloids, as well as their derivatives, are being studied extensively for the treatment of colon and lung cancers [34].

Pyridine and piperidine alkaloids are another two major types of alkaloids that are L-lysine derivatives. Piperidine alkaloids, which feature a saturated piperidine ring and are usually produced from lysine, have been found. In most cases, lysine is the site of α-side chain attachment for simple α-substituted piperidines. The Apiaceae (family of mostly aromatic flowering plants), Solanaceae (family of flowering plants, which also include herbs and trees), Chenopodiaceae (a subfamily of the flowering plant family Amaranthaceae), Fabaceae (bean family), Crassulaceae (stonecrop family or the orpine family), Lycopodiaceae (a family of vascular plants), and Asteraceae (composite family of the flowering plant order Asterales) include this type of alkaloids. Pilocarpine, whose production may involve histidine and threonine, is the most significant alkaloid from the category of histidine derivatives. *Pilocarpus jaborandi*, a neotropical plant in the Rutaceae family native to Brazil and which is grown there, produces it.

1.2.2.2 Nonheterocyclic alkaloids

Nonheterocyclic alkaloids make up a significant portion of the alkaloid family. Nonheterocyclic nitrogen-containing compounds are those made from amino acids or biogenic amines. Capsaicin and ephedrine are two of the most prominent members of this class. The compounds like hordenine from *Hordeum distochon* (Poaceae) and mescaline from *Lophophora williamsi* are also included in this protoalkaloid family [23].

1.2.2.3 Properties of alkaloids

For the most part, the salts of organic acids, esters, or tannins (Cinchona bark) are present in plant tissues as water-soluble salts of the alkaloids. The majority of alkaloids are found in the plant matrix as crystalline, amorphous, nonodorous, and nonvolatile compounds. It is possible to find liquid alkaloids of low molecular weight, such as arecoline and pilocarpine, and alkaloids without an oxygen atom in their structure. There are a few exceptions to this rule, including berberine and colchicine, the orange-yellow alkaloids betaine and sanguinarine, the red-colored sanguinarine, and the orange-yellow canadine. Tonic water still contains quinine as a bittering agent. Alkaloids with optically active counterclockwise isomers are more pharmacologically active than their racemic mixtures, which are less active or have dramatically differing activity, such as morphine's enantiomers.

Alkaloids, in general, dissolve in acidic water, whereas their salts dissolve in water. In other words, they are soluble in water or dilute acids but not in organic solvents. Organic solvents (chloroform, ether, methylene chloride) can dissolve alkaloids' free forms, but water cannot (exceptions include ephedrine and caffeine). Pharmaceutical companies take use of the structural variations in alkaloids' solubility to separate them from complex plant matrices and produce pharmaceutically acceptable products [32].

1.2.3 Steroids

Plants, animals, and microbes all produce steroid hormones, physiologically essential secondary metabolites. They usually have a tetracyclic carbon skeleton (1,2-cyclopentenoperhydrophenanthrene (5- or 5-gonane)) with methyl substituents at C-10 and C-13 and an alkyl substituent (side chain) at C-17. The oxidation states of the carbons in the tetracyclic core and methyl groups, as well as the structure of the side chain, give steroids their enormous chemical variety. Phytosterols (structural elements of plant biologic membranes), withanolides (commonly found in nightshade genera), brassinosteroids (necessary for optimal plant growth and development), phytoecdysteroids (for defense against phytophagous), steroidal saponins (commonly found in plants with hemolytic and toxic characteristics), steroidal alkaloids (nitrogen-containing derivatives of natural steroids), cardiac glycosides (medicine for heart failure and some irregular heartbeats.), and mammalian steroidal hormones are the seven primary categories of plant steroids based on taxonomic considerations and biologic roles and/or structures.

Steroids have a vital role in plant function. Phytosterols are part of the lipid bilayer that governs the fluidity and permeability of the plant cell membrane [35]. Withanolides are steroidal lactones whose role in plants is unknown, but they have important biologic actions in mammals. Brassinosteroids are plant hormones that play an indispensable role in plant growth. Ecdysteroids, the insect hormones, are structurally identical to phytoecdysteroids [36]. Insect repellents and chemical barriers against infections are recognized properties of steroidal alkaloids.

Phytosterols are steroidal alcohols found in a wide range of plants. Phytosterols have recently received a lot of interest due to reports that they can lower cholesterol levels [37]. Withanolides are a class of steroidal lactones formed by oxidizing C-22 and C-26 to generate a lactone or a prospective lactone ring on an unaltered or modified ergostane skeleton. They are primarily found in the genera *Acnistus*, *Discopodium*, *Dunalis*, *Deprea*, *Datura*, *Exodeconus*, *Hyoscyamus*, *Nicandra*, *Iochroma*, *Jaborosa*, *Larnax*, *Lycium*, *Physalis*, *Physalis*, *Salpichroa*, *Tubocapsicum*, *Trechonaetes*, *Vassobia*, and *Withania* in the Solanaceae family [38]. Aside from the Solanaceae family, withanolides may be found in Fabaceae, Lamiaceae, Myrtaceae, and Taccaceae plants. More than 70 members of the brassinosteroids family of plant growth hormones are steroidal plant growth hormones. These brassinosteroids may be divided into three subgroups depending on the number of carbon atoms in the side chain at position 17: (C27), (C28), and (C29). Substitutes on the A/B rings and on the side chain provide them with a wide range of structural options.

In several countries, herbal formulations containing phytoecdysteroids have been licensed as tonics in phytomedicine, while in others, the same plants are employed in folk medicine. Athletes who want to bulk up can take phytoecdysteroids in specific formulations for this reason. It is notable because phytoecdysteroids' anabolic effects are not accompanied by androgenic, antigonadotropic, or thymolytic (destructive) adverse effects [39].

Antitumor, antiviral, antifungal, and embryotoxic properties of steroidal glycoalkaloids of the solanidine and spirosolane kinds have been documented. Antibacterial, antiviral, antifungal, antimalarial, glutathione S-transferase inhibitory, and cholinesterase inhibitory actions are all demonstrated by steroidal alkaloids with a pregnane structure. S-transferases are detoxifying enzymes that may generate adducts with electrophilic compounds like glutathione. Anticancer medicines with electrophilic centers create adducts with glutathione S-transferase that are easily eliminated from the body, reducing the drug's effectiveness. As a result, glutathione S-transferase inhibitors are crucial in cancer treatment [40]. The breakdown of acetylcholine is carried out by cholinesterases, including acetyl- and butyl-cholinesterases. Alzheimer disease is thought to be caused by a lack of acetylcholine in the brain. As a result, powerful cholinesterase inhibitors are therapeutic options for Alzheimer disease [40].

1.2.4 Terpenes

Originally, the name terpenes was derived from the term turpentine. A sticky, sweet-smelling balsam that pours when pine tree bark and fresh wood are chopped or carved, turpentine is the so-called "resin of pine trees" (Pinaceae). "Resin acids" and hydrocarbons, once known as terpenes, are found in turpentine. The term terpene has traditionally been used to refer to all-natural chemicals derived from isoprene monomers and originating from plants.

Many plants or portions of plants (roots, rhizomes, stems, leaves, blooms, fruits, seeds) smell nice, taste spicy, or have special pharmacologic effects. These qualities are influenced mainly by terpenes. However, terpenes can also be enhanced by carving or steam distillation of plants, such as creating incense from balm trees or myrrh from myrtle trees; in most cases, terpenes are extracted or steam distilled from certain fragrant rose flowers. Ethereal or essential oils are steam-distilled extracts and steam distillates that are employed in the production of excellent fragrances, fine-tuning of food and beverage flavors and aromas, and herbal medicines. Terpenes are yet to be extensively studied in their ecologic and biologic roles. A variety of plants emit volatile terpenes to either attract pollinating insects or repel animals that could be attracted to the plants' food supply. Some plants are protected against animal consumption by terpenes that are less volatile but have a pronounced bitter or poisonous flavor. Lastly, preliminary studies have demonstrated that terpenes play a vital role in developing plants as signaling chemicals and growth regulators. Various insect hormones and pheromones are synthesized from the terpenes they ingest into their diet. It is via the use of these odorous molecules that insects and other species communicate with one another, e.g., warning each other of dangers, identifying food sources, and marking their locations and forming social groups, as well as attracting sex partners for mating and reproduction. Because pheromones do not hurt the environment, they may be used instead of traditional pesticides to catch destructive and deadly insects like bark beetles [41].

Currently, there are around 30,000 recognized terpenes in the scientific literature. It is based on a fundamental principle: the carbon skeleton of terpenes is made up of 2-methylbutane residues known as (C5)n isoprene units. In this way, terpenes might be referred to as isoprenoids, as well. Hydrocarbons, glycosides, alcohols, carboxylic acids, aldehydes, esters, and ketones are the most common forms of terpenes found in nature.

1.2.5 Pigments

In plants, pigments are the chemical components that give fruits and vegetables their brilliant hues and appealing appearances. Metabolic and light harvesting in photosynthesis, growth and defense regulation, and prevention from photooxidative damage are just some of the functions that these chemicals perform in plants. Their ingestion has been linked to a lower risk of acquiring a variety of ailments in people. Plants' inherent brilliant color is caused by pigments. The most frequent pigments present in plants and fruits are red-yellow betalains, red-purple anthocyanins, green chlorophylls, and yellow-orange carotenoids. These plant pigments have potential health-promoting benefits in addition to their coloring capabilities. Agricultural leftovers constitute a significant source of natural pigments that are increasingly being recognized as fundamentally sustainable. Using them to recover natural pigments might assist in alleviating the environmental issues associated with their management. Although the seeds and peels of certain fruits and vegetables are removed during processing, they may still contain large amounts of pigments, often in higher quantities [42,43].

Chlorophylls are the well-known photosynthetic greenish pigments found in algae, plants, and cyanobacteria, and they belong to the tetrapyrrole family. Chlorophyll is a widely dispersed natural pigment that plays a vital role in photosynthesis. The catabolic process of chlorophyll degradation is essential for leaf senescence and fruit ripening. Due to its unique features, it can be used in a variety of sectors of research and industrial technology. The five primary classes of chlorophyll are a, b, c, d, and f. Chlorophyll is found primarily in plants, mainly green fruits and vegetables

[44]. The porphyrin macrocycle, which consists of four pyrrole rings, is the basic structure of chlorophylls. Magnesium (Mg) is the most abundant element in chlorophyll [45] Chlorophyll has a hydrophilic porphyrin ring edge, but the phytol chain side chain has a strong hydrophobic side chain. Using this structure, the phospholipid bilayer membrane's chlorophyll may be more efficiently arranged. Chlorophyll's capacity to absorb visible light is enhanced by a variety of conjugated double bonds [46].

In nature, carotenoids are lipid-soluble natural pigments that may be found in yellow, red, and orange hues. Plants, microalgae, bacteria, and fungi are among the natural sources of carotenoids. Two kinds of carotenoids may be distinguished based on their functional groups: carotene, xanthophylls, and lycopene, which include just the parent hydrocarbon chain, and carotene, which contains oxygen-containing functional groups like lutein and zeaxanthin. When carotenoids are oxidized, they are destroyed, but when they are geometrically isomerized, the fraction of Z isomers increases. In the isoprenoid family, carotenoids are found. The chemical structure of conjugated carbon—carbon double bonds is crucial to the production of color. A conjugated system is one that alternates between double and single bonds [47].

Flavonoids are polyphenolic chemicals with a 2-phenylchromane nucleus with a wide range of medicinal, pharmacologic, and biochemical applications. Anthocyanins are water-soluble pigments of the flavonoids family that give plants their red, purple, and blue hues and play important roles in plant growth and defense. Anthocyanins are flavylium cation ($C_{15}H_{11}O^+$) derivatives that have been glycosylated, polyhydroxylated, or polymetoxylated. The oxygen atom in the C-ring of the basic flavonoid structure is positively charged in flavylium cation, with a molecular weight of 207.24724 g/mol. Cyanidin, pelargonidin, delphinidin, malvidin, peonidin, and petunidin are some of the most often found anthocyanidins in plants, but there are dozens more to choose from. Anthocyanin conjugated connections are crucial to the creation of plants with red, blue, and purple hues [48].

Tyrosine-derived water-soluble nitrogenous plant pigments known as betalains are made up of betalamic acid [4-(2-oxoethylidene)-1,2,3,4-tetrahydropyridine-2,6-dicarboxylic acid]. There are two primary betalains: betaxanthin (yellow) and betacyanin (red). The leaves, blossoms, and stems of plants, as well as their edible parts, contain betalains. It is the most frequent betacyanin found in plants, and red beet is the most abundant source. Yellow beets and cactus pears contain vulgaxanthin and indicaxanthin. The combination of betaxanthins and betacyanins in the same regions of the plants results in an orange to red hue, depending on the pigment percentage. The absorbance peaks of betacyanins and betaxanthins are located at $\lambda_m = 536$ nm and $\lambda_m = 480$ nm, respectively. Although the hydroxyl groups in betacyanins and betaxanthins have been found to be glycosylated, this has not been seen in betaxanthins [49].

1.2.6 Others

Secondary metabolites having sugar moieties linked to some nonsugar bioactive substances are classified as glycosides (aglycone) [50]. Therefore, glycosides may be categorized based on their glycogen constituent, glycosidic linkage, and aglycone constituents [51]. The inert glycosidic form of a chemical component or aglycone can be activated by hydrolysis with enzymes in various plant sections [52]. It is possible to classify these glycosides as "pro-drugs," as they may be hydrolyzed to release aglycone, the active ingredient that can be employed as medicine [53].

There are several therapeutic qualities associated with glycosides, which are found in various forms, including phenolic glycosides and alcoholic glycosides, cardiac glycosides, and flavonoid glycosides. These include cardiac glycosides, alcoholic glycosides, and flavonoid glycosides, all of which have antiinflammatory, analgesic, and antipyretic properties [54,55]. Aside from the water-soluble nature of glycosides, they are also known to be more soluble in water than their glycocone counterparts. Pharmacokinetic characteristics of the aglycone portion are influenced by the connected glycosidic unit, which increases its hydrophilicity. Hydrophilicity, on the other hand, has the most significant impact on the membrane transport system [56]. Some glycosides, for example, may be carried into brain tissue via the glucose transport system. Another notable example of glycosylation in action is the placental barrier, which prevents intoxication by preventing many glucuronides from entering the fetal tissues [56,57].

Isothiocyanates, indoles, allylic sulfur compounds, sulforaphane, and other organosulfur phytochemicals are found chiefly in plants of the *Allium* and *Brassica* genera, such as garlic, leek, shallot, onion, cauliflower, broccoli, brussels sprouts, cabbage, kale, and so on [58]. Compounds of the *Allium* genus, such as cysteine sulfoxides, impart taste and strong odor to its species, such as onion and garlic, when hydrolyzed [59]. Alliin (found in garlic), isoalliin (found in onions and shallots), methiin (found in garlic, onions, shallots, and leeks), and propiin (only in shallots) are the several types of cysteine sulfoxides [60]. Isothiocyanates, which are produced by the hydrolysis of glucosinolates, are commonly found in brassica crops [61].

Due to its potential pharmacologic actions, garlic, including alliin, is extremely helpful to human health. An enzyme called alliinase converts alliin to allicin (activated by disruption of cellular membranes) [62]. When extracted using aqueous solutions, allicin can be transformed into more stable molecules such as diallyl sulfides or S-allyl cysteine [63]. Garlic oil contains diallyl sulfide, which is thought to be an anticarcinogenic agent that prevents tumor development by metabolically activated carcinogens [64]. Because of their antioxidant, antibacterial, antithrombic, and lipid-lowering capabilities, allicin-based substances protect against a variety of chronic illnesses such as atherosclerosis, hypertension, obesity, and associated disorders [65]. Garlic also increases allicin levels in the blood, lowering systolic blood pressure in hypertensive patients [66]. The relevance of allium organosulfur compounds to human health is enormous. They work as antioxidants, preventing free radical damage to cellular membranes and lowering the risk of certain malignancies, neurologic illnesses, and cardiovascular ailments.

1.3 Analytical approaches for determining bioavailability and bioaccessibility of bioactive compounds

The term "bioaccessibility" refers to the amount or proportion of a substance liberated from the plant matrix and made accessible for absorption. This involves the breakdown of the food into assimilation-ready material, which is then taken up by intestinal epithelial cells, where it undergoes presystemic metabolism before being transported to the bloodstream.

In certain cases, the beneficial effects of nonabsorbed nutrients (such as bile salt binding by calcium in the colon) may be overlooked by absorption-based definitions of nutrients. In vitro digestion methods, which mainly simulate stomach and small intestine digestion, are used to assess bioaccessibility, which is occasionally followed by Caco-2 cell uptake [67]. In vitro, bioaccessibility tests do not replace in vivo testing, although they are useful for determining the impact of gastrointestinal digestion and dietary matrices on compound systemic bioavailability. Since only components absorbed in the small intestine are able to become available and have positive effects on the body, bioaccessibility of phenolic compounds and other antioxidants is crucial. Mastication reduces meals to minute particles, increasing the surface area available to digestive enzymes, resulting in improved digestion and gastrointestinal absorption of antioxidants. In the colon, only the antioxidants liberated from the food matrix as a result of digestion enzymes and bacterial microflora activity are accessible, hence bioavailable.

It is important to note that the word "bioavailability" encompasses the use of nutrients as well as the number of nutrients absorbed into the bloodstream and utilized. Bioavailability encompasses gastrointestinal digestion, absorption, metabolism, tissue distribution, and bioactivity as a whole. As a result, when a claim is made in terms of bioavailability, it must be proved that the component being studied is easily digested and assimilated and that once absorbed, it has a good influence on human health. However, because quantifying bioactivity presents practical and ethical challenges, the word "bioavailability" is widely used to describe the fraction of a chemical or its metabolite that enters the systemic circulation without considering bioactivity [68]. Bioavailability is defined as the area under the curve (plasma concentration) of an isolated chemical or compound-containing meal in animals or humans when an acute or chronic dosage is administered [69]. When it comes to calculating bioavailability, in vivo procedures are employed to determine the proportion of nutrients or phytochemicals that are digested, absorbed, and metabolized before reaching and entering the systemic circulatory system. To make studies easier, the word "bioavailability" is often defined as the proportion of a chemical or its metabolites that reaches the systemic circulation without taking into account bioactivity. Thus, the in vivo plasma concentration of a chemical-containing meal or substance influences bioavailability.

Bioactivity is the impact that a substance has when it is exposed to it. It comprises tissue uptake and the physiologic reaction (such as antioxidant, antiinflammatory) [70]. Bioactivity can be examined in vivo, ex vivo, or in vitro. In contrast, digestibility refers to the percentage of dietary components that are transformed into potentially accessible elements during digestion. Meanwhile, assimilation refers to the uptake of bioaccessible material across the epithelium via a transepithelial absorption process [71].

1.4 Commercialization of naturally occurring bioactive compounds

According to the World Health Organization, there are roughly 20,000 medicinal plants in 91 nations worldwide, including 12 mega-biodiversity countries [72]. For both research and development as well as market concerns, the extensive extraction techniques required to extract bioactive phytochemicals from crops provide considerable obstacles. Similarly, the pharmaceutical/medical business is motivated by the market to introduce novel plant crops with medicinal relevance. When it comes to determining which plants and chemicals are suitable for commercialization-oriented research, it is a lengthy and complex process that demands great skill and consideration of several market-related issues, including rigorous extraction and product development procedures [73,74]. Several plant species are suitable for use in the pharmaceutical and food industries for the production of commonly prescribed pharmaceutical drugs and consumer goods including energy drinks, health supplements, and food additives, among other things. These species include *Azadirachta indica* (Indian lilac), *Curcuma longa* (turmeric), *Brassica juncea* (mustard greens), *Cuminum cyminum* (cumin), *Trigonella foenum-graecum* (fenugreek), *Allium sativum* (garlic), *Ocimum tenuiflorum* (basil), *Santalum album* (Indian sandalwood), *Syzgium aromaticum* (clove), *Withania somnifera* (ashwagandha), and *Zingiber officinale* (ginger) to name a few, each of which includes a significant amount of a phytochemical with medicinal potential. Dietary supplements, food goods, cosmetics, medications, and dentistry products include Panax ginseng extracts. *Curcuma longa* is traditionally used as a food or in medical formulations. *Mentha* sp. is utilized in the pharmaceutical, cosmetic, and flavoring industries, among other things. *Azadirachta indica* oil is used as a pesticide, lubricant, and therapy for diabetes and tuberculosis, among other things. Medicines, tonics, and cosmetics have all been made with *Ocimum sanctum* in the cosmetic and pharmaceutical sectors. Skincare and cosmetics items contain *Bacopa monnieri*. Extracts of *Withania somnifera* are utilized in cosmetics and personal care products [75].

With the widespread adoption of modern medicines, traditional remedies like those found in countries like India have been widely accepted and practiced alongside them. In the United States, over-the-counter drugs containing herbal treatments and nutritional supplements that have been proven to be safe and effective are widely used by medical experts. Herbal medications, herbal drug preparations, and herbal medical goods now have guidelines authorized by the European Agency for the Evaluation of Medicines. For many developing nations, medicinal plants are an important source of foreign cash, and the global market for herbs and medicinal plants is worth several billion dollars annually. Plant-based medicines and raw materials for foreign medicinal plant businesses are crucial exports in Bulgaria, Germany, Poland, and others in Africa and Asia. The herbal medicine business is estimated to be worth between $43 billion and $60 billion yearly, according to a slew of studies. China's Traditional Chinese Medicines were sold for over $2.4 billion, with 400 million dollars in sales going abroad; Malaysia's herbs generated 60 million dollars for the country's economy in 1996 [76]. Ethno-veterinary medicine and human health benefit significantly from using medicinal plants and other natural substances, particularly in treating heart disease, cancer, and infections caused by microbes [76]. However, there is a lack of essential public and private sector infrastructure (such as universities and other government institutions) and governmental interest and financial support that severely hampers medicinal plant research, development, and commercial production, especially in developing countries. There has been no concurrent development of methodologies for assessing traditional and complementary alternative medicines to fulfill national or international criteria since they have emerged within diverse cultures in different parts of the world. As a result, there are great misgivings and even outright skepticism regarding their supposedly beneficial properties. It is still debatable, for example, whether traditional medications, which have been shown to stimulate the immune system, can be used to combat AIDS.

1.5 Conclusions and future perspectives

Phytochemicals include pigments, phenolics, flavonoids, nonflavonoids, alkaloids, glycosides, saponins, steroids, and terpenoids, among other bioactive molecules. Some of these compounds have a chemical structure that is unique, and they have biologic activity that has never been seen before. Pest repellents and growth control are only a few of the critical activities they play in the plant's secondary metabolism. They are generally present in small concentrations and have pharmacologic properties. Furthermore, these unique chemical entities have led to discoveries in the realm of drug development and have opened up new domains of fundamental research. In vitro and cell culture studies, animal studies, and human epidemiology all support the beneficial roles of phytochemicals in the treatment of cancer, cardiovascular disease, diabetes, hypertension, inflammation, microbial, viral, and parasitic infections, psychosis, spasmodic conditions, ulcers, and other diseases.

Bioaccessibility, bioavailability, and bioactivity may be studied using a wide range of analytical approaches available today. Bioavailability and bioaccessibility are often studied using in vivo and in vitro methodologies, respectively. The bioactivity of phytochemicals may be studied using three different methods: in vivo, ex vivo, and in vitro. However, a distinction must be noted between the sorts of knowledge that may be gleaned from in vitro, animal, and human investigations. Although in vitro studies are necessary to determine the mechanisms of action, the efficacy of these same substances must also be proved in vivo, as well. It is imperative that food and pharmaceutical industries face new challenges in dealing with public concerns about supplement efficacy and safety, government regulations on product labeling and health claims, and the manufacturing of foods with varying qualities, stability, and shelf life, all of which are impacted by the rapid growth in the use of phytochemicals in nutraceutical and functional foods. Moreover, additional study into the molecular processes of bioactive phytochemicals is critical to have a better understanding of how they might be used to benefit human health.

References

[1] T.N. Baite, B. Mandal, M.K. Purkait, Ultrasound assisted extraction of gallic acid from Ficus auriculata leaves using green solvent, Food and Bioproducts Processing 128 (2021) 1−11.
[2] V.L. Dhadge, M. Changmai, M.K. Purkait, Purification of catechins from Camellia sinensis using membrane cell, Food and Bioproducts Processing 117 (2019) 203−212.
[3] N.M. Daud, et al., Valorisation of plant seed as natural bioactive compounds by various extraction methods: a review, Trends in Food Science & Technology 119 (2022) 201−214.
[4] D. Haldar, M.K. Purkait, Lignocellulosic conversion into value-added products: a review, Process Biochemistry 89 (2020) 110−133.
[5] B.V. da Silva, J.C. Barreira, M.B.P. Oliveira, Natural phytochemicals and probiotics as bioactive ingredients for functional foods: extraction, biochemistry and protected-delivery technologies, Trends in Food Science & Technology 50 (2016) 144−158.
[6] C. Leitzmann, Characteristics and health benefits of phytochemicals, Complementary Medicine Research 23 (2) (2016) 69−74.
[7] M. Sharma, P. Kaushik, Vegetable phytochemicals: an update on extraction and analysis techniques, Biocatalysis and Agricultural Biotechnology 36 (2021) 102149.
[8] S. Quideau, et al., Plant polyphenols: chemical properties, biological activities, and synthesis, Angewandte Chemie International Edition 50 (3) (2011) 586−621.
[9] D.M. Pereira, et al., Phenolics: from chemistry to biology, Molecules 14 (6) (2009) 2202−2211.

[10] D. Beconcini, et al., Antioxidant and anti-inflammatory properties of cherry extract: nanosystems-based strategies to improve endothelial function and intestinal absorption, Foods 9 (2) (2020) 207.

[11] P. Duarah, D. Haldar, M.K. Purkait, Technological advancement in the synthesis and applications of lignin-based nanoparticles derived from agro-industrial waste residues: a review, International Journal of Biological Macromolecules 163 (2020) 1828–1843.

[12] J.B. Harborne, Methods in plant biochemistry, Plant phenolics 1 (1989).

[13] A. Belščak-Cvitanović, et al., 1 - overview of polyphenols and their properties, in: C.M. Galanakis (Ed.), Polyphenols: Properties, Recovery, and Applications, Woodhead Publishing, 2018, pp. 3–44.

[14] C.S.-M. González, Compuestos polifenólicos: estructura y clasificación. Presencia en alimentos y consumo. Biodisponibilidad y metabolismo, Alimentaria: Revista de tecnología e higiene de los alimentos 329 (2002) 19–28.

[15] G.G. Duthie, P.T. Gardner, J.A. Kyle, Plant polyphenols: are they the new magic bullet? Proceedings of the Nutrition Society 62 (3) (2003) 599–603.

[16] L. Bravo, Polyphenols: chemistry, dietary sources, metabolism, and nutritional significance, Nutrition Reviews 56 (11) (1998) 317–333.

[17] C.S. Yang, et al., Inhibition of carcinogenesis by dietary polyphenolic compounds, Annual Review of Nutrition 21 (1) (2001) 381–406.

[18] H. Adlercreutz, W. Mazur, Phyto-oestrogens and Western diseases, Annals of Medicine 29 (2) (1997) 95–120.

[19] K.P.L. Bhat, J.M. Pezzuto, Cancer chemopreventive activity of resveratrol, Annals of the New York Academy of Sciences 957 (1) (2002) 210–229.

[20] D. Haldar, M.K. Purkait, Thermochemical pretreatment enhanced bioconversion of elephant grass (*Pennisetum purpureum*): insight on the production of sugars and lignin, Biomass Conversion and Biorefinery 12 (2020).

[21] V. Preininger, Chapter 5 the pharmacology and toxicology of the Papaveraceae alkaloids, in: R.H.F. Manske (Ed.), The Alkaloids: Chemistry and Physiology, Academic Press, 1975, pp. 207–261.

[22] Alkaloids, In Medicinal Natural Products, 2009, pp. 311–420.

[23] T. Aniszewski, Alkaloidssecrets of life, Alkaloid Chemistry, Biological Significance, Applications and Ecological Role 56 (710) (2007) 182–189.

[24] L. Grycová, J. Dostál, R. Marek, Quaternary protoberberine alkaloids, Phytochemistry 68 (2) (2007) 150–175.

[25] E.V. Leitao da-Cunha, et al., Protoberberine alkaloids, in: G.A. Cordell (Ed.), The Alkaloids: Chemistry and Biology, Academic Press, 2005, pp. 1–75.

[26] P.W. Jeffs, Chapter 2 the protoberberine alkaloids, The Alkaloids: Chemistry and Physiology 9 (1967) 41.

[27] M. Gadzikowska, G. Grynkiewicz, Tropane alkaloids in pharmaceutical and phytochemical analysis, Acta Poloniae Pharmaceutica - Drug Research 59 (2) (2002) 149–160.

[28] G. Grynkiewicz, M. Gadzikowska, Tropane alkaloids as medicinally useful natural products and their synthetic derivatives as new drugs, Pharmacological Reports 60 (4) (2008) 439–463.

[29] B. Dräger, Analysis of tropane and related alkaloids, Journal of Chromatography A 978 (1) (2002) 1–35.

[30] M.E. O'Leary, J.C. Hancox, Role of voltage-gated sodium, potassium and calcium channels in the development of cocaine-associated cardiac arrhythmias, British Journal of Clinical Pharmacology 69 (5) (2010) 427–442.

[31] B. Avula, et al., Characterization and screening of pyrrolizidine alkaloids and N-oxides from botanicals and dietary supplements using UHPLC-high resolution mass spectrometry, Food Chemistry 178 (2015) 136–148.

[32] W.A. Kukula-Koch, J. Widelski, Chapter 9 - alkaloids, in: S. Badal, R. Delgoda (Eds.), Pharmacognosy, Academic Press, Boston, 2017, pp. 163–198.
[33] A. Emam, M. Eweis, M. Elbadry, A new furoquinoline alkaloid with antifungal activity from the leaves of Ruta chalepensis L, Drug discoveries & therapeutics 4 (6) (2010) 399–404.
[34] N. Guilbaud, et al., Marked antitumor activity of a new potent acronycine derivative in orthotopic models of human solid tumors, Clinical Cancer Research 7 (8) (2001) 2573–2580.
[35] W. Kreis, F. Müller-Uri, Biochemistry of Sterols, Cardiac Glycosides, Brassinosteroids, Phytoecdysteroids and Steroid Saponins. Annual Plant Reviews Volume 40: Biochemistry of Plant Secondary Metabolism, 2010, pp. 304–363.
[36] A. Bajguz, A. Tretyn, The chemical characteristic and distribution of brassinosteroids in plants, Phytochemistry 62 (7) (2003) 1027–1046.
[37] M.H. Moghadasian, Pharmacological properties of plant sterols: in vivo and in vitro observations, Life Sciences 67 (6) (2000) 605–615.
[38] L.-X. Chen, H. He, F. Qiu, Natural withanolides: an overview, Natural Product Reports 28 (4) (2011) 705–740.
[39] B. Gunaherath, G. K., A.L. Gunatilaka, Plant Steroids: Occurrence, Biological Significance and Their Analysis. Encyclopedia of Analytical Chemistry: Applications, Theory and Instrumentation, 2006, pp. 1–26.
[40] A. Ata, B.J. Andersh, Buxus steroidal alkaloids: chemistry and biology, The Alkaloids - Chemistry and Biology 66 (2008) 191–213.
[41] E. Breitmaier, Terpenes: Flavors, Fragrances, Pharmaca, Pheromones, John Wiley & Sons, 2006.
[42] S. Ghosh, et al., Micro and nanoencapsulation of natural colors: a holistic view, Applied Biochemistry and Biotechnology 193 (11) (2021) 3787–3811.
[43] M. Sharma, et al., Valorization of fruits and vegetable wastes and by-products to produce natural pigments, Critical Reviews in Biotechnology 41 (4) (2021) 535–563.
[44] S. Jurić, et al., Sources, stability, encapsulation and application of natural pigments in foods, Food Reviews International (2020) 1–56.
[45] S. Pareek, et al., Chlorophylls: chemistry and biological functions, Fruit and Vegetable Phytochemicals 29 (2017) 269.
[46] A.K. Singh, H.K. Rana, A.K. Pandey, Analysis of chlorophylls, in: Recent Advances in Natural Products Analysis, Elsevier, 2020, pp. 635–650.
[47] S. Shilpa, et al., Factors affecting bioaccessibility and bio-efficacy of carotenoids, in: Carotenoids: Properties, Processing and Applications, Elsevier, 2020, pp. 41–73.
[48] M.E. Eker, et al., A review of factors affecting anthocyanin bioavailability: possible implications for the inter-individual variability, Foods 9 (1) (2020) 2.
[49] E.A. Hussain, Z. Sadiq, M. Zia-Ul-Haq, Betalains: Biomolecular Aspects, Springer, 2018.
[50] A. Bhattacharya, Chapter 5-High-Temperature Stress and Metabolism of Secondary Metabolites in Plants. Effect of High Temperature on Crop Productivity and Metabolism of Macro Molecules, Academic Press, 2019.
[51] A. Onaolapo, O. Onaolapo, Herbal beverages and brain function in health and disease, in: Functional and Medicinal Beverages, Elsevier, 2019, pp. 313–349.
[52] D. Haldar, M.K. Purkait, A review on the environment-friendly emerging techniques for pretreatment of lignocellulosic biomass: mechanistic insight and advancements, Chemosphere 264 (2021) 128523.
[53] C.G. Awuchi, The biochemistry, toxicology, and uses of the pharmacologically active phytochemicals: alkaloids, terpenes, polyphenols, and glycosides, Journal of Food and Pharmaceutical Sciences 7 (2019).

[54] N. Tawfeek, et al., Phytochemistry, pharmacology and medicinal uses of plants of the genus Salix: an updated review, Frontiers in Pharmacology (2021) 50.
[55] A.F.M. Botelho, et al., A review of cardiac glycosides: structure, toxicokinetics, clinical signs, diagnosis and antineoplastic potential, Toxicon 158 (2019) 63–68.
[56] L. Weignerová, V. Křen, Enzymatic processing of bioactive glycosides from natural sources, in: Carbohydrates in Sustainable Development II, Springer, 2010, pp. 121–146.
[57] L. Ziberna, et al., Bioavailability of flavonoids: the role of cell membrane transporters, in: Polyphenols in Human Health and Disease, Elsevier, 2014, pp. 489–511.
[58] R.T. Ruhee, et al., Organosulfur compounds: a review of their anti-inflammatory effects in human health, Frontiers in Nutrition 7 (2020) 64.
[59] M.M. Poojary, et al., Stability and extraction of bioactive sulfur compounds from Allium genus processed by traditional and innovative technologies, Journal of Food Composition and Analysis 61 (2017) 28–39.
[60] E. Block, Garlic Other Alliums, RSC publishing, Cambridge, 2010.
[61] D. Angelino, E. Jeffery, Glucosinolate hydrolysis and bioavailability of resulting isothiocyanates: focus on glucoraphanin, Journal of Functional Foods 7 (2014) 67–76.
[62] L.D. Lawson, S.M. Hunsaker, Allicin bioavailability and bioequivalence from garlic supplements and garlic foods, Nutrients 10 (7) (2018) 812.
[63] D.A. Ramirez, et al., Analytical methods for bioactive sulfur compounds in Allium: an integrated review and future directions, Journal of Food Composition and Analysis 61 (2017) 4–19.
[64] S. Melino, R. Sabelli, M. Paci, Allyl sulfur compounds and cellular detoxification system: effects and perspectives in cancer therapy, Amino acids 41 (1) (2011) 103–112.
[65] J. Sharifi-Rad, et al., Therapeutic potential of allicin-rich garlic preparations: emphasis on clinical evidence toward upcoming drugs formulation, Applied Sciences 9 (24) (2019) 5555.
[66] V. Londhe, et al., Role of garlic (*Allium sativum*) in various diseases: an overview, Angiogenesis 12 (2011) 13.
[67] J. Courraud, et al., Stability and bioaccessibility of different forms of carotenoids and vitamin A during in vitro digestion, Food Chemistry 136 (2) (2013) 871–877.
[68] B. Holst, G. Williamson, Nutrients and phytochemicals: from bioavailability to bioefficacy beyond antioxidants, Current Opinion in Biotechnology 19 (2) (2008) 73–82.
[69] M.J. Rein, et al., Bioavailability of bioactive food compounds: a challenging journey to bioefficacy, British Journal of Clinical Pharmacology 75 (3) (2013) 588–602.
[70] D.I. Santos, et al., Methods for determining bioavailability and bioaccessibility of bioactive compounds and nutrients, in: Innovative Thermal and Non-thermal Processing, Bioaccessibility and Bioavailability of Nutrients and Bioactive Compounds, Elsevier, 2019, pp. 23–54.
[71] J.M. Carbonell-Capella, et al., Analytical methods for determining bioavailability and bioaccessibility of bioactive compounds from fruits and vegetables: a review, Comprehensive Reviews in Food Science and Food Safety 13 (2) (2014) 155–171.
[72] S. Sasidharan, et al., Extraction, isolation and characterization of bioactive compounds from plants' extracts, African Journal of Traditional, Complementary and Alternative Medicines 8 (1) (2011).
[73] B. Debnath, D. Haldar, M.K. Purkait, A critical review on the techniques used for the synthesis and applications of crystalline cellulose derived from agricultural wastes and forest residues, Carbohydrate Polymers 273 (2021) 118537.
[74] B. Debnath, D. Haldar, M.K. Purkait, Potential and sustainable utilization of tea waste: a review on present status and future trends, Journal of Environmental Chemical Engineering 9 (5) (2021) 106179.

[75] J.K. Patra, et al., Selected commercial plants: a review of extraction and isolation of bioactive compounds and their pharmacological market value, Trends in Food Science & Technology 82 (2018) 89–109.
[76] B.Y. Muhammad, A. Awaisu, The need for enhancement of research, development, and commercialization of natural medicinal products in Nigeria: lessons from the Malaysian experience, African Journal of Traditional, Complementary and Alternative Medicines 5 (2) (2008) 120–130.

CHAPTER 2

Utilization of various parts of the plant for the extraction of phytochemicals and high-throughput screening techniques

2.1 Introduction

In recent years, there has been a growing appreciation for the therapeutic properties of plants, which constitute a great source of potential medicines. Over 50,000 species of plants are utilized in herbal medicine preparation around the world, with Asia providing the majority of the medication. Many bioactive compounds play a role in decreasing blood pressure, avoiding cardiovascular disease, lowering cancer risk, and regulating blood sugar levels [1].

Bioactive compounds, which are also known as "phytochemicals," may be found in the roots, leaves, bark, and blooms of mangrove species, which are used to treat a variety of human disorders. Within the same plant, various portions might have distinct active compounds. This can result in one part of a plant being toxic while another part is completely benign. The protective exterior coating of a tree trunk, shaped by deposits of living cells above the timber, is known as bark. The bark has more significant amounts of active compounds. Quinine bark, willow bark, pepper bark, and oak bark are types of bark utilized for therapeutic purposes. A bulb is a fleshy structure composed of numerous layers of leaf bases, also referred as bulb scales, which are arranged in a radial pattern. The therapeutic properties of onion species and garlic bulbs are well known. In traditional medicine, plant blossoms have long been valued. Clove and chamomile blossoms are two excellent instances of this occurrence. Saffron stamens, maize stigmas, and pollen are among the flower components utilized. Fruits, too, have

Advances in Extraction and Applications of Bioactive Phytochemicals
ISBN 978-0-443-18535-9
https://doi.org/10.1016/B978-0-443-18535-9.00004-1

long been used for medical purposes. The fruits of several members of the carrot family, such as fennel and anise, are used in medicine. The plant's leaves also contain a large number of bioactive phytochemicals. Leaves can be utilized by themselves or combined with twigs, stems, and buds. Maidenhair tree is one example. The roots, whether fleshy or woody, are employed for therapeutic reasons. Seeds are a collection of bioactive phytochemicals that might be solid (ginseng), fibrous (stinging nettle), or squishy (devil's claw).

Seeds can be found within a fruit or utilized on their own. Juniper berries appear to be fruits, but they are seeds encased in lovely woody cones [2]. Fig. 2.1 illustrates the occurrence of bioactive compounds in various parts of plants, with examples of major bioactive compounds. As seen, curcumin, desmethoxycurcumin, and bisdemethoxycurcumin are some examples of bioactive compounds found in turmeric (root). Similarly, benzoic acid, hexadecane, terpenoids, and a few flavonoids can be found in almonds (seed). Catechin, epicatechin, flavonol glycosides, and caffeine are some of the major bioactive components of tea leaves. Similarly, some of

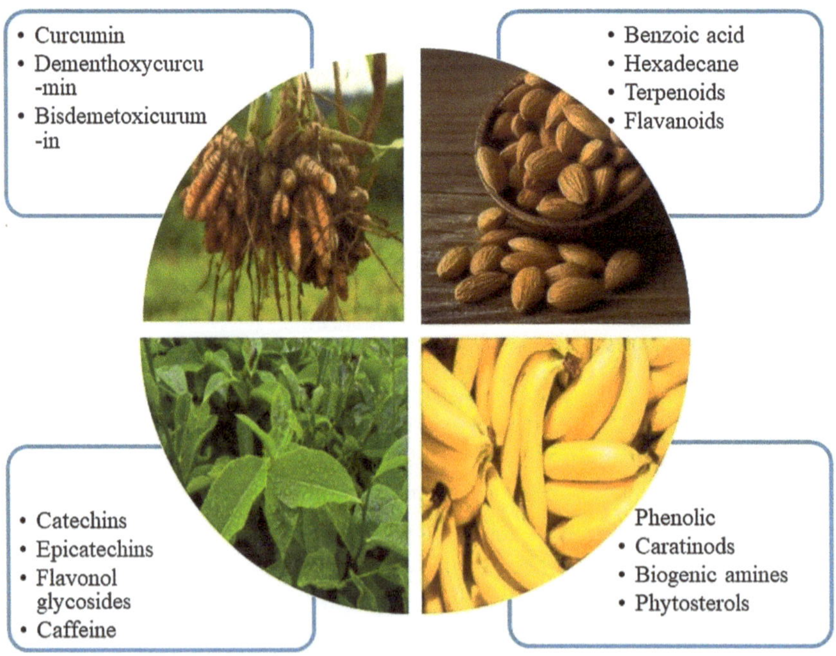

Figure 2.1 Examples of the presence of bioactive compounds in different parts of plants.

the major bioactive components found in bananas (fruit) are phenolics, carotenoids, buiogenic amines, and phytosterols.

Terpenes and terpenoids (about 25,000 varieties), alkaloids (roughly 12,000 types), and phenolic compounds (about 8,000 types) are the three primary classes of bioactive substances. The quest for innovative pharmaceutical candidates involves the development of reliable screening methodologies for natural goods' bioactive components due to a large number of bioactive compounds present in plant sources. A high-throughput screening (HTS) technique that allows for identifying potentially active ingredients in natural goods will significantly improve screening and play a crucial role in natural product pharmacologic assessment and quality control. The occurrence of bioactive compounds in various portions of plants, as well as HTS approaches for bioactive phytochemicals, will be discussed in this chapter.

2.2 Different parts of plants used to produce the pharmaceutically active compound

It has already been noted that different parts of plants, such as the leaves, roots, stems, seeds, and flowers, are utilized to extract bioactive compounds for use in a variety of pharmaceutical applications. This section provides a brief summary of the instances of how different areas of plants have been used.

2.2.1 Extracted from leaves

Leaf extracts have been utilized for medical purposes for many decades. For example, traditional medicine has long utilized olive leaf extract to treat colds and the flu. Antibacterial, antiinflammatory, and antioxidant activities of oleuropein may be found in the olive leaf extract. Table 2.1 lists a few instances of bioactive phytochemicals found in leaves, as well as how they were extracted under various conditions. Olive leaf (*Olea europaea*) extract also contains other complex chemicals that may be useful against influenza viruses and some bacteria. These are present in the leaves. Olive leaf extract has been shown to have antiviral properties, which may help prevent colds and flu as well as other illnesses. Inflamed sore throats may be soothed by gargling with olive leaf extract. The use of olive leaf extract for a limited period of time is usually believed to be safe. Olive leaf extract's long-term safety has yet to be proved. Patients with early-stage rheumatoid arthritis who received dehydrated olive leaf extract and methotrexate for 6 weeks

Table 2.1 Examples of extraction of bioactive phytochemicals from leaf extracts under various conditions.

Leaf	Phytochemicals	Extraction process	Extraction conditions			References
			Temperature (°C)	Time (hours)	Solvent	
Olea europaea	Phenolic	Solid-liquid maceration	23	6	Ethanol	[3]
	Oleuropein, luteolin-7-O-glucoside, apigenin-7-O-glucoside, quercetin, and verbascoside mannitol	Pressurized liquid extraction	190	0.083	Ethanol-water	[4]
Camellia sinensis	Polyphenols (threefold), catechins (twofold), and flavonoids (twofold)	Ultra-sonication extraction	80	0.33	Double distilled water	[5]
		Agitation extraction	80	0.33	Double distilled water	
Melastomastrum capitatum	Saturated fatty acid esters and phthalate acid derivatives	Cold maceration	–	48	Methanol	[6]
Ceratonia siliqua	Total phenolic and flavonoids content	Maceration	–	–	Ethanol-water	[7]
Nauclea latifolia	Antioxidant compounds	–	–	24	Methanol	[8]
Cynara cardunculus var. *scolymus*	Caffeoylquinic acid and flavones	Solvent extraction	Room temperature	1	Methanol	[9]
Cymbopogon *Salvia officinalis* *Psidium guajava*	Antioxidant, phenol, and flavonoid	Solvent extraction	Room temperature	48	Ethanol	[10]

Crocus sativus L.	Flavonols and flavones		Room temperature	5	Methanol	[11]
Beta vulgaris L.	Total phenolic compounds, betacyanins, and betaxanthins		30–80	24	Ethanol-water	[12]
Curcuma longa L.	Flavonoids, anthocyanins, and tannins	Soxhlet method	–	–	Methanol	[13]

saw a faster reduction in cell damage, restoration of antioxidant balance, and an improvement in IL-6 suppression throughout high disease activity. However, long-term rheumatoid arthritis sufferers did not see these improvements [14]. There are several bioactive compounds in olive leaf ethanolic extracts, including phenolic derivatives, pentacyclics, and alditols triterpenes, all of which have fascinating pharmacologic properties. The primary triterpene found in olive leaves is oleanolic acid (3.0%–3.5% DW), which is followed by maslinic acid and tiny amounts of erythrodiol, ursolic acid, and uvaol [15].

In recent decades, polyphenols found in green tea leaves have drawn a lot of interest. Green tea extracts have a high concentration of polyphenols, flavonoids, caffeine, amino acids, phenolic acids (especially hydroxybenzoic acids), carbohydrates, lipids, and volatile chemicals in their biomolecules. Catechins, such as (−)-catechin (C), (−)-epigallocatechin gallate (EGCG), (−)-epicatechin gallate (ECG), (−)-epicatechin (EC), (−)-epigallocatechin (EGC), (−)-gallocatechin gallate (GCG), and (−)-gallocatechin (GC), are the most important cumulative polyphenolic components [5]. There are two more varieties of tea: black tea and oolong tea. Catechins, such as epigallocatechin and epigallocatechin gallate, are abundant in green tea. Black tea is made from the fermentation of leaves, during which catechins are converted and which gives it its color. Fermentation significantly reduces the catechin concentration in black tea [16]. The bioactive chemicals profile and biologic characteristics of stigmas, spathes, tepals, tunics, and leaves from the saffron plant (*Crocus sativus*) were examined by Lahmass et al. [11]. The biologic features of stigmas (saffron spice) are linked to a high level of crocins. Despite having greater total phenolic and flavonoid content, the antioxidant activity of saffron's main product was lower than that of spathe and leaf extracts. There are three possible explanations for these findings: first that leaves have unusually rich content in glycosylated derivative luteolin; second, it contains glycosylated derivative kaempferol; and third, they have uncommonly rich content in glycosylated derivative of spaths, which contain crocins and other malvidin derivatives [11]. In comparison to other vegetables, beet (*Beta vulgaris* L.) has a large quantity of biomass that goes unused, and the leaves are thrown away as trash. Beet leaf extracts with high concentrations of total phenolics, betacyanins, and betaxanthins were produced by Bengardino et al. [12] using an improved method for simultaneous recovery of phytochemicals. Beet pigments betacyanins and betaxanthins (betalins) contain nitrogen and are water soluble. They have been described in the literature as having bioactive properties [12]. Turmeric (*Curcuma longa* L.) cultivation is restricted to the rhizomes, with the leaves as the primary by-product. This is similar to beet agriculture. The nutritional makeup and bioactive components of turmeric leaves were studied by Braga et al. [13]. Researchers found only minimal levels of nitrate and no cyanogenic chemicals on the leaves, which led them to believe that they could safely eat them. In addition, they noted that microwave drying was the best method for drying turmeric leaves, enhancing the antioxidant potential of both fresh and dried leaves [13]. Hundreds of more examples of the extraction of bioactive chemicals from leaf extracts may be found in the literature in addition to those already listed [17,18].

2.2.2 Extracted from flower and seed

Oil has been extracted from plant seeds for culinary, medical, and industrial applications. As a by-product of industrial fruit processing, it can be obtained directly. For the isolation of bioactive phytochemicals from the plant, preextraction and extraction techniques are critical. Separation and sifting techniques are used to recover the seed from fruit pomace, which is a mixture of the fruit's vascular tissues and skin. Seeds have the highest concentration of bioactive compounds of any fruit component and are commonly regarded as trash in the agro-industry; hence, using seeds will significantly decrease difficulties with ultimate disposal [19].

Cleaning, seed coat removal, grinding, and preheating are all steps in the extraction process that must be completed before the oil can be extracted. To separate arils, the outermost covering of seeds, the selected plant seed must be rinsed and dried. Arils must be removed because they clump together with seeds, causing fermentation and moisture absorption. Grinding of seed ensures that any oil embedded in the fibrous layers is disturbed, thereby allowing for the release of oil from the seed. As the surface area increases, more solvents will enter, allowing the oil to be extracted more effectively. Microwave pretreatment of seeds can improve oil extraction efficiency and enhance the quantity of tocopherols and phytosterols. However, due to the breakdown process, pretreating seeds with microwave irradiation can reduce the polyunsaturated fatty acid concentration [20].

Various examples of the isolation of phytochemicals from seed extracts are listed in Table 2.2. Plant oils are a rich source of fat-soluble vitamins and essential fatty acids, as well as other bioactive constituents such as volatile organic compounds. The features of antioxidant, antibacterial,

Table 2.2 Examples of extraction of bioactive phytochemicals from seed extracts under various conditions.

Plant source	Extraction condition				Outcomes		
	Method	Solvent	Temperature (°C)	Time (hours)		*n*-hexane	Ethanol
Passion fruit (*Passiflora edulis* Var. *Flavicarpa*)	Soxhlet	*n*-hexane ethanol	50	4	Oil yield (%)	26.12 ± 0.74	20.46 ± 1.36
					Fatty acid composition (linoleic, oleic, and α-linolenic acid) (%)	84.07	86.63
					Total tocopherol content (α-, γ-, δ-) (mg/100 g)	8.22 ± 0.01	2.98 ± 0.03
					Antioxidant activities (%)	53.57 ± 0.30	82.81 ± 0.49
Grapevine	Soxhlet	Hexane	70	–	Linoleic acid = 68.10–78.18 g/100 g oil. Oleic acid (MUFA) = 8.82 g/100 –16.92 g/100 g		
Almond	Hydrodistillation	–	N/S	2.5	Oil yield = 0.7%, benzaldehyde (62.52%), benzoic acid (14.80%), hexadecane (3.97%)		
Apricot	Hydrodistillation	–	N/S	3	Benzaldehyde = 90.6%, mandelonitrile = 5.2%, benzoic acid = 4.1%		

Anise *(Pimpinella anisum)*	Soxhlet	*n*-hexane	70	8	Oil yield = 7.40 ± 3.03% β-Sitosterol = 4034.53 ± 3.21% Total phenolics = 0.42 ± 0.04 mg GA/g oil DPPH = 3.44 ± 0.29 μmol TEAC/g
	Hydrodistillation	–	N/S	1, 2, and 3	*Pimpinella* in essential oils = A1: 94.4%, A2: 93.7% and A3: 97.3% Estragole = A1: 2.00%, A2: 3.39%, A3: 5.51% *trans*-Anethole = A1: 88.3%, A2: 87.0%, A3: 89.9%) γ-Himachalene = A1: 2.53%, A2: 2.90%, A3: 1.31%
Coriander	Soxhlet	*n*-hexane	70	8	Oil yield = 20.00 ± 3.25% β-Sitosterol = 997.97 ± 8.07% Total phenolics = 0.17 ± 0.15 mg GA/g oil DPPH = 2.24 ± 0.21 μmol TEAC/g
	Hydrodistillation	–	N/S	4	Oil yield at 160 min = 0.358% Linalool at 240 min = 68% Antioxidative capacity at 240 min = 35.9 μmol TEAC/g

Continued

Table 2.2 Examples of extraction of bioactive phytochemicals from seed extracts under various conditions.—cont'd

Plant source	Extraction condition				Outcomes
	Method	Solvent	Temperature (°C)	Time (hours)	
Nutmeg (*Myristica fragrans*)	Soxhlet	*n*-hexane	70	8	Oil yield = 7.43 ± 2.25% β-Sitosterol = 1203.19 ± 1.67% Total phenolics = 1.19 ± 0.12 mg GA/g oil DPPH = 16.46 ± 0.77 μmol TEAC/g
	Hydrodistillation	—	—	4	Oil yield = 5.811% Sabinene = 25.6%, Limonene = 5.84%, Myristicin = 13.16%

Reproduced with permission from Daud et al. [2].

antiinflammatory, anticancer, antiviral, and antidiabetic properties may be identified by seed extraction. Seed extracts' antidiabetic properties can help to control blood glucose levels by blocking the carbohydrate-digesting enzyme. Postprandial glucose levels are increased by digestive enzymes such as amylase and glucosidase in humans. Because bulky molecules such as starch are unable to cross the blood—brain barrier, alpha-amylase is responsible for starch hydrolysis, which results in the formation of low-molecular-weight compounds such as glucose units [21]. The blood sugar level will rise if glucose is converted to sugars at an excessive rate. Then, the extra sugar metabolized by the cells and stored as glycogen for energy is made possible by insulin. Because of its substantial suppression of glucosidase enzyme activity (98.4%), *Swietenia macrophylla* seeds extract could be utilized as an antidiabetic medicine. However, it has a modest inhibition of amylase enzyme activity (34.9%). Plant herbs' capacity to deploy antiviral activity is crucial in the treatment of viral illnesses. As an alternative to antiviral research, several pharmaceutical establishments are inclined to produce medications extracted from herbal plants. An inhibitory impact on Asia's most extensively transmitted dengue virus (DENV-2) was discovered in the seeds of *Swietenia macrophylla*'s triterpenoid phytochemical, limonoid. Grape seed extract, which is high in proanthocyanins, has recently been discovered to have the capacity to combat the hepatitis A virus and the Tulane virus when combined with heat treatment [22].

Bioactive compounds in plant seeds have the ability to cause cytotoxicity in cancer cells, making them a useful source of bioactive chemicals. As much as 70% of the polyphenols found in high quantities in the seeds of grapes have cytotoxic characteristics, according to research. A concentration- and time-dependent approach of inhibiting cell growth using extracts from grape seeds was shown to be more effective than extracts from the grape peel in limiting mesothelioma cell proliferation [23]. Jurkat cells, which are utilized as a model for human T cell acute lymphoblastic leukemia (ALL), can undergo apoptosis when exposed to avocado seeds (acute lymphocytic leukemia). Mitochondrial dysfunction and the release of phosphatidylserine from the cytoplasm membrane are hallmarks of apoptosis or programmed cell death. The seeds of the grape, avocado, and *Swietenia macrophylla* have been found to offer medicinal promise in the pharmaceutical, nutraceutical, and food industries, according to the literature reviewed. Waste seeds must undergo a variety of pretreatments, and extraction procedures must be chosen carefully. Extraction of the seeds into the oil, which is easy to eat, improves their quality [2]. Antibacterial efficacy against Gram-positive bacteria, including methicillin-resistant *Staphylococcus aureus*, as well as modest anticancer activity in vitro were found in the whole extract of oligostilbene chemicals from chi shao seed shell, according to Zhang et al. [24].

The availability of bioactive compounds in flowers has been discovered in the same way that it has been found in seeds. Trigonelline, gallic acid, caffeine, protocatechuic acid, as well as melanoidins make up the phenolic profile of coffee flowers. Nguyen et al. [25] used a green technique to produce bioactive chemicals such as high phenolic content, melanoidins, and bio-sugars from coffee flowers. Coffee pulp antioxidant potential as well as its high polyphenol and flavonoid concentration have been extensively discussed in the literature. Caffeic acid is the most abundant hydroxycinnamic acid ingredient in this coffee by-product, followed by chlorogenic, ferulic acids, and p-coumaric.

2.2.3 Extracted from stem bark

Extraction of bioactive phytochemicals from the stem bark of numerous plants has been described, similar to plant leaves. Table 2.3 describes examples of phytochemical extraction from stem bark. Various tree barks have traditionally been used to cure a variety of ailments. Willow tree bark, for example, has been used to treat fever, discomfort, and inflammation for thousands of years. Salicin, a related component to aspirin that reduces pain and inflammation, is found in the bark of the willow tree. Cascara buckthorn barks have also been used to treat constipation and hemorrhoids and as a recto-anal postoperative therapy in the past. The bark of *Rhamnus purshiana* (cascara sagrada) includes laxative anthranoid derivatives, which can be found in the form of free anthraquinones, dianthrones, anthrones, and/or O- and C-glycosides formed from these chemicals in a variety of laxative herbs [26]. In recent decades, many researchers have worked on the isolation of bioactive compounds from bark stems. For instance, several second metabolites, including scoparone, β-sitosterol, fraxidin, fraxetin, 3-acetylaleuritolic acid, and sitosterone from the stem bark of *Jatropha podagrica* have been reported by several researchers [27]. Thengyai et al. identified the stem bark of *V. glabrata* as the most bioactive part of the plant, and six known compounds (lupeol, betulinic acid, β-amyrin, scopoletin, α-amyrin, and betulin) were extracted using bioassay-guided fractionation [28]. Similarly, Minh et al. identified and isolated bioactive compounds (gallic acid, methyl gallate, fraxetin, and tomentin) from *Jatropha podagrica* [27].

Table 2.3 Examples of extraction of bioactive phytochemicals from bark stem extracts under various conditions.

Plant source	Bioactive phytochemicals	Extraction method/ detection	Extraction conditions			References
			Temperature (°C)	Time (hours)	Solvent	
Jatropha podagrica	Gallic acid, methyl gallate, fraxetin, and tomentin	Solvent extraction	25	168	Methanol	[27]
Cynara cardunculus var. *scolymus*	Caffeoylquinic acid and flavones	Solvent extraction	Room temperature	1	Methanol	[9]
Bruguiera gymnorrhiza	Phenols and terpenoids	Solvent extraction	—	—	Ethyl acetate	[29]
Vitex glabrata R.	Lupeol, β-amyrin, α-amyrin, betulin, betulinic acid, and scopoletin	Solvent extraction	50–55	48	Ethanol	[28]
Asimina triloba	Asimicin, Bullatacinone, N-trans- feruloyltyramine, (+)-syringaresinol, N-p-coumaroyltyramine	—	—	—	Ethanol	[30]
Albizia coriaria	Lupeol, lupenone, betulinic acid, acacic acid lactone, (+)-catechin and benzyl alcohol	—	Room temperature	48	Ethyl acetate, methanol, and water	[3[illegible]]
Juglans mandshurica	Ethyl gallate, aromadedrin, naringenin, juglone, menadione, and plumbagin	Ultrasonic-assisted solvent extraction	Room temperature	—	Methanol	[31]

2.2.4 Extracted from the root

Many plant roots have been used all over the world due to their medicinal properties. Some of the most popular roots that have been used for decades include ginger (*Zingiber officinale*), maca (*Lepidium meyenii*), kava kava (*Piper methysticum*), turmeric (*Curcuma longa*), valerian (*Valeriana officinalis*), echinacea (*Echinacea purpurea*), goldenseal (*Hydrastis canadensis*), Ashwagandha (*Withania somnifera*), and licorice (*Glycyrrhiza glabra*).

The volatile oils zingerone, shogaols, and gingerols are found in the root of the ginger plant. In many parts of the world, ginger root is sold as a spice, oral solution, capsules, and dried powdered root. Ginger is used to treat and prevent nausea from a variety of sources, including motion sickness, morning sickness, and other illnesses. Ginger contains antiinflammatory effects and can be used to treat rheumatoid arthritis, osteoarthritis, and muscle and joint discomfort. Ginger's bioactive chemicals, particularly the gingerol and shogaol classes, interact with multiple pathways that cause chemotherapy-induced nausea and vomiting. Furthermore, ginger's active ingredients have antiinflammatory capabilities. Ginger inhibits chemokine synthesis from synoviocytes, chondrocytes, and leukocytes directly, most likely by reduced TNF- and PGE-2 production, with NF–B and IBalpha mechanisms inhibiting their activation [32]. Turmeric root contains a phenolic molecule of the curcumin class (2%–9% of the overall composition) known as curcumin (70%–75%), which is followed by demethoxycurcumin (10%–25%) and bisdemethoxycurcumin (5%–10%) as the most important bioactive components [33]. One of the six primary kavalactones found in kava kava roots, kavain, has been shown to have antithrombotic properties in human platelets. Apart from that, 18 kavalactones and three chalcones, bornyl ester of cinnamic acid derivatives, and many flavanones have been found in kava roots to date. The pharmacologic and biologic benefits of kava roots might be due to a synergistic impact of all the chemicals found in the root. However, most kava research has focused on kavain, 7,8-dihydrokavain, methysticin, dihydromethysticin, desmethoxyyagonin, and yagonin, as well as the three dihydrochalcones, with little attention made to additional kava lactones and components in kava roots [34,35]. Likewise, alkylamides, phenolics, and glycoproteins/polysaccharide are the principal bioactive components found in *Echinacea* root extract. Echinacoside, cynarin, cichoric acid, caftaric acid, and chlorogenic acids are phenolics with antioxidant and antimicrobial properties [36,37]. Regarding phytoconstituents, ashwagandha's bioactive activities are due to two secondary metabolites: withanolide A and withaferin A. Other pharmaceutically important chemicals include withastramonolide, 27-hydroxywithanone, 20-deoxywithanolide A, somnine, tropine, somniferine, and somniferinine [38].

In recent decades, a number of other roots have been discovered that can be used to extract bioactive chemicals. Black carrot (*Daucus carota* L. ssp. *sativus* var. *atrorubens*), for example, is commonly employed for the recovery of these colorful chemicals and produces a lot of bagasse. Despite the extraction of the main pigment, Kumar et al. [39] claim that bagasse is a rich source of total phenolic content, flavonoid, and anthocyanin, resulting in a significant antioxidant potential. When compared with other traditional extraction approaches, the bioactive potential of microwave-aided extraction has doubled, according to researchers.

2.2.5 Other parts of the plant

A few plants' skins and husks are also high in bioactive compounds. In recent years, coffee silverskin has been intensively studied for its biologic properties, revealing a significant antioxidant capacity and phenolic content. This useful by-product has an interesting phenolic profile that is high in chlorogenic acids (mostly 5-O-caffeoylquinic acid), caffeic acid, and caffeine. All of the chemicals discussed above have a high bioavailability and are hence connected with a variety of bioactive characteristics [40]. In in vitro (human skin cells) and in vivo (*C. elegans* under UV-C treatment) oxidative stress models, Iriondo-DeHond et al. [41] discovered that coffee silverskin extract (1 mg/mL) was capable of protecting skin health and minimizing the risk of accelerated aging and skin illnesses. It has been suggested that coffee husk and silverskin may have a role in adipogenesis-related inflammation and insulin resistance, although this has yet to be proven [42]. Adipogenesis problems and inflammation from infiltrating macrophages—adipocytes interaction were reduced by the aforementioned coffee by-products. By-product biologic activities have been shown to be significantly influenced by chlorogenic acid and kaempferol.

Bioactive phytochemicals are abundant in vegetables and fruits, which we consume in our daily lives. Tomatoes are one of the most extensively grown vegetable crops, and they are consumed either raw or cooked. Tomato peels and their water-insoluble components are rich in lycopene, the principal tomato bioactive ingredient, which has been linked to a variety of health benefits. Tomato pomace, a mixture of tomato skin and seeds with a tiny portion of the pulp, is the most common residue produced by this sector. Due to the high proportion of tomato skins, tomato pomace possesses significant quantities of carotenoids, primarily lycopene, lutein, and carotene. It also includes important fatty acid derivatives that our bodies require [43]. Onions are the second most significant horticultural crop in the world, and their largest by-product is dried skin, which results from the peeling of the bulbs in an industrial setting. The flavonoid profile of dried onion skin is particularly rich in quercetin and its derivatives, as well as kaempferol and protocatechuic acid. Flavonoids and phenolic chemicals were more readily extracted from samples using supercritical carbon dioxide and subcritical water extractions than with other methods [44,45]. Likewise, artichoke is a source of bioactive substances such as phenolic compounds and inulins, as well as cyclitols and sesquiterpenes. Moreover, there is a modest amount of bioactive phytochemicals in all of the fruits and vegetables we consume on a daily basis.

2.3 High-throughput screening techniques for bioactive phytochemicals

Many people throughout the world have relied on natural products for thousands of years for the treatment of human ailments, and this trend has lately picked up steam. There are hundreds of chemical elements in natural products, making it challenging to determine the active ingredients responsible for their performance. The search for novel medication candidates necessitates the creation of accurate screening procedures for natural products' bioactive components. Natural product libraries benefit greatly from the discovery of new components. Natural products are challenging to screen for because of their many targets and combinatorial activities.

As a standard procedure, the pharmacologic activity of compounds of interest, followed by studies on the pharmacokinetics of such compounds, is used to identify bioactive components in natural products. However, long hours of experimentation and labor intensity are two major drawbacks of the conventional approach. An HTS approach that enables the identification of potentially active elements in natural goods will significantly enhance screening and play a key role in the pharmacologic assessment and quality control of natural products.

To rapidly identify active compounds, antibodies, or genes that modulate a specific biomolecular pathway, HTS uses a combination of robotics, liquid handling devices, software, and sensitive detectors to quickly run thousands of chemical, genetic, or pharmaceutical tests. Target interrogation is expedited with an HTS technique, allowing enormous libraries to be screened fast and affordably [46]. Biologic activity approaches, such as small compounds (including phytochemicals), siRNA, and shRNA, are initially separated into full-scale HTS libraries, which can contain tens of thousands of constructs. Further, smaller libraries are created based on the specificity or biologic family. All libraries are organized onto micro-well plates, allowing for screening in 96-, 384-, and, in some cases, 1536-well plates. Any HTS experiment has several phases, which may be broadly divided into three sets: (1) preparation of sample, (2) handling sample, and (3) readouts and data gathering.

HTS is a feasible approach for investigating a large number of phytochemicals in miniaturized in vitro experiments to find phytochemicals or compounds capable of regulating activity at the biologic target of interest. Identifying new therapeutic targets beyond the capabilities of manual pipetting and assaying was one impetus for enhancing throughput. To stay up with Pfizer's commercial rivals, hundreds of thousands of compounds had to be reviewed for successful screening; the interview with Sills [47] is particularly instructive for understanding the background behind the effort at Pfizer. Due to the commercial sensitivity of this information, comparable methodologies were not released for many years. Beggs [48] and Fox et al. [49] prompted academic and nonprofit groups to embrace it. An essential read is a firsthand account of the origins of the HTS idea at Pfizer Global Research and Development. This is given in three separate phases: (1) idea creation and philosophical implementation options, (2) practical implementation and technologic development, and (3) logical expansion to encompass adjacent fields in drug development [50].

2.3.1 High-throughput screening platforms

In HTS, the microtiter plate is the most significant reaction or testing medium. A typical configuration is a small rectangular container, typically made of machined or molded disposable plastic, which is populated with a grid of smaller, open invaginations or divots, known as "wells," that are spaced at regular intervals down the length of the container. Microtiter plates were first used during an influenza outbreak in Hungary in the early 1950s when standard laboratory equipment was in short supply due to a lack of available supplies. This terrible occurrence prompted Gyula Takátsy (1914–80), a Hungarian surgeon, to design machined leucite micro-well plates in 1951 (6 × 12, 10 × 10 wells) and a 96-well V-bottom machined plate the following year. There has been a brief history of the microplate and its early evolution written. Modern HTS microplates (created after 2013) often include 384, 1536, or 3456 wells, depending on the intended use. All are multiples of 96 (following the original 96-well microplates); the examples can be seen in Fig. 2.2. To get an idea of what plates are now available, investigators can review commercial literature. When conducting an experiment, the majority of the wells carry either test or control materials. Purified or, in the case of natural materials, plant extracts are dissolved in an aqueous solution with the supersolvent dimethyl sulfoxide. Wells commonly include all of the solubilized components needed to perform a test, such as proteins, DNA, cells, or even embryos in certain cases.

A translucent bottom is necessary for luminescence or fluorescence measurements on plates. Thus, the contents of the microplates may be easily examined, and transmitted light measurements can be made. When doing cell-based tests, these plates may be inspected directly under a microscope.

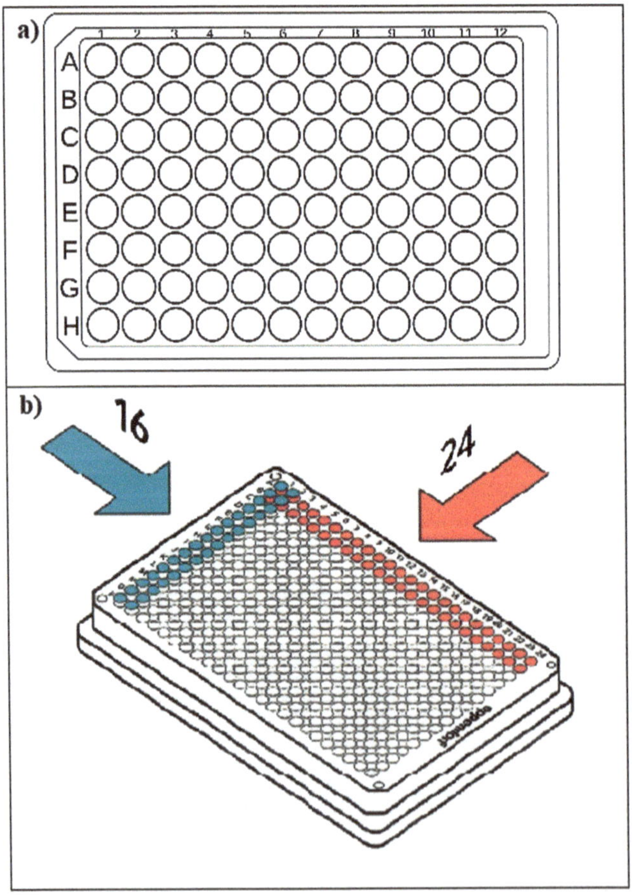

Figure 2.2 Symmetric diagram of (A) 96-well microplate and (B) 384-well microplate.

Additionally, the top structure's pigmentation helps to reduce inter-well cross-talk. Nontreated surfaces, immunoassay surfaces, and cell culture surfaces can all be found in a variety of sizes and shapes. In addition to sterile and nonsterile microplates, immunoassay plates and cell culture plates with clear bottoms are all readily accessible.

Phytochemicals, natural product extracts, and fractions of natural products may now be tested using HTS methods, which were originally developed to support the current drug discovery process by generating "lead" compounds from synthetic libraries created by classical and/or combinatorial synthesis. The extraction, isolation, and structural elucidation processes have been revolutionized by computational and mathematical modeling, which has reduced the total time and effort required to create dereplicated phytochemical libraries or other natural products libraries. Natural product collections or libraries are thought to be able to reach even the most difficult screening objectives due to their structural variation, complexity, stereogenic centers, and drug-like properties. Targeted or focused phytochemical libraries rely on the combinatorial synthesis and computational chemistry. Phosphochemical libraries targeting specific types of chemicals or therapeutic targets have been attempted in various papers, including the creation of alkaloid- and flavonoid-like libraries, for instance. Natural sources, such as bacteria, fungi, microalgae, and plants, can provide a wide range of microbial diversity.

Natural product samples are being prepared for testing in a variety of ways. When it comes to processing phytochemical samples manually, the procedure may be time consuming and cumbersome. Some of these problems can be solved by using a unique, automated sample preparation technique based on solid-phase extraction (SPE). A customized Zymark RapidTrace SPE workstation (Hopkinton, MA) developed by Schmid et al. [51] allowed for quick incorporation into high-throughput drug discovery campaigns, as detailed by Pereira et al. [50]. A comprehensive list of commercial solutions to this problem is beyond the scope of this discussion. Automatic SPE and filtering systems such as SPEEDY can handle SPE plates and cartridges. The samples are diluted and dispensed by separate probes once the column has been preconditioned. With software-controlled vacuum and/or positive pressure, reproducible and predictable outcomes may be accomplished (nitrogen or air). All commercially available filter plates, columns, and cartridges (1, 3, and 6−10 mL) are compatible. Filter disks control extraction, optional heating and cooling, pH testing, automated vial closing, evaporation, and sample processing (plasma, sera, cell culture materials, viscous samples).

It is difficult to isolate and identify active molecules in HTS natural product drug discovery programs, despite the abundance of unexplored potential medicines and molecular diversity. Bioassay-guided fractionation has become an essential economic element in the separation and identification of desired bioactive components of natural product mixtures. Both metabolomics and natural product discovery emphasize various parts of metabolite analysis, which may be seen by comparing the two. It is the former that makes sense of enormous amounts of data, whereas the latter concentrates on discovering specific bioactive metabolites that are of relevance. Bioprospecting is now a term for these kinds of searches because of the expected value of new finds. Both methods focus on identifying metabolites and use the same analytical techniques to identify them [52]. The methods of choice include chromatographic separation followed by mass spectrometry (MS) analysis and nuclear magnetic resonance (NMR). Despite significant technical breakthroughs in separation and analysis (Ultra Performance Liquid Chromatography, High-performance liquid chromatography, ion mobility), natural product structural variety and complexity as well as their physiochemical behavior remain as barriers. When spectrum databases are queried using physicochemical characteristics derived for complicated mixtures of isolated metabolites, metabolomics and natural product identification come together. The accessibility of comprehensive spectrum databases is completely dependent on the quality of peak annotation in metabolomics studies and dereplication in natural product screening. As a result, it is desirable, if not essential, to employ trustworthy spectrum databases in identification operations. Databases have been built for 13C NMR spectra, which are less affected by solvent influences than 1H NMR spectra.

One such database, which has 13C NMR spectrum information for over 6000 natural substances, makes it possible to identify known molecules in a short amount of time. It offers some insight into the structure of unknown molecules. Unlike NMRShiftDB, NAPROC-13 generates visuals using Cartesian coordinates, enhancing structural representations, and allowing for more straightforward stereocenter attribution in line with the International Union of Pure and Applied Chemistry (IUPAC) principles. In 2014, the number of compounds in the collection had risen to 21,000 [53]. Before recently, natural product researchers depended mainly on paper-based libraries, disks, and subsequently online commercial databases (such as the NIST Standard Reference MS Database and Aldrich Spectral Viewer NMR Library) for their study. NAPROC-13, a database for dereliction of natural product mixture, is useful because the placement of 13C NMR peaks is less solvent dependent than proton spectra. As a result, a number of pharmaceutical firms have built private internal databases with limited or even no public access to remain competitive. Real-time data analysis, open-access databases, and annotation/commenting are all encouraged in metabolomics in contrast to other domains of bioinformatics, from sample monitoring to online and real-time data analysis tools and algorithms. If present trends continue, open access, not-for-profit platforms will eventually replace commercial libraries as the primary source of natural product research information. On the web, Johnson et al. [54] created a collection of open access metabolomics datasets for natural product research.

2.3.2 Assay development and optimization

Numerous drug research initiatives have relied on plant extracts as a primary source of bioactive compounds, many of which have been isolated and found in prominent pharmaceuticals. Isolation programs that aim to produce medicine or a lead chemical must use bioassay screening or pharmacologic evaluation to identify the pure bioactive component. The target syndrome and the amount of information available about the plant being examined both go into the decision of which biologic test to conduct. Using a bioassay approach that can forecast a plant's purported therapeutic action, for example, would logically leverage an ethnopharmacologic history of usage against a certain illness to extract the lead responsibility for this biologic activity. Traditionally, plant extracts were studied exclusively in laboratory mice and rats. Disk diffusion antimicrobial test is now in use. However, this method has a number of drawbacks. There are several bioactive components in the phytochemical extracts, making them very variable. To get a specific biologic reaction, it may be necessary to combine many bioactive substances rather than relying just on one. Although new bioassay techniques have been created, they are still expensive and time consuming, as well as technologically difficult at this moment, despite this. Bioassay procedures have the significant drawback of requiring the use of living creatures such as mice and rats, which is impractical due to the high rate of animal sacrifice. Bioassays can be cumbersome to use when trying to identify and quantify certain bioactive compounds. As a result, this method is losing its luster.

2.3.3 Primary and secondary screening

Phytochemical screening is another name for this process. These extracts are made from plant samples rich in secondary metabolites such as the leaves and stems, roots, and bark of the plants studied. The secondary metabolites, such as alkaloids, terpenes, and flavonoids, are then examined in the plant extracts. Compounds can be analyzed using standard assays found in the literature. An analysis technique such as thin-layer chromatography is commonly used to determine how many and what kind of components are present in a mixture. The extracts are placed on a glass dish coated with silica gel or another adsorbent. The dish is then placed in a chromatographic chamber containing a suitable solvent for thin-layer chromatography. Using this method, the compounds are separated by polarity from one another in two distinct phases: the mobile phase and the stationary phase. After the plate is removed from the chromatographic chamber, a developing solvent may also be employed to identify the compounds. In developing nations, this strategy has been engaged in the past and is still being used now. Due to the time and effort required to isolate pure bioactive components, this method allows the extraction of known metabolites from the extracts, making it more cost effective. Even though it is a straightforward test, it is ineffective in sorting out the various components of the sample, making it difficult to identify even small amounts of them in the final product.

2.4 Summary

The present chapter ascertains the richness of bioactive compounds present in various parts of the plants from root to seed. Many parts of the plant have great nutritional and nutraceutical value, in addition to their well-documented biologic activities, including antioxidant, anticarcinogenic, antimicrobial, antiinflammatory, antiadipogenesis, antidiabetic, antiaging, and antihypertensive properties. The literature makes it clear that screening for bioactive phytochemicals is a major priority for researchers to find their usefulness in pharmaceutical industries. An HTS approach for identifying potentially active chemicals in natural products would considerably enhance screening and play an essential role in natural product pharmacologic assessment and quality management. This chapter primarily gave an overview of the distribution of bioactive phytochemicals in various plant sections. A summary of the HTS approach was also presented.

References

[1] P. Wangchuk, Therapeutic applications of natural products in herbal medicines, biodiscovery programs, and biomedicine, Journal of Biologically Active Products from Nature 8 (1) (2018) 1–20.

[2] N.M. Daud, et al., Valorisation of plant seed as natural bioactive compounds by various extraction methods: a review, Trends in Food Science & Technology 119 (2022) 201–214.

[3] P.R. Das, J.-B. Eun, A comparative study of ultra-sonication and agitation extraction techniques on bioactive metabolites of green tea extract, Food Chemistry 253 (2018) 22–29.

[4] C.A. Ukwubile, et al., Cytotoxic effects of new bioactive compounds isolated from a Nigerian anticancer plant *Melastomastrum capitatum* Fern. leaf extract, Scientific African 8 (2020) e00421.

[5] A.B. Hsouna, et al., Characterization of bioactive compounds and ameliorative effects of *Ceratonia siliqua* leaf extract against CCl4 induced hepatic oxidative damage and renal failure in rats, Food and Chemical Toxicology 49 (12) (2011) 3183–3191.

[6] O.S. Ajayi, et al., Bioactive compounds from *Nauclea latifolia* leaf extracts, Journal of King Saud University Science 32 (4) (2020) 2419–2425.

[7] G. Pandino, S. Lombardo, G. Mauromicale, Globe artichoke leaves and floral stems as a source of bioactive compounds, Industrial Crops and Products 44 (2013) 44–49.

[8] M.A. Elchaghaby, S.F. Abd El-Kader, M.M. Aly, Bioactive composition and antibacterial activity of three herbal extracts (lemongrass, sage, and guava leaf) against oral bacteria: an in vitro study, Journal of Oral Biosciences 64 (2022).

[9] I. Lahmass, et al., The waste of saffron crop, a cheap source of bioactive compounds, Journal of Functional Foods 35 (2017) 341–351.

[10] M.B. Bengardino, et al., Recovery of bioactive compounds from beet leaves through simultaneous extraction: modelling and process optimization, Food and Bioproducts Processing 118 (2019) 227–236.

[11] M.C. Braga, E.C.S. Vieira, T.F. de Oliveira, *Curcuma longa* L. leaves: characterization (bioactive and antinutritional compounds) for use in human food in Brazil, Food Chemistry 265 (2018) 308–315.

[12] A. Čabarkapa, et al., Dry olive leaf extract in combination with methotrexate reduces cell damage in early rheumatoid arthritis patients—a pilot study, Phytotherapy Research 30 (10) (2016) 1615–1623.

[13] Á. Guinda, et al., Determination of major bioactive compounds from olive leaf, LWT - Food Science and Technology 64 (1) (2015) 431–438.

[14] A.L.S. Oliveira, et al., Olive leaf phenolic extract from two Portuguese cultivars – bioactivities for potential food and cosmetic application, Journal of Environmental Chemical Engineering 9 (5) (2021) 106175.

[15] A. Lama-Muñoz, et al., Content of phenolic compounds and mannitol in olive leaves extracts from six Spanish cultivars: extraction with the Soxhlet method and pressurized liquids, Food Chemistry 320 (2020) 126626.

[16] A.F. Korystova, et al., Black tea is more effective than green tea in prevention of radiation-induced oxidative stress in the aorta of rats, Biomedicine & Pharmacotherapy 142 (2021) 112064.

[17] D. Haldar, M.K. Purkait, A review on the environment-friendly emerging techniques for pretreatment of lignocellulosic biomass: mechanistic insight and advancements, Chemosphere 264 (2021) 128523.

[18] D. Haldar, M.K. Purkait, Lignocellulosic conversion into value-added products: a review, Process Biochemistry 89 (2020) 110–133.

[19] E. Gómez-Mejía, et al., Valorisation of black mulberry and grape seeds: chemical characterization and bioactive potential, Food Chemistry 337 (2021) 127998.
[20] B. Fathi-Achachlouei, et al., Microwave pretreatment as a promising strategy for increment of nutraceutical content and extraction yield of oil from milk thistle seed, Industrial Crops and Products 128 (2019) 527–533.
[21] P. Agarwal, R. Gupta, Alpha-amylase inhibition can treat diabetes mellitus, Research Review Journal of Medical and Health Science 5 (4) (2016) 1–8.
[22] M. Patwardhan, et al., Heat sensitization of hepatitis A virus and Tulane virus using grape seed extract, gingerol and curcumin, Food Microbiology 90 (2020) 103461.
[23] F. Di Meo, et al., Anticancer activity of grape seed semi-polar extracts in human mesothelioma cell lines, Journal of Functional Foods 61 (2019) 103515.
[24] Y. Zhang, et al., Paeonia veitchii seeds as a promising high potential byproduct: proximate composition, phytochemical components, bioactivity evaluation and potential applications, Industrial Crops and Products 125 (2018) 248–260.
[25] T.M.T. Nguyen, et al., Use of coffee flower as a novel resource for the production of bioactive compounds, melanoidins, and bio-sugars, Food Chemistry 299 (2019) 125120.
[26] T.N. Minh, et al., Isolation and purification of bioactive compounds from the stem bark of *Jatropha podagrica*, Molecules 24 (5) (2019) 889.
[27] N. Nurjanah, et al., Bioactive Compounds and Antioxidant Activity of Lindur Stem Bark (*Bruguiera gymnorrhiza*), 2015.
[28] S. Thengyai, et al., α-Glucosidase and α-amylase inhibitory activities of medicinal plants in Thai antidiabetic recipes and bioactive compounds from *Vitex glabrata* R. Br. stem bark, Journal of Herbal Medicine 19 (2020) 100302.
[29] G. Zhao, et al., Additional bioactive compounds and trilobacin, a novel highly cytotoxic acetogenin, from the bark of *Asimina triloba*, Journal of Natural Products 55 (3) (1992) 347–356.
[30] R. Byamukama, et al., Bioactive compounds in the stem bark of *Albizia coriaria* (Welw. ex Oliver), International Journal of Brain and Cognitive Sciences 9 (2) (2015) 1013–1024.
[31] D. Medan, C. Schirarend, Rhamnaceae, in: Flowering Plants·Dicotyledons, Springer, 2004, pp. 320–338.
[32] B. Ozola, et al., Bioactive compounds in fresh and dried ginger root (*Zingiber officinale*), Food Belt 50 (1) (2019) 265–268.
[33] J.G. de Oliveira Filho, et al., Bioactive compounds of turmeric (*Curcuma longa* L.), in: H.N. Murthy, K.Y. Paek (Eds.), Bioactive Compounds in Underutilized Vegetables and Legumes, Springer International Publishing, Cham, 2021, pp. 297–318.
[34] D. Wu, M.G. Nair, D.L. DeWitt, Novel compounds from piper methysticum forst (kava kava) roots and their effect on cyclooxygenase enzyme, Journal of Agricultural and Food Chemistry 50 (4) (2002) 701–705.
[35] T.D. Xuan, et al., Efficacy of extracting solvents to chemical components of kava (*Piper methysticum*) roots, Journal of Natural Medicines 62 (2) (2007) 188.
[36] R. Bruni, et al., Analytical methods for the study of bioactive compounds from medicinally used Echinacea species, Journal of Pharmaceutical and Biomedical Analysis 160 (2018) 443–477.
[37] J.L. Parsons, et al., Echinacea biotechnology: advances, commercialization and future considerations, Pharmaceutical Biology 56 (1) (2018) 485–494.
[38] A.G. Namdeo, D.K. Ingawale, Ashwagandha: advances in plant biotechnological approaches for propagation and production of bioactive compounds, Journal of Ethnopharmacology 271 (2021) 113709.

[39] M. Kumar, et al., Valorisation of black carrot pomace: microwave assisted extraction of bioactive phytoceuticals and antioxidant activity using Box–Behnken design, Journal of Food Science & Technology 56 (2) (2019) 995–1007.
[40] S.M. Bessada, et al., Coffea canephora silverskin from different geographical origins: a comparative study, Science of the Total Environment 645 (2018) 1021–1028.
[41] A. Iriondo-DeHond, et al., Coffee silverskin extract protects against accelerated aging caused by oxidative agents, Molecules 21 (6) (2016) 721.
[42] M. Rebollo-Hernanz, et al., Phenolic compounds from coffee byproducts modulate adipogenesis-related inflammation, mitochondrial dysfunction, and insulin resistance in adipocytes, via insulin/PI3K/AKT signaling pathways, Food and Chemical Toxicology 132 (2019) 110672.
[43] K. Szabo, et al., Antimicrobial and antioxidant properties of tomato processing byproducts and their correlation with the biochemical composition, Lebensmittel-Wissenschaft & Technologie 116 (2019) 108558.
[44] M. Munir, et al., Subcritical water extraction of bioactive compounds from waste onion skin, Journal of Cleaner Production 183 (2018) 487–494.
[45] L. Campone, et al., Response surface methodology to optimize supercritical carbon dioxide/co-solvent extraction of brown onion skin byproduct as source of nutraceutical compounds, Food Chemistry 269 (2018) 495–502.
[46] A. Dove, High-throughput screening goes to school, Nature Methods 4 (6) (2007) 523–532.
[47] M.A. Sills, Future considerations in HTS: the acute effect of chronic dilemmas, Drug Discovery Today 3 (7) (1998) 304–312.
[48] D.H. Pereira, et al., Intake and total and partial digestibility of nutrients, ruminal pH and ammonia concentration and microbial efficiency in beef cattle fed with diets containing sorghum (*Sorghum bicolor* (L.) Moench) silage and concentrate in different ratios, Livestock Science 107 (1) (2007) 53–61.
[49] S.L. Robinette, et al., NMR in metabolomics and natural products research: two sides of the same coin, Accounts of Chemical Research 45 (2) (2012) 288–297.
[50] F.M.D. Ismail, L. Nahar, S.D. Sarker, Chapter 6 - high-throughput screening of phytochemicals: application of computational methods, in: S.D. Sarker, L. Nahar (Eds.), Computational Phytochemistry, Elsevier, 2018, pp. 165–192.
[51] S.L. Johnson, et al., Consistent age-dependent declines in human semen quality: a systematic review and meta-analysis, Ageing Research Reviews 19 (2015) 22–33.
[52] M. Beggs, A. Long, High throughput genomics and drug discovery–, Drug Discovery (2002) 75.
[53] S. Fox, et al., Increasing the chances of lead discovery, Drug Discovery World Spring 2001 (2001) 35–44.
[54] I. Schmid, et al., Natural products in high throughput screening: automated high-quality sample preparation, SLAS Discovery 4 (1) (1999) 15–25, https://doi.org/10.1177/108705719900400104.

CHAPTER 3

Conventional approaches for the extraction of bioactive compounds for pharmaceutical applications

3.1 Introduction

Extraction is a word used in the pharmaceutical industry to describe separating bioactive compounds of animal or plant tissues from inert or inactive constituents using standard extraction techniques, such as the use of specific solvents. Plant-derived products, such as liquids, semisolids, and powders, are designed for oral or external use exclusively. As a general rule, they fall into one of six categories: decoctions, tinctures, fluid extracts, pilulars (semisolid), infusions, and powdered extracts. Preparations like this are commonly referred to as "galenicals" in honor of the second-century Greek physician Galen [1].

The solubility, the presence of different substances in the plant matrix, and the solvent used to solubilize the bioactive elements all influence the extraction process. Before being extracted, the plant tissue should be thoroughly homogenized to enhance the extraction rate. Bioactive phytochemicals come from a variety of sustainable sources, including plants, animals, microorganisms, and aquatic species. Natural sources always have a small quantity of bioactive natural chemicals that are concentrated in the plant matrix. Plant parts including exudates, fruits, flowers, twigs, and even the entire plant emit active substances that are known as "phytochemicals" in various concentrations [2—4]. To optimize the extract from tissues, choosing the correct extraction procedure is critical. Several essential factors, such as extraction method, plant component matrix characteristics, pressure, extraction solvent, temperature, and time, all influence extraction efficiency [5].

Advances in Extraction and Applications of Bioactive Phytochemicals
ISBN 978-0-443-18535-9
https://doi.org/10.1016/B978-0-443-18535-9.00006-5

Bioactive phytochemicals may be extracted using a variety of methods. These methods can be classified as both traditional and advanced [6,7]. Traditional procedures use organic solvents or water and operate at barometric pressure, but advanced strategies use pressure and/or extreme temperatures. Using adequate solvents is required to distinguish active components of plant tissues from the originating components utilizing extraction methods. The solvents travel into the solid plant components and solubilize the chemicals with identical polarity throughout this process. It is crucial to choose a solvent as well as an extraction method that is compatible with the targeted bioactive compound. The solvent selection follows the "like dissolves like" adage. Therefore, polar solvents can isolate polar compounds, whereas nonpolar solvents may isolate nonpolar molecules. Soxhlet extraction, maceration, decoction, percolation, and hydrodistillation are typical procedures for extracting bioactive chemicals from plants. Traditional extraction procedures, such as maceration, percolation, and Soxhlet extraction, employ organic solvents and need a significant volume of solvents and a long extraction period. In contrast, decoction and hydrodistillation use water as a solvent [1].

There are several conventional methods for extracting bioactive phytochemicals from plants, and this chapter attempts to offer a complete assessment of these approaches and highlight their merits and limitations.

3.2 Conventional approaches for the extraction of bioactive compounds

3.2.1 Soxhlet extraction

In 1879, German scientist Franz Ritter von Soxhlet devised the Soxhlet extractor (SE). It was first employed for lipid extraction; it has since been used for a wide range of extraction. SE is used in a variety of experimental approaches to extract necessary phytochemicals from a variety of natural sources. It entails the continual extraction of phytochemicals from a solid mixture. A conventional setup for the SE is illustrated in Fig. 3.1A. During the extraction process boiling solvent vapors climb via the larger side arm. Condensed droplets of solvent dropping into a porous cup dissolve the needed component of a solid mixture, and the solid mixture is no longer required. Whenever the smaller side arm becomes overfilled to the point of overflowing, a syphoning motion occurs. The solvent, which contains the dissolved component, is poured into the distillation flask. In the process of

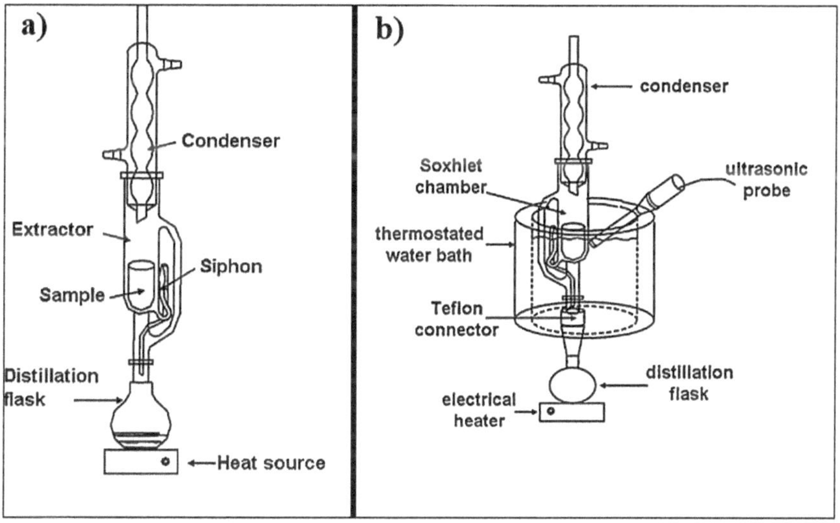

Figure 3.1 (A) Conventional Soxhlet extractor. (B) Ultrasound-assisted Soxhlet extractor. *(A) Reproduced with permission from Castro et al. [8] (B) Reproduced with permission from Garcia et al. [9].)*

fresh solvent droplets falling into the porous cup, remaining solvent drains away, and the cycle is repeated once again.

It may be used to compare the effectiveness of different extraction methods. SE has several advantages, including minimal upfront costs and the ability to operate at extreme temperatures (which increases kinetics), as well as no filtering or minimal filtration-related expenditures. To maintain a reasonable extraction temperature, the solvent is repeatedly brought into contact with the solid matrix. This causes a shift in the transfer equilibrium. The extract does not need to be filtered. One of the key drawbacks of the SE technique is that it is restricted due to its low extraction efficiency, lengthy operation, and several solvents. Solvents cause target compounds to evaporate and decompose, along with an increase in extraction kinetics, resulting in the loss of thermolabile molecules when substances boil at elevated temperatures. The Soxhlet does not allow for agitation. Because extraction usually takes place at the boiling point of the solvent for an extended period, the risk of thermal degradation of the target compounds must be overlooked.

Some variations were created based on the advantages and drawbacks associated with the standard SE, and these were then improved upon to address the flaws while also maintaining and even increasing the advantages.

The majority of the advancements documented in recent decades have aimed to bring SE closer to more modern solid sample preparation processes by reducing leaching times and automating the extraction assembly [8]. High-pressure SE, ultrasonic-assisted SE, and microwave-assisted SE are examples of modified SE techniques.

3.2.1.1 High-pressure Soxhlet extraction

Supercritical fluid SEs commercially available or custom-built laboratories can obtain SE at high pressure by installing the extractor within a circular stainless-steel autoclave. Extractants in high-pressure SE do not reach supercritical temperatures. They can include low-boiling solvents or gases under normal pressure and temperature, but under high pressure and temperature, they must be liquid. Time and solvent consumption should be cut in half with the advancement of the Soxhlet process at high pressure (1000−1500 psi). Using high-pressure SE, pesticides such as organochlorines and polychlorinated biphenyls have been isolated before being tested in lyophilized fish tissue, potato, olive oil, carrot, and oil samples. At the height of its popularity, carbon dioxide was employed as an extractant medium in this application. Condensation of the extractant was achieved by submerging the extraction apparatus in a water bath at a temperature of 0°C [8,10].

The major downside of these extraction devices is the way they are operated. The Soxhlet process should not be hindered by the extractors' reduced robustness and increased complexity when operating at high pressure.

3.2.1.2 Ultrasound-assisted Soxhlet extraction

The researchers' strategies developed and used an extractor based on Soxhlet's physical-chemical principles that used ultrasonic effects to extract total fat from oilseeds such as sunflower and soybean. Fig. 3.1B illustrates an experimental setup for ultrasound-assisted Soxhlet extraction. The technique employs traditional Soxhlet glassware, but the Soxhlet chamber is housed in a thermostatic bath through which ultrasound is administered through an ultrasonic probe. There are no significant differences in performance between conventional SE and ultrasound on the sample cartridge. But it considerably decreases the number of Soxhlet cycles necessary in conventional procedures. When ultrasonics are used, they provide a decompression effect that saves the usual grinding steps between Soxhlet cycles, which are typically required to minimize the increased compactness caused by the lowering extractant. Despite the fact that ultrasound has been shown to have an oxidative impact at extreme settings, the low conditions utilized in this extractor do not harm the extracted oil [9,11].

3.2.1.3 Microwave-assisted Soxhlet extraction

The most effective endeavor to increase Soxhlet performance has been microwave, which has allowed a wider choice of techniques. In reality, microwave-assisted SE is still the most intriguing advancement above normal SE.

Microwave-assisted SE differs from other microwave-assisted extraction techniques primarily in four ways: (a) under normal pressure where the vessel is kept open, (b) by focused microwave irradiation on the sample compartment, (c) as in the typical SE, the extraction stage is completed entirely or partially, and (d) excluding subsequent filtration. As a consequence, these approaches maintain the advantages of classical SE while also overcoming its constraints, notably in terms of speed, automaticity, and the ability to quantitatively extract heavily retained analytes [8].

3.2.2 Maceration

Maceration is another conventional extraction method that is carried out at room temperature. To ensure that the food and solvent are properly mixed in during the extraction process, the entire or coarse foodstuff is ground or chopped into smaller pieces. Menstruum serves as the solvent in a sealed container during this procedure. This is accompanied by compressing the solid residue, termed "marc," to collect the greatest amount of occluded solution possible from the extraction process once the extraction procedure is complete. The combined pressed liquid with strained solvent is filtered to eliminate any unwanted components from the mixture [12,13]. The use of more delicate powder is generally avoided in this process as it complicates the process of clarification. The menstruum must have adequate time to penetrate through the cell wall to disintegrate and disperse the constituents of vegetal medicines. The extraction process allows for molecular diffusion because the solution is stationary except for periodic shaking. The concentrated solution that builds upon the surface of the particles can be dispersed by shaking them every now and then, which aids diffusion and brings new menstruum to the surface of the particles for further extraction. Because the menstruum is extracted in a sealed container, there is no batch-to-batch variance. Extractive activities are aided by frequent agitation during maceration by two ways, i.e., by encouraging diffusion and by increasing extraction yield by adding additional solvent to the menstruum and separating the concentrated solution from the sample surface. In spite of its simplicity, this extraction process has the disadvantages of a long extraction time and low extraction efficiency. A thermolabile component might be extracted using this method. Anthraquinone, a phenolic compound, was effectively isolated from *Rheum emodi* using the maceration approach by Arvindekar et al. [14]. Ethanol was the extraction solvent, and it took 24 h to complete. It might take anywhere from a few hours to a few weeks for some plant materials to be macerated. As a result, it takes a long time to complete this procedure [14]. When the source material is not completely depleted, the extraction process is incomplete. Despite the lengthy processing time, this method is suggested for extracting heat-labile compounds. Similarly, by Ćujić et al. [15], total phenols and anthocyanins were extracted from chokeberry fruit using maceration, a simple and effective approach, at a 50% ethanol, a solid—solvent ratio of 1:20, and a particle size of 0.75 mm, which indicated that maceration was a good method for extracting these chemicals [15]. Maceration is considered to be an economical process compared with the other traditional and advanced processes. Albuquerque et al. [16] extracted catechin was from *Arbutus unedo* L. fruits utilizing three different extraction methods: maceration, microwave-assisted, and ultrasound. The results showed that microwave-assisted extraction was the most effective, but maceration used a lower temperature and produced remarkably similar extraction efficiency, which can be translated into financial gains [16]. Similarly, to extract Serpylli herba polyphenols, Jovanovi et al. [17] performed maceration, heat-assisted extraction, and ultrasonic-aided extraction methods. Ultrasonic-aided extraction yielded the highest total flavonoid output relative to total polyphenol content, and no significant difference was observed between maceration and heat-assisted extraction during the experiment [17].

The marc is squeezed during the maceration of phytochemicals because a significant amount of liquid clings to it and cannot be separated in any other way. As a result, the volume of the marc does not change since there is a variable amount of liquid containing soluble substances in it. A subpar product will be produced if the amount is changed. Without adjusting, the amount of liquid expressed affects the product yield and the percentage of soluble materials; no matter what type of press it is pressed in, the strength of the product is unaffected. Vinegar of squill (British Pharmaceutical Codex, BPC), tincture of orange (Indian Pharmacopoeia, IP), oxymel of squill (BPC), tincture of capsicum (BPC), tincture of lemon, compound tincture of gentian, and tincture of squill (BPC) are all examples of preparations formed using this method. The marc is not squeezed in the maceration of disorganized pharmaceuticals because the preferred substance is dissolved, and the residual marc is sticky and slimy. As a result, pressing it is not practical nor essential. In addition, the volume may be modified since the upper, transparent layer can be readily separated from the bottom layer by filtration. The drug's soluble components are nearly all present in the solution; the minor quantity that remains attached to the gummy matrix is removed from the marc during the filter's menstrual fluid wash. As a result, volume adjustments lead to homogeneity. Tolu tincture, BPC tincture, and compound tincture of benzoin are only some of the products that may be manufactured using this method.

Because some of the active ingredients is left behind in the first pressing of the marc, repeated maceration may be more effective than a single maceration operation. It is common to practice utilizing double maceration when the active ingredients are especially important and volatile oil is also present. Moreover, researchers have modified the maceration process in many other ways to improve the efficiency of the process [18].

3.2.2.1 Modified maceration process

There may be a large quantity of active principle retained in the marc after the initial pressing; hence it may be more effective to use multiple maceration than a single maceration technique, as described earlier. It is the usual procedure to apply twofold maceration when the active components are highly significant and volatile oil is also present. To obtain more juice out of the marc when pressing is not a possibility, some people resort to a procedure known as triple maceration [19]. However, the total amount of solvent utilized is large, and the second and third macerates are generally mixed and evaporated prior to becoming given to the first macerate.

Certain alterations are required for industrial extraction on a wide scale. A modest amount of solvent (500—1000 mL) can be shaken without causing any harm. However, for industrial activity involving a big volume of solvent and large containers, shaking the containers is difficult. There are, of course, less-complicated approaches to the agitation that are just as powerful. Another essential goal is to limit the amount of solvent used during extraction, lowering the amount of evaporation required for highly concentrated products. The advantage of reducing evaporation costs reduces heat damage to thermolabile substances.

When using a maceration procedure, it is possible to increase extraction efficiency by circulating solvent through the drug, as shown in Fig. 3.2. By use of spray nozzles, the solvent is pushed from the bottom of the vessel and spread over the drug More quickly, local concentrations are reduced due to a more uniform dispersion of the solvent [18,20].

As mass transfer stops when equilibrium is attained in the typical maceration phase, extraction is partial. A multistage approach can be used to solve this issue. It requires a vessel for the crude medicine, a pump, spray distributors, and many tanks to hold the extracted solution for this process to work properly. Using the pipework and valves illustrated in Fig. 3.3, the extractor may be linked to any of the tanks to transfer the solution. Each batch of medication is subjected to a series of solvent treatments, with the strongest solution in receiver 1 and the weakest solution in receiver 3 [18,21].

3.2.3 Infusion

The infusion procedure usually requires a shorter time to accomplish than the maceration. This organic solvent extraction method produces plant

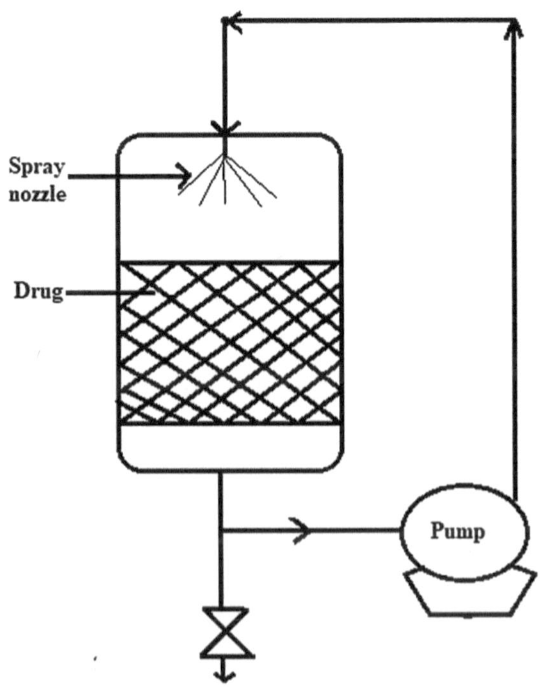

Figure 3.2 Experimental setup for circulatory extraction.

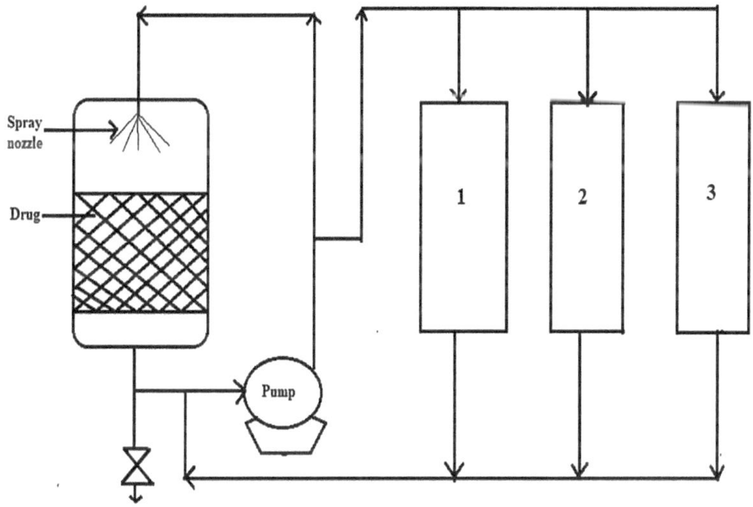

Figure 3.3 Experimental setup for multistage extraction.

extracts that are volatile and quickly dissolve or release their active components [22]. The plant material is macerated in boiling or cold water then steeped for a few hours. To concentrate the liquid, a rotating evaporator is utilized, which usually has a vacuum. The quantity of herb and solvent used will vary depending on the herb used and the strength of the infusion. Ergen et al. [23] used infusion to extract bioactive chemicals from medicinal plants, increasing yield from 12.46% to 35.39%.

Dilute solutions containing the easily soluble components of crude medications are known as infusions. Fresh infusions were originally utilized and reduced to eight volumes by macerating the medicine for a brief time in cold or boiling water, but nowadays, infusions are commonly made by diluting one volume of a concentrated infusion to 10 volumes using water. A modified percolation or maceration procedure is used to make concentrated infusions. After diluting with water, concentrated infusions have the same potency and aroma as fresh infusions. For this reason, infusions should be administered within 12 h of preparation to avoid the growth of germs and fungi.

Generally, this technique is performed in an appropriate container with a lid, where 50 mL cold water is added to the coarsely powdered crude drug (50 g) and left to stand for 15 min. After that, 900 mL of hot water is poured into the vessel, and it is let to stand for 30 min with the lid snugly on. After the combination has been filtered, the infusion is given a final volume of 1000 mL by adding more water. Drugs that are delivered in muslin bags for infusion preparation are precise enough to be utilized for this purpose. Cold water should be used if the boiling water affects the infusion's activity. Due to the limited shelf life of fresh infusions, they should only be prepared at the time of usage [18,24].

Another type of infusion is referred to as "concentrated infusion." In this process, a 25% alcohol solution is added either during the infusion operation or after the operation and then diluted according to pharmacopeial criteria. When the active and desirable constituents of the drug are equally soluble in water and menstruum, concentrated infusions are generally used in those scenarios.

3.2.4 Decoction

Plant parts that are tougher to process, for instance barks, roots, and seeds, are typically utilized in decoctions. Preparing the decoction begins with the grinding or crushing of the entire root and bark, as well as the seeds. It is important to boil the targeted portions for 30 min, or just until 50% of the water has dissipated, to produce the necessary chemicals. To prevent the evaporation of essential components, the vessel must be covered while being heated. After the extract is removed from the heat and filtered through a filter, the decoction can be utilized whole or diluted. This extraction method is useful for extracting thermally stable and water-soluble components from raw plant matter. This method is used to make ayurveda extracts called "quath" or "kwath." The extract is concentrated before being filtered or further treated [25]. In most cases, decoctions are consumed orally. They are the most readily absorbed and have the most potent impact of all the standard forms of preparations available. In general, target chemicals in decoction are oil soluble [26]. Decoction and infusion of *Teucrium polium* L. from the Lamiaceae family also possessed greater levels of phenolic compounds and antioxidant activity, according to Ozer et al. [27]. The decoction has various drawbacks, such as the fact that it takes a long time to make. They do not always have a pleasant or perceptible flavor. It is tough to carry and store them. Many of the active elements of plants do not dissolve well in water. The procedures are straightforward, but a huge volume of solvent is required.

3.2.5 Percolation

In contrast to maceration, which is a batch operation, percolation utilizes a continuous flow of new solvent to replenish the saturated solvent. As the solvent passes through the percolator, the medication is structured into a powdered form that may be easily dispersed [28]. The use of a solvent during the process causes the dried material to swell, and the extent of this swelling increases as the aqueous nature of the solvent increases. Because of the reduced or blocked flow of solvent caused by the swelling, the extraction process is adversely affected. If the dry powder is packed, fine particles may move via the column and settle at lower levels, diminishing its porosity and making it nonuniform. A washout of the column's finer particles is possible. To avoid these challenges, the raw material should be soaked in menstruum for 4 h in a separate, closed container. This procedure is known as imbibition. During this time, the raw drug is allowed to reach its full swelling potential. In other words, if you are extracting using aqueous solvents, you will require more menstruum in the imbibition process. It is possible that the substance will be more evenly packed, and the menstrual flow will be more constant if the air in the medicinal powder is replaced by the vapor of the solvent used to dissolve it. Uneven packing causes inefficient extraction because it allows more solvent to flow via channels with less resistance to the flow of the solvent than is intended. The medicine is equally distributed into the percolator once it has been ingested. It is packaged in a loose plug of tow or other appropriate material that is been soaked in the solvent. An even packing process may be performed by layer-by-layer introduction of material and pressing with an appropriate tool to provide an even compression, which is dependent on the kind of material and its capacity to withstand pressure. To prevent the top layer of the medication from being disturbed during extraction, a layer of filter paper and clean sand are put on the surface once packing is complete. The medication is now saturated with enough menstruum, and the tap at the bottom is left open, so the occluded gases between particles may be released. As long as the tap is open, obstructing air might flow from the top and disrupt the bed. When the menstrual flow starts, the tap is closed, and enough menstrual flow is added to keep a thin coating of menstrual fluid over the medication, which is then left to stand for 24 h. Drying of the top layer of the bed is prevented by the menstrual layer above it, which might lead to fractures appearing on the bed's surface. The drug's components are solubilized, and soluble material is removed during a 24-h maceration phase. A more efficient extraction can be achieved if the maceration period is included [26,29].

3.2.6 Hydrodistillation

Extracting phytochemicals and essential oils from fruit fragments or plants using hydrodistillation is one of the oldest methods currently in use. There are no organic solvents employed in this process, and it may be done before the plant materials are dried. Raw materials are placed into a chamber, and then enough water is added to bring the mixture to a boil. Alternatively, the plant sample can be injected with direct steam. The vapor mixture is condensed by cooling the vapor mixture of water and oil with water. The condensed mixture is sent to a separator, which automatically separates the oil and bioactive compounds from the water [30,31]. The primary physicochemical processes involved in the hydrodistillation of plant material are hydrodiffusion, hydrolysis, heat induced, and decomposition. When essential oils and hot water are mixed together, they diffuse through plant membranes, and this process is known as hydrodiffusion. Steam distillation does not penetrate the dry cell membranes. Due to the significant comminution of the oil-bearing cells, dry plant material can only be exhausted with dry steam after the volatile oil has been freed from the cells. However, when the plant material is submerged in water, the permeability of the tissue determines the rate of vapor exchange. In plant cells, the membranes are nearly impenetrable to volatile oils. A little amount of volatile oil gets dissolved in the water in the gland and then permeates through its dilated membranes to reach the outside surface, where it is vaporized by passing steam. This is the real process, and it occurs at the temperature of boiling water. Essential oil ingredients are hydrolyzed in this context, which is a chemical reaction between water and essential oil molecules. Aromatic essential oils include ester compounds, which react with water to generate acids and alcohols, especially when heated. Equilibrium concentrations of molal concentrations of various components can be expressed in terms of the following equation:

$$(\text{alcohol}) \times (\text{acid})K = (\text{ester}) \times (\text{water})$$

In which K represents the equilibrium constant. Consequently, if there is a lot of water in distillation, the amount of alcohol and acid will also be considerable, resulting in a lower yield of essential oil. Hydrolysis progress also depends on the length of time oil and water are in contact, as this reaction takes place over time. This is a drawback of the water distillation process [32].

Essential oils lose their potency when heated over a certain point. Distillation at low temperatures yields the highest quality oil. Steam distillation's temperature is solely governed by the operating pressure, whereas atmospheric pressure is typically used in water distillation and water and steam distillation. Hydrodiffusion, hydrolysis, and thermal degradation all take place simultaneously and interact with one another: the solubility of essential oils in water increases as the temperature rises. Also, hydrolysis proceeds at the same rate and scale. As a result, it is feasible to increase the production and quality of the oils by (1) keeping the temperature low, (2) using as little water as possible, and (3) fully comminuting the plant material before distillation to ensure a uniform distribution of oil.

To separate essential oils from plant sources, three different hydro-distillation methods are used: water distillation, steam distillation, and direct steam distillation.

3.2.6.1 Water distillation

In this method, the material is immersed fully in hot water, followed by boiling them in a steam jacket, a closed steam jacket, or an open or closed steam coil. The fundamental feature of this method is that boiling water comes into direct contact with the plant material. Proper precautions must be taken to avoid the charge from overheating while the chamber is being heated by direct fire. When a steam jacket or closed steam coil is utilized, the risk of overheating is reduced; with open steam coils, this risk is eliminated. When using open steam, however, caution must be exercised to avoid the build-up of condensed water within the still. As a result, they still must be thoroughly insulated. As the water heats up, it is necessary to agitate the plant material in the chamber; otherwise, thick clumps of dense material would develop on the bottom of the chamber and get thermally affected. In order for the charge to disperse freely in water, some mucilage-rich plant materials, such as cinnamon bark, must be pulverized prior to being used. It is certain that when the water temperature rises, the mucilage extracted from the crushed cinnamon will seep out. The water-charge mixture's viscosity is substantially increased. As a result, it is allowed to burn. It is thus necessary to do a small-scale water distillation in glassware prior to conducting actual field distillations to determine whether any variations exist throughout the distillation process. The production of oil from a known weight of plant material may be calculated using the results of this laboratory study.

In order for this to be possible, the distillation material must be charged loosely and allowed to remain loose in the boiling water, which can only be accomplished by agitating the distillation material. Using live steam to treat finely powdered material or plant parts would typically create lumps, making it impossible to use water distillation. This is the one benefit water distillation has. Water distillation stills are inexpensive, easy to assemble, and suited for use in the field, among other advantages. In several countries, they are still commonly utilized with portable tools. Only partial extraction may be achieved using the process of water distillation, which is a major drawback of this process. Aldehydes and other sensitive compounds like esters polymerize when exposed to hydrolysis. More stills, room, and fuel are needed to perform water distillation. It necessitates a high degree of expertise and familiarity. There is no way to totally vaporize the oil components due to their high boiling points and water solubility. As a result, the procedure becomes unprofitable. Consequently, when the plant material cannot be processed by steam distillation or direct steam distillation due to the nature of the material, water distillation is used as a last alternative.

3.2.6.2 Water and steam distillation

Steam can be produced in a satellite boiler or within the still during the water and steam distillation, despite the fact that it is separate from the plant material. A frequent technique in rural areas involves both water and steam distillation. The setup for the process takes very little investment to get started. It is similar to water distillation, with the exception that the plant material is suspended on a perforated grid above the boiling water. The combination of water distillation and steam distillation is becoming increasingly popular among those who begin with water distillation. As a result, rural distillers recognize that the quality of oil produced by water distillation is not excellent because of its still notes (subdued aroma). A few alterations have been made as a result. Similar to a perforated grid or plate, plant material rises above the water in a similar way. The still's capacity is reduced, but the oil it produces is of higher quality. This method ensures that no matter how much water is consumed in the distillation, it will never run out since a condensation tube is attached and condensate water is manually reintroduced into the still. Reusing the condensate water also has the potential to reduce the loss of dissolved components, such as oxygenated compounds. This is because more oil will be dissolved in the condensate water once it has gotten saturated with the dissolved components [31].

3.2.6.3 Direct steam distillation

A satellite steam generator, often referred to as a boiler, is used to generate steam for direct steam distillation. Like previous distillation systems, the raw materials are positioned on a perforated grid above the steam input. Satellite steam generating allows for variable steam output, which is a huge benefit. A satellite boiler generates steam that heats the materials up to 100°C, which keeps plant materials from being overheated and causing thermal degradation. Steam distillation is the most often used method for the large-scale production of essential oils. As far as the flavor and fragrance business is concerned, direct steam distillation is standard operating practice for these industries.

An obvious drawback of steam distillation is that it requires a much more significant capital investment. Large-scale production of low-cost oils (for example, citronella and lavender) may not be able to justify steam distillation production without amortizing the cost of the plant over a period of 10 or more years due to low market pricing of the oils on the global market [32].

3.3 Limitations associated with the conventional techniques

Extraction methods encompass a variety of ways, each of which is used to extract biologically active chemicals from plant material for a distinct purpose. The extraction capacity of the different solvents utilized as well as the method of heating and/or stirring are used to develop these procedures. Table 3.1 summarizes the strengths and limitations of traditional approaches for extracting bioactive chemicals from plants. When compared to other procedures, such as maceration, the SE method uses less solvent. SE, on the other hand, has its downsides, including the potential for hazardous emissions during extraction and the risk of exposure to harmful and flammable liquid organic solvents. Using high-purity solvents may raise the expense of the extraction method. Compared with more modern techniques like supercritical fluid extraction, this procedure is considered environmentally unfriendly and might result in pollution. A dry, finely separated solid is the best sample for SE, and different factors such as temperature, solvent-to-sample ratio, and agitation speed must be considered. These conditions limit the selectivity of the process. Maceration has become popular in the study of medicinal herbs. The goal of this technique is to soften and dissolve the plant's cell wall, so the soluble phytochemicals can be released. There are various advantages to this method, such as the absence of organic solvents, simpler separation, and faster extraction periods. Due to limitations on high-temperature applications, the use of heat-sensitive phenolic compounds is limited, which is a major disadvantage of this method.

Table 3.1 Advantages and limitations of conventional methods for the extraction of bioactive compounds.

Conventional methods	Parameters	Advantages	Limitations	References
Soxhlet extraction	Solid to solvent ratio, temperature, extraction time	Simplicity and application at high temperatures improves the kinetics of the process	Poor extraction efficiency, significant energy use, and a lengthy method	[33,34]
Maceration	Transport of solvent into the mass, solubilization rate, the rate of transport of solution out of the insoluble material	The low initial investment, selectivity modification by solvent choice	Some compounds are destroyed by temperature	[18]
Infusion	Transport of solvent into the mass, solubilization rate, the rate of transport of solution out of the insoluble material	Since extraction takes less time and has a lower latent heat of vaporization than water, less heat is required to concentrate and extract	A substantial amount of solvent is required	[18]
Decoction	Solvent, contact method, temperature, number of washes	Methods of operation are simple	A substantial amount of solvent is required; only suitable for thermally stable and water soluble	[12]
Percolation	Transport of solvent into the mass, solubilization rate, the rate of transport of solution out of the insoluble material	It improves the extraction yield by increasing the contact time between the solvent and the plant material	A substantial amount of solvent is required, and a long extraction time	[18]
Hydrodistillation	Temperature, time	The water naturally separates bioactive compounds from them; no organic solvent is used	If the extraction temperature is excessively high, certain volatile components may be lost	[12]

Samples are occasionally combusted. The same concept applies to infusion and decoction as it does to maceration. The sample is cooked in a certain volume of water (e.g., 1:4 or 1:16) for a predetermined duration for decoction, although the maceration period for infusion is shorter. Only heat-stable molecules from hard plant materials may be extracted via decoction, which often results in a higher concentration of oil-soluble substances. Percolation is a time-consuming and solvent-intensive method. Hydrothermal distillation, like the other technologies, has gained popularity due to its simplicity. However, the technique has a number of major flaws, including the fact that the plant material near the bottom of the still comes into direct contact with the furnace's fire, which can cause it to char and lend an unpleasant odor to the essential oil. Furthermore, heat regulation is problematic, which may result in fluctuating distillation rates.

3.4 Summary

Extraction is the initial step in isolating and purifying bioactive chemicals from plant material. Due to their insoluble nature, secondary metabolites, including phenolic acids and flavonoids are difficult to extract. While traditional extraction methods, namely, SE, maceration, decoction, and distillation, are effective ways for extracting bioactive chemicals, the equipment used in each process is different. These approaches, however, have numerous drawbacks in terms of thermal stability, time consumption, selectivity, and toxicity. When it comes to extracting bioactive compounds from plant parts, it is important to choose an effective extraction approach that strikes a balance between quality of product, operational efficiencies, cost of production, and environmentally friendly processes. According to the literature, modifications of traditional processes have just recently been introduced, and the amount of research into the extraction of bioactive compounds utilizing these modified processes is growing. However, process improvement of the bioactive compound extraction method is still required to address the growing market demand.

References

[1] M. Manzoor, et al., Valorization of natural colors as health-promoting bioactive compounds: phytochemical profile, extraction techniques, and pharmacological perspectives, Food Chemistry 362 (2021) 130141.

[2] N.M. Daud, et al., Valorisation of plant seed as natural bioactive compounds by various extraction methods: a review, Trends in Food Science & Technology 119 (2022) 201–214.
[3] P. Duarah, D. Haldar, M.K. Purkait, Technological advancement in the synthesis and applications of lignin-based nanoparticles derived from agro-industrial waste residues: a review, International Journal of Biological Macromolecules 163 (2020) 1828–1843.
[4] V.L. Dhadge, M. Changmai, M.K. Purkait, Purification of catechins from *Camellia sinensis* using membrane cell, Food and Bioproducts Processing 117 (2019) 203–212.
[5] C. Drosou, et al., A comparative study on different extraction techniques to recover red grape pomace polyphenols from vinification byproducts, Industrial Crops and Products 75 (2015) 141–149.
[6] M. Changmai, et al., Uses of ceramic membrane-based technology for the clarification of mosambi, pineapple and orange juice, in: V. Katiyar, R. Gupta, T. Ghosh (Eds.), Advances in Sustainable Polymers: Processing and Applications, Springer Singapore, Singapore, 2019, pp. 459–483.
[7] B. Debnath, D. Haldar, M.K. Purkait, Potential and sustainable utilization of tea waste: a review on present status and future trends, Journal of Environmental Chemical Engineering 9 (5) (2021) 106179.
[8] M.D. Luque de Castro, F. Priego-Capote, Soxhlet extraction: past and present panacea, Journal of Chromatography A 1217 (16) (2010) 2383–2389.
[9] J.L. Luque-Garcia, M.D. Luque de Castro, Ultrasound-assisted Soxhlet extraction: an expeditive approach for solid sample treatment: application to the extraction of total fat from oleaginous seeds, Journal of Chromatography A 1034 (1) (2004) 237–242.
[10] J.L. Bernal, M.J. del Nozal, J.J. Jiménez, Use of a high-pressure Soxhlet extractor for the determination of organochlorine residues by gas chromatography, Chromatographia 34 (9) (1992) 468–474.
[11] M.P. Cañizares-Macías, J.A. García-Mesa, M.D. Luque De Castro, Determination of the oxidative stability of olive oil, using focused-microwave energy to accelerate the oxidation process, Analytical and Bioanalytical Chemistry 378 (2) (2004) 479–483.
[12] N. Srivastava, et al., Chapter 21 - advances in extraction technologies: isolation and purification of bioactive compounds from biological materials, in: R.p. Sinha, D.-P. Häder (Eds.), Natural Bioactive Compounds, Academic Press, 2021, pp. 409–433.
[13] R.S. Jackson, Wine Science: Principles and Applications, Academic press, 2008.
[14] A.U. Arvindekar, G.R. Pereira, K.S. Laddha, Assessment of conventional and novel extraction techniques on extraction efficiency of five anthraquinones from *Rheum emodi*, Journal of Food Science & Technology 52 (10) (2015) 6574–6582.
[15] N. Ćujić, et al., Optimization of polyphenols extraction from dried chokeberry using maceration as traditional technique, Food Chemistry 194 (2016) 135–142.
[16] B.R. Albuquerque, et al., Catechin-based extract optimization obtained from Arbutus unedo L. fruits using maceration/microwave/ultrasound extraction techniques, Industrial Crops and Products 95 (2017) 404–415.
[17] A.A. Jovanović, et al., Optimization of the extraction process of polyphenols from Thymus serpyllum L. herb using maceration, heat-and ultrasound-assisted techniques, Separation and Purification Technology 179 (2017) 369–380.
[18] J.P.M. Singh, Percolation and Infusion Techniques of Extraction of Medicinal and Aromatic Plants (MAPs), 2007.
[19] S.A. Anatolyevna, et al., Method of obtaining of extract by the method of modified maceration, Research Journal of Pharmacy and Technology 12 (12) (2019) 5956–5958.
[20] Sharma, K.S., J. Sahoo, and A. Rajput, Extraction Techniques for Herbal Drugs.

[21] S. Both, F. Chemat, J. Strube, Extraction of polyphenols from black tea—conventional and ultrasound assisted extraction, Ultrasonics Sonochemistry 21 (3) (2014) 1030—1034.
[22] N. Harbourne, et al., Conventional extraction techniques for phytochemicals, in: Handbook of Plant Food Phytochemicals: Sources, Stability and Extraction, 2013, pp. 397—411.
[23] N. Ergen, et al., Evaluation of the lifespan extension effects of several Turkish medicinal plants in *Caenorhabditis elegans*, Turkish Journal of Biology 42 (2) (2018) 163—173.
[24] Indian Pharmacopoeia, C., Pharmacopoeia of India : (The Indian Pharmacopoeia), Manager of Publications, Delhi, 1955.
[25] M.K. Hussain, M. Saquib, M.F. Khan, Techniques for extraction, isolation, and standardization of bio-active compounds from medicinal plants, in: Natural Bio-Active Compounds, Springer, 2019, pp. 179—200.
[26] N. Azwanida, A review on the extraction methods use in medicinal plants, principle, strength and limitation, Medicinal & Aromatic Plants 4 (196) (2015), pp. 2167—0412.
[27] Z. Özer, et al., Investigation of phenolic compounds and antioxidant activity of *Teucrium polium* L. decoction and infusion, Balıkesir Üniversitesi Fen Bilimleri Enstitüsü Dergisi 20 (1) (2018) 212—218.
[28] G. Füleky, I. Czinkota, Hot water percolation (HWP): a new rapid soil extraction method, Plant and Soil 157 (1) (1993) 131—135.
[29] B. Rathi, S. Bodhankar, A. Baheti, Evaluation of Aqueous Leaves Extract of Moringa Oleifera Linn for Wound Healing in Albino Rats, 2006.
[30] J. Azmir, et al., Techniques for extraction of bioactive compounds from plant materials: a review, Journal of Food Engineering 117 (4) (2013) 426—436.
[31] C. Boutekedjiret, et al., Extraction of rosemary essential oil by steam distillation and hydrodistillation, Flavour and Fragrance Journal 18 (6) (2003) 481—484.
[32] S. Tandon, 7 Distillation Technology for Essential Oils, Extraction technologies for medicinal and aromatic plants, 2008, p. 115.
[33] W.A.d. Costa, et al., Supercritical CO_2 extraction and transesterification of the residual oil from industrial palm kernel cake with supercritical methanol, The Journal of Supercritical Fluids 147 (2019) 179—187.
[34] S. Zhao, D. Zhang, Supercritical CO_2 extraction of Eucalyptus leaves oil and comparison with Soxhlet extraction and hydro-distillation methods, Separation and Purification Technology 133 (2014) 443—451.

CHAPTER 4

Advancement in bioactive compound extraction from natural products for pharmaceutical applications

4.1 Introduction

The process of extracting bioactive phytochemicals from medicinal plants is critical in supplying customers with a high-grade herbal product, with contemporary "advanced" extraction methods outperforming traditional ones. Extraction is regarded as one of the most important procedures in the production of herbal products, since it has a qualitative and quantitative impact on the active components in the sample. Given the diverse spectrum of physiologically active compounds and plant species, screening methods must be both reliable and exhaustive. Only adequate extraction processes allow for further separation, identification, and characterization of physiologically active chemicals [1,2].

Novel extraction processes have been created in the last 50 years that are more ecologically sound due to minimized use of organic and synthetic chemicals, reduced operating time, and increased extract yield and quality. Novel extraction methods are gaining popularity to increase the selectivity and overall yield of bioactive phytochemicals recovered from plant sources [3]. A number of alternative extraction processes have been developed to circumvent some of the constraints of conventional extraction methods. Some of the advances in extraction processes are referred to as "green technologies" since they make use of nontoxic organic solvents, consume less energy, and are environmentally friendly. Aided advanced extraction techniques like ultrasound-assisted, membrane-assisted, infrared-assisted, flash extraction, enzyme-assisted, microwave-assisted, supercritical fluid, and pressurized liquid extraction are of interest to the pharmaceutical

Advances in Extraction and Applications of Bioactive Phytochemicals
ISBN 978-0-443-18535-9
https://doi.org/10.1016/B978-0-443-18535-9.00011-9

industry. Combining advanced extraction technologies has been proven in several researches to be helpful for speedy and efficient extraction [4–8].

The current chapter emphasizes the advanced methods that have been developed to isolate phytochemicals, as well as the advantages and disadvantages of each method. Moreover, the latest advancements in the extraction methods of phytochemicals are given the most attention.

4.2 Different extraction approaches

4.2.1 Microwave-assisted extraction

Extraction of water-soluble compounds from various materials employing microwave radiation is an innovative procedure to separate the soluble compounds from the plant matix. Electromagnetic energies with a frequency ranging from 300 MHz to 300 GHz are called microwaves. They are formed by two oscillating fields that are perpendicular to one another, the magnetic and electric fields. The theory of microwave heating is based on the fact that it directly influences polar materials. Ionic conduction and dipole rotation processes convert electromagnetic energy to heat. The resistance of the medium to the movement of ions generates heat during the ionic conduction mechanism. Ions, on the other hand, maintain their orientation along constantly changing field indications. Because of the rapid changes in direction, molecules collide, causing heat to be generated. Alupului et al. [9] describe three sequential steps in the extraction mechanism of microwave-assisted extraction (MAE): first is thermal and pressure-induced separation of solutes from the sample matrix; second is solvent diffusion in the sample matrix; and third is solvent-mediated solute release from a sample matrix. Cravottoa et al. [10] mention several advantages of MAE, including faster heating for the extraction of bioactive compounds from plant materials, lower temperature gradients, smaller equipment, and higher extract yield. Using this method, more complete organic and organometallic compounds may be extracted. Using MAE instead of organic solvents makes it an environmentally friendly process. Conventional extraction methods cannot match the speed and efficiency of MAE when it comes to extracting bioactive compounds. For instance, MAE extracts a greater number of polyphenols and caffeine from green tea leaves in 4 min than any other extraction process that requires 20 h at room temperature. Extracting ginsenosides in 15 min using the focused MAE approach was more efficient than extracting ginsenosides in a solvent for 10 h. Extraction of flavolignin and silybinin from *Silybum marianum* enhanced the extraction efficiency of MAE, as demonstrated by Dhobi et al. [11] compared with standard extraction methods like Soxhlet and maceration. Asghari et al. [12] showed that MAE is a quicker and simpler approach to extract bioactive chemicals (E- and Z-guggulsterone, cinnamaldehyde, and tannin) from diverse plants than traditional extraction procedures. Chiremba et al. [13] used MAE to liberate bound phenolic acids from sorghum and maize bran and flour fractions of varying hardness. Maximizing the recovery of flavonoids and phenolics and improving the extracts' capacity to donate electrons were the primary goals of the MAE technique developed from *Chaenomeles Sinensis* [14].

4.2.1.1 Important parameters

Efficiencies of microwave heating for organic extraction were originally published in 1986. Soil, food, seeds, and feed may all be extracted in a few milliliters of solvent and irradiated for 30 s seven times in a household oven (1140 W). These methods have been documented in the literature for optimizing extraction conditions, such as altering each element in isolation or using factorial and central composite and Box-Behnken designs, or employing a response surface approach. It allows for a reduced number of manipulations to determine influence variables on the extraction process and optimal extraction settings through experiment design. The MAE procedure can be influenced by a wide range of factors: the solvent composition, the power supplied, the extraction temperature, the solvent-to-feed ratio, and the size and moisture of the plant material. Solubility, stability, and volatility of target compounds influence the selection of parameters and their values. It is also dependent on the interaction of other substances in the plant material [15].

As a general rule, all extraction methods use temperature as a crucial parameter to enhance yield. With a rise in temperature, solubilization capacity, surface tension, and viscosity of the solvent decrease, resulting in improved sample wetting and matrix penetration. High extraction recoveries are achieved by efficient desorption of chemicals from the matrix active site. The dielectric constant of the solvent in MAE determines the ability of a solvent to absorb microwaves and the amount of microwave energy delivered. The boiling point of the solvent might be exceeded in a sealed container. Once the temperature rises over the boiling point and pressure becomes a factor, the process can be accelerated. Extraction vessels need to be sealed to prevent volatile solutes from dissolving and spilling out into the headspace; however, this can significantly lengthen extraction time.

When using a closed vessel, it is imperative that the power be selected so the temperature may be reached in the shortest amount of time possible while avoiding overheating and overpressure. Increased power and longer exposure times may lead to solvent loss through evaporation, which is a potential problem. For closed systems, the maximum power consumption is in the region of 600–1000 W, whereas for open systems, it is closer to 250 W [6].

Depending on the type of matrix in which the solutes are found, extraction yields can be significantly reduced or increased. Microwave radiation is strongly absorbed by water molecules, whether they are already in the sample or introduced to it. Water molecules have a large dipole moment. The increased polarity of the extraction solvent and/or capacity to heat the sample are made possible by water's influence on microwave absorption capabilities. It is common for extraction recoveries to improve when the matrix moisture is higher. Solute–matrix interactions may also be affected by the expansion of the matrix, making solutes more accessible to the extracting solvent. The dielectric characteristics of a dry raw material can be altered by rehydrating it before extraction to speed up the heating process and increase extraction efficiency. It is possible to soak the sample in water for a variety of lengths of time. Depending on the amount of time spent soaking, the extraction rate might rise from 10 min to 24 h [16].

MAE's effectiveness is generally affected by the size and dispersion of plant particles. Typical particle size ranges from 100 to 2 mm for the components that are removed. The diffusion of chemicals from the plant matrix to the surrounding solvent is frequently the limiting step in extraction, so fine powders can assist the extraction process since they have a reduced diffusion depth. Fine powder has a higher surface area than coarse powder, and smaller particles penetrate less deeply into plant tissue, which results in a more uniform microwave exposure.

4.2.2 Ultrasound-assisted extraction

Ultrasound is a sound wave that is higher than the human ear's maximum audible range. In chemistry, the frequency range is usually 20 kHz to 100 MHz. It travels across a medium by compressing and expanding, much like other waves. This results in a phenomenon known as cavitation, which refers to the formation, development, and collapse of bubbles (as shown in Fig. 4.1). The transfer of kinetic energy of motion into heating the bubble's contents can yield a significant quantity of energy. Bubbles have a

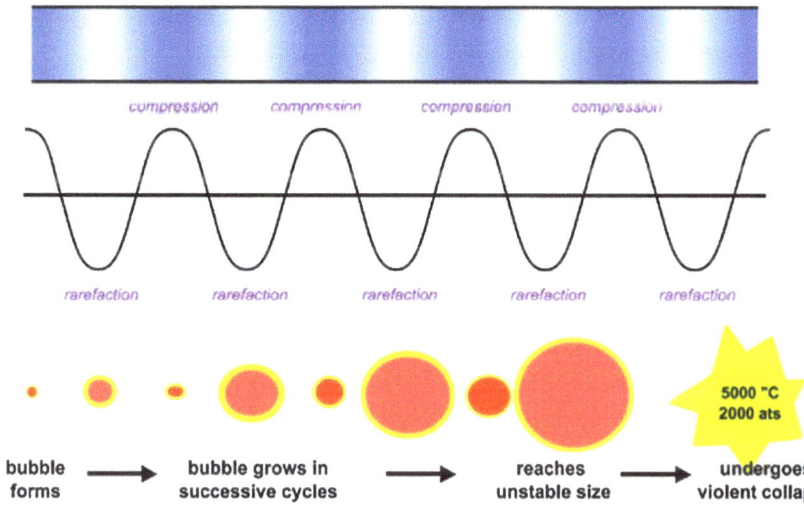

Figure 4.1 The formation and collapse of cavitation bubbles. *(Reproduced with permission from Vinatouru et al. [17].)*

temperature of around 5000 K, a pressure of 1000 atm, and a heating and cooling rate of more than 1010 K/s, according to the researchers. Ultrasound-assisted extraction (UAE) has been built on this premise. There is no cavitation impact on solids or liquids that include solids. The primary effect of UAE is seen in solid plant samples since ultrasonic energy accelerates the leaching of organic and inorganic components from the plant matrix. The most likely mechanism is that ultrasound intensifies mass transfer and accelerates solvent access to plant cell components. Ultrasound extraction comprises two distinct physical operations: (a) cell wall diffusion and (b) washing the contents of the cell once the walls have been shattered. The moisture content of the sample, the degree of milling, the particle size, and the solvent are all critical components in attaining an efficient and successful extraction. Additionally, the temperature, frequency, pressure, and duration of sonication all play a role in how ultrasound works. UAE has also been included with many traditional procedures due to its purported ability to increase the efficiency of a conventional system. An ultrasonic device is positioned appropriately in a solvent extraction machine to maximize extraction efficiency. Reduced extraction time, energy consumption, and solvent use are all benefits of using UAE. More efficient mixing, quicker transmission of energy, lower thermal gradients, extraction temperature, and selective extraction are only some of the advantages that may be gained by using ultrasound energy for extracting.

Extraction of bioactive compounds from herbal plants may benefit from the UAE approach. Daidzin, genistin, malonyl genistin, and glycitin were successfully extracted from soybeans utilizing the mix-stirring technique, which involved different extraction durations and solvents, according to Rostagno et al. [18]. Based on the kind of solvent utilized, researchers found that ultrasonic can boost extraction yields. Strawberry phenolic components including rutin, quercetin, naringin, naringenin, ellagic acid, and kaempferol were extracted utilizing a semiautomatic process based on ultrasounds by Herrera et al. [7]. Li et al. [19] reported that UAE, under optimal conditions (70% methanol, sample ratio, 20:1 solvent, and 30 min duration), was able to extract chlorogenic acid from fresh leaves, dried bark, and fresh bark of *Eucommia ulmodies* Oliv. Extraction of bioactive chemicals from *Euonymus alatus* (Thund.) Sieb using optimal sonication conditions proved to be more efficient than standard approaches, according to Yang et al. [20]. *Catharanthus roseus* has three alkaloids (vindoline, catharanthine, and vinblastine) that may be extracted using ionic liquid–based UAE. Optimum solvent, temperature, and time were all considered for extracting anthocyanins and phenolic components from grape peel using the UAE method. Chemical compounds such as carnosic acid, phenolic acids, and rosmarinic acid were extracted from *Rosmarinus officinalis* utilizing an ionic liquid–based UAE extraction method that proved to be more efficient and quicker than standard extraction procedures [21].

4.2.2.1 Important parameters

Aside from the factors intrinsic to the ultrasonic device (including the wavelength, frequency, and amplitude of the wave), ultrasonic intensity and power have an influence on extraction and may be improved. The form of the probe, as well as the design of the reactor, can have an impact on the procedure. When extracting, time, temperature, and solvent type all have an influence on the extraction yield and composition, so it is important to consider these factors. As a parameter, the raw material matrix and target molecules for UAE should be carefully evaluated. The meticulous examination of those affecting parameters is critical to get the optimum extraction effectiveness and yield possible. However, it is important to remember that the maximum yield is not necessarily the only goal of an extraction process; it is also important to consider the least amount of nonrenewable resources and energy used. As a result, to translate experimental laboratory settings to industrial sizes, those characteristics must be optimized [22].

As ultrasound is a mechanical wave, the wavelength, frequency, and amplitude of the ultrasound can all affect the cavitation bubbles. In a similar vein, pH is a crucial factor influencing the extraction yield and characteristics of bioactive compounds throughout the UAE process. Polysaccharides (pectin) were extracted from fruit and vegetable byproducts in a pH range of 1—5, and the results were analyzed. When the pH is kept at a low level, the recovery of pectin is high. Cell wall fragmentation is improved by using a highly acidic media, which also hydrolyzes the insoluble pectin into a soluble form and decreases the molecular weight of the pectin, boosting solubility into the surrounding medium and therefore promoting recovery. Pectin clumps, when exposed to a high pH value, prevent them from being released into the extraction medium. Pectin extraction from pomegranate peel has been shown to be most effective at pH 1.2, with pH 1.5 recorded for orange peel, jackfruit peel, and pomegranate seed extracts, and pH 3.2 reported for banana peel and sunflower head extraction [22].

4.2.3 Pressurized liquid extraction

At temperatures over the boiling point, solvents are used to dissolve solid matrices while maintaining their liquid state using pressurized extraction, commonly known as hot pressurized liquid extraction (HPLE). A sample extraction with ethanol or water at high pressure (4—20 MPa) and moderate heat (50—250°C) breaks secondary bonds, resulting in faster desorption and solubilization of matrix-bound species. This is the green solvent method. As a result, the solid sample and solvent are kept separate in a jar and extracted statically over short time intervals. HPLE can also be carried out in dynamical runs, in which the extraction chamber is continually supplied with solvent. HPLE is a low-solvent-consumption method that does not require filtering and can be used with food-grade solvents, making it an excellent choice for ecologically conscious businesses [23]. As a result, HPLE is perfect for automation since commercial equipment can be set to run in automated mode, which increases repeatability and quality control and makes HPLE superior to ultrasound or microwave alternatives. When compared with typical extraction methods, HPLE uses less solvent and produces cleaner extracts, which may eliminate the need for further filtering and/or purification of crude preparations. Furthermore, due to the matrix's ion-suppression actions, the increased purity raises the signal-to-noise ratio, and the decreased background boosts the dependability of downstream processes, particularly liquid chromatography—mass spectrometry (LC-MS) separation and analytical screens. As a result, HPLE provides advantages in extraction quality as well as favorable properties for expanding plant waste valorization. HPLE, however, has certain drawbacks in addition to its advantages. Its most prominent drawback is its poor selectivity, which is less than desirable in many applications because of the frequent co-extraction of undesirable compounds from various intricate matrices with the targeted compounds. Dilution is another undesirable side effect of HPLE, especially if the extraction is carried out in many cycles. Furthermore, the requisite instrumentation is costly, yet its exceptional capabilities might quickly outweigh the original investment.

HPLE applications employ high pressures that cause sample disruption including pore formation. The viscosity and surface tension of solvents drop while they remain liquid, whereas matrix penetration and desorption kinetics improve. As a result, particle size decreases, and solubilized polyphenol species' mass transfer rates rise. These pressure-mediated actions allow thermolabile species to be extracted in less time and at lower temperatures, preserving their integrity and biologic potential. It should be noted that keeping the solvent liquid is adequate under optimum HPLE settings since pressing over this level does not result in further improvements. HPLE's performance is also influenced by temperature. The temperature increases the diffusivity and solubility of polyphenols by disrupting sample-analyte bonds and lowering solvent viscosity [24]. When it comes to thermal extractability, there is a threshold beyond which the temperature compromises chemical stability and polyphenols degrade into undesired products such as Maillard chemicals and 5-(hydroxymethyl)furfurals [25]. Polyphenol extractions commonly use temperatures between 40 and 60°C because of this reason [26]. Temperatures of 80—120°C were employed in pressurized solvent extraction of anthocyanins from red cabbage since temperatures below 80°C resulted in unsatisfactory yields, while temperatures over 120°C resulted in polyphenol degradation [5]. Similarly, anthocyanins from red grape skins degrade by 50% in 100-atm HPLE water extracts at temperatures over 100°C [27]. Thermal degradation of phenolic antioxidants extracted in 30% ethanol from grape stems was prevented when temperatures did not exceed 120°C and extraction periods were short (up to 10 min). However, because phenolics deteriorate at high temperatures, the chemical condition in which they are retrieved must be determined. In this regard, nine phenolic compounds isolated from grape seeds and skins in superheated methanol at 100°C and 100 atm deteriorated by 10%, including the most oxidizable catechins, which only degraded at 150°C [28]. HPLE has also been used to extract phenolics from apple skin and pulp, with considerable time and sample handling savings (up to 100% efficiency in hydromethanolic combinations). Similarly, extracting phenolic-rich fractions from banana passion fruit seeds using a 100% ethanol in acethyl acetate mixture at high pressure and temperature yielded the best results in terms of extracting flavanols, flavonoids, and abundant proanthocyanidins, as well as antioxidant activity.

Pressure and temperature have a significant impact on the solvent's dielectric constant/polarity. To be clear, HPLE's ability to extract an extensive range of phytochemicals is reliant on ad hoc combinations of the temperature—pressure—solvent triad. Because of their solubilization capabilities, selectivity, and ecologic neutrality, the use of water and hydroalcoholic mixtures is recommended in HPLE tracks [25]. Water stays liquid but much less polar under high pressure and temperatures over its boiling point (about 200—275°C) owing to the breaking of intermolecular hydrogen bonds. As a result, the molecule may dissolve fewer polar molecules in the same manner as traditional solvents like ethanol or methanol can under normal atmospheric conditions. Furthermore, pressured water disrupts internal matrix bonds, which increases analyte diffusivity and extractability. Depending on these improved aptitudes, extraction methods based on pure water have been found to be appropriate for phenolic of plant wastes. In this regard, an eco-friendly approach for extracting phenolic compounds from pomegranate peels was demonstrated using a combination of hot water at 70°C and ultrasound (480 W) [29]. Protic ethanol lowers polarity and promotes the solubilization of polyphenolic chemicals in hydroethanolic solutions, whereas water facilitates their desorption from the matrix, improving yield of extraction. Furthermore, ethanol reduces thermal hydrolysis and polyphenol degradation in hazardous compounds as a co-solvent. A hydroethanol extraction system is highly suggested, not only for HPLE but also in circumstances when HPLE is combined with ultrasound, microwave, or other technologies. The extraction yield of thermolabile phenolics from defatted passion fruit bagasse was enhanced by 60% using an efficient and eco-friendly hydroethanolic HPLE technique combined with ultrasound [30]. HPLE has also been used to fractionate cranberry pomace and isolate the polyphenolic and lipophilic fractions, the latter of which contains anthocyanins and procyanidins, using supercritical carbon dioxide extraction (SC-CO_2). Further, in the same research, response surface methodology (RSM) is used, which allowed for the optimization of operational conditions to gradually enhance yields and antioxidant activity after each extraction phase, as well as the configuration of a "zero waste" by-product platform for biorefining cranberry pomace at a commercial scale. Studying the chemical profile of sweet cherry (*Prunus avium*) stems, researchers discovered that HPLE was more effective than SC-CO_2 in releasing a wide range of distinct phenolic acids and flavonoids with various polarity (37.31% vs. 4.42%, respectively) [31].

For more than 2 decades, scientists have been using HPLE to extract plant biocompounds more quickly, increase yields and quality, and minimize or eliminate the environmental effect of phytochemical extraction. Short pulse cycles (100−1000 MPa) and subsequent relaxation are used in ultra high pressure extraction (UHPE) to operate at ultra-high pressures, resulting in cell shape deformations. When the plant's cell wall is broken by a solvent, active chemicals diffuse more readily, and mass transfer is expedited. It is possible to operate at moderate temperatures (20−50°C) because of the intense pressure, which improves the recovery of thermolabile bioactive substances. Several plant byproducts have been recovered and upcycled using UHPE, which has been approved by the US Federal Drug Administration as ecologically benign. So, a combination of UHPE and an electric-pulse pretreatment appeared to result in permanent holes in plant membranes and the deactivation of enzymes that degrade them. When combined with 3 kV cm-1 pulses, 70°C UHPE with 3 kV cm-1 pulses enhanced the extractability by 17% and doubled the antioxidant capacity of anthocyanins extracted from grape byproducts. It was shown that high hydrostatic pressure (600 MPa) and ultrasound-aided extraction delivered three times and two times more total phenolic content than control extraction in hot water, respectively.

UHPE (70% ethanol, 295 MPa) revealed a higher yield of total procyanidins, flavonoids, and phenolics from the lychee pericarp compared with conventional extraction and UAE. *Chenopodium formosanum* was extracted in a successful UHPE setup that yielded a higher antioxidant activity than traditional extraction of the same solvent at 25°C for 12 h. For example, The UHPE extracts' antioxidant properties and the amount of phenolics and flavonoids, particularly gallic and rutin acid, showed that this plant waste might be a valuable source of antioxidants for the food and cosmetics industries.

Rapid solid-liquid dynamic extraction (RSLDE) is another environmentally friendly pressurized extraction technique that uses cyclic pressure to pressurize the extractant onto a solid matrix. RSLDE is basically a solid-liquid extraction method that results in faster extraction at room temperature. Novel RSLDE preserves the yield and extraction time advantages of high-pressure extraction while allowing the release of structurally unchanged thermolabile polyphenols under low temperatures. Extracting over two dozen polyphenols from grape peel with water is effective and reproducible at low temperatures. RSLDE, which has been proposed as a feasible alternative to maceration, enables green extractions with little energy need and without putting targeted species under heat stress.

4.2.4 Supercritical carbon dioxide extraction

SC-CO_2 is a low-impact method that guarantees bioactive chemicals are preserved as much as possible. Many of these benefits stem from carbon dioxide's features, particularly its low critical temperature (31.1°C) and nonoxidative medium, which favors the extraction of thermally unstable and quickly oxidized chemicals. In comparison to its counterparts generated using organic solvents, SC-CO_2 extracts have shown efficacy as antibacterial, antiproliferative, and antioxidant agents [2].

The capacity to change the CO_2 density, which regulates solubility, by altering pressure or temperature is the main benefit of this technology. Another advantage of SC-CO_2 extraction is the ability to produce solvent-free extracts. Because CO_2 is a gas at room temperature, it is removed by depressurizing the system when the extraction is complete. Because it avoids the energy-intensive methods necessary to remove solvents, this step has the potential to save money and energy. Nonpolar to mid-polar chemicals, such as essential oil, are the subject of most investigations on SC-CO_2's ability to extract high-value compounds from various plant sources. SC-CO_2 has a limited capacity to extract more polar molecules; hence co-solvents are added in modest amounts to boost extraction efficiency. A knowledge of the SC-CO_2 thermodynamic and kinetics is required for high extraction selectivity and minimal co-extraction of nontarget compounds like waxes. Finally, due to the significant energy consumption for compression and decompression, large capital investment is necessary. Energy costs related to recycling methods can be reduced if recycling procedures are implemented at an industrial scale [4].

$SC-CO_2$ performs well because solvating power of CO_2 changes a lot when it is heated and pressurized. Phase equilibrium, mass transfer by diffusion and convection, and displacement of the solution by expansion are the parts of this process that make it work. The low viscosity as well as high diffusivity make it easy for the fluid to move through the plant matrix, like a gas, and help dissolve the solute like a liquid, so it can get through. When this process is done, how well it works depends on the pressure, flow rate, temperature, density, extraction time, and co-solvents that are used.

4.2.4.1 Important factors

$SC-CO_2$ is highly sensitive to changes in pressure. $SC-CO_2$ density is directly related to the solubility of target solutes, resulting in a greater extraction yield at any given temperature. The carotenoid concentration of citrus byproduct extracts increased with pressure, according to Ndayishimiye et al. [32]. In both trials, extraction yields decreased as pressure climbed to 30 MPa (300 bar). As a result of the co-extraction of other compounds at higher pressures, the target compound recovery decreased, which was attributable to lesser volatility. Although this impact is plant and compound specific, a study by Zkal et al. [33] found that increasing pressure by as much as 60 MPa increased flaxseed oil recovery.

As the solvation power of $SC-CO_2$ decreases due to a rise in temperature in an isobaric process, extraction rates fall. It is important to note that the vapor pressure of solutes increases as the temperature increases, whereas the density of CO_2 decreases. Retrogradation is a pressure-controlled phenomenon that occurs when the temperature rises, gradually encroaching on itself. Crossover or inversion pressure is the name given to the pressure that exists at that location. In the investigation on *Lupinus albescens* extracts, Confortin et al. [34] found that extraction yield increased when pressure was below the inversion pressure. Temperature increases favor extraction rate if it is higher than inversion pressure, which is common in aqueous solutions. It will be necessary to compromise between these two conflicting effects to find an appropriate temperature for a high extraction yield.

Extraction yield can be improved by altering the affinity of CO_2 for molecules that have low solubility in fluids, such as polar chemicals, by adding co-solvent. According to Lima et al. [35], compared with utilizing only CO_2, adding 5% methanol increased pipercallosidine yields from pepper leaves by 40%. Between the supercritical fluid and the molecule being extracted, Srinivas et al. [36] observed that adding volatile co-solvents can help the process. We chose ethanol because it is less harmful and easier to get rid of than other solvents despite its poor CO_2 miscibility. However, there are no published studies on the impact of pH of co-solvents on the yield and purity of target compounds, which are additional factors. Co-solvent selection should be based on the sample's physical qualities and the chemical composition of its targets.

Besides all these factors, particle size, solvent flow rate, and time also influence the extraction efficiency of the process.

4.2.5 Subcritical water extraction

Hot water at a pressure sufficient to sustain the liquid state between 100°C (the boiling point of water) and 374°C (the critical point of water) at critical pressure (1–22.1 MPa) is referred to as subcritical water extraction (SWE). Its dielectric constant, viscosity, and surface tension diminish over time as temperature rises, while its diffusivity improves. Water may be kept liquid at high temperatures by applying enough pressure. When water is at 25°C, the water's dielectric constant has an initial value of 80. At a pressure of 25 bar and a temperature of 250°C, the dielectric constant lowers to 25, which is between methanol's dielectric constant and ethanol's dielectric constant at 25°C. As a result, water's characteristics can be compared to those of organic solvents capable of dissolving a wide variety of medium- and low-polarity molecules. In SWE, the dielectric constant may be adjusted across a wide range by changing the temperature and pressure. This is a wonderful feature. In addition, the diffusion and convection processes of SWE lead to mass transfer. By decreasing the activation energy required for desorption, subcritical water can disrupt adhesive–cohesive interactions and aid extraction by allowing water to enter into matrices where it is hard to do so under normal conditions. A reduction in the polarity of subcritical water occurs as the temperature increases. Because of this, the polar, medium-polar, low-polar, and nonpolar molecules may be identified [37].

SWE's extraction process is comprised of four distinct phases. The first step is to pressurize and heat the sample matrix to desorb the solute from different active sites. The diffusion of the extracts into the matrix is the primary focus of the second stage. The solutes may separate from the sample matrix and enter the extraction fluid on their own in the third stage, which is dependent on the matrix of the sample. By chromatography, the sample solution is extracted from the extraction cell and collected. Previous research has revealed that the SWE process follows the thermodynamic model [38]. To extract a chemical from a matrix in this paradigm, two stages are required. (1) The chemicals must be desorbed from the sample matrix's initial binding location. (2) The chemicals must be extracted from the sample using a method similar to front elution chromatography.

The following two factors sum up the rationale for enhancing SWE efficiency: solubility and mass transfer effects have improved, whereas surface balance has been damaged. Subcritical water's characteristics alter constantly as its temperature rises and thus boosts the analyte's dissolving capacity [39]. As the viscosity decreases and the diffusibility increases, the matrix particles are able to penetrate deeper into the solution. Fresh water is continuously fed into the subcritical water dynamic extraction process to improve mass transfer efficiency and extraction yield. In addition, the material's surface can be damaged under high temperatures and pressures. Hydrogen bonds, van der Waals forces, active spots in the matrix, and dipole attraction of solute molecules can be overcome by increasing the temperature. In order for water to remain liquid at a temperature over the boiling point, it is required to exert a significant amount of pressure. In the presence of high pressure, analytes can be more easily dissolved from the matrix pores [1,25].

4.2.5.1 Important parameters

Temperature is the most important factor affecting extraction efficiency and selectivity in SWE. Temperature affects both the physicochemical properties of water and the degradation of thermally labile analytes. During SWE, the temperature frequently exceeds the boiling point of the fluid that is being used. At high temperatures, subcritical water has great diffusivity, low viscosity, and low surface tension. The vapor pressure and rapid thermal breakdown of target compounds can increase SWE efficiency [40]. As the temperature rises, the nature of subcritical water changes, and the property of the water shifts from polar to nonpolar. Less polar substances will dissolve faster in water as a result of this. However, high temperatures can cause compound breakdown as well as the amplification of processes like oxidation and hydrolysis. Between 200 and 250°C, the quantity of terpene extracted from basil and oregano leaves using subcritical water did not rise, and there was a considerable deterioration. When subcritical water reaches temperatures beyond 300°C, it has a very low dielectric constant, which increases the solubility of nonpolar chemicals and hence improves extraction efficiency [41,42]. When extracting diverse compounds with subcritical water, it is vital to pick the appropriate extraction temperature based on the individual chemicals [43].

Changing the pressure can also have the effect of altering the water phase. Maintaining the liquid condition of water requires a medium pressure of 15 bar at 200°C and 85 bar at 300°C. The pressure is normally maintained between 10 and 80 bar during the SWE process to keep the water in a liquid form under the extraction temperature. When using subcritical water, pressure has no effect on the recovery of phytochemicals, unlike temperature [44].

If the solubility of a chemical in a solvent determines the extraction kinetics, then raising the flow rate will increase the extraction rate. High-temperature water can be extracted more effectively because of the shorter residence time of the compounds and the greater flow rate of the water used in the process. It is essential to keep in mind that if the flow rate of the extractant is too high, the extracts will be diluted too much, necessitating a further stage of concentration. Extraction efficiency cannot be improved by increasing the flow rate if it is constrained simply by the resolution and diffusion of chemicals within the sample matrix' pores. Furthermore, the maximum flow rate (4 mL/min) yielded the optimum essential oil extraction yield from coriander seeds (*Coriandrum sativum* L.), owing to the fact that mass transfer of essential oils from the solid phase's surface to the water phase governed the majority of the extraction process. As a result, the extraction time and solid-to-liquid ratio must be adjusted during the dynamic SWE process. The extraction duration and solid-to-liquid ratio must also be taken into account in the static phase of SWE [45].

A significant influence on the extraction process is exerted by particle size in SWE. For small particle sizes, the extraction yield is generally high, whereas for larger particle sizes, the extraction efficiency is poor, and the extraction time must be increased. Reduced diffusion distance and the increased contact area between extractant and sample matrix are two advantages of smaller particle sizes in a matrices' extraction process [46].

4.2.6 Enzyme-assisted extraction

Several phytochemicals have recently been extracted using enzyme-aided extraction (EAE). Additionally, it is seen as an eco-friendly approach of extracting phytochemicals that is both effective and delicate. Polysaccharides and lignin are frequent binders of phytochemicals in plant tissue, making it difficult to separate them using a standard technique. Enzymatic preextraction has been increasingly popular in recent years since it liberates bound components and boosts yield. It is common practice to supplement the extraction process with enzymes such as cellulolytic enzymes, amylase, and pectinase, to improve extraction efficiency and permit full biomass extraction. An array of critical variables, including but not limited to pH, enzyme/substrate ratio, extraction duration, and temperature, can influence the enzyme's ability to degrade and disrupt cell wall structure and release bioactive compounds. Researchers can use two approaches to extract physiologically active components from plant tissues: enzyme-assisted aqueous extraction and enzyme-assisted cold pressing [47].

For the extraction of different seed oils, oil extraction procedures are commonly used. EAE cannot and does not want to hydrolyze the entire plant cell wall, so this is not an option [48]. Enzyme-based extraction of physiologically active chemicals from plant materials has already been documented in scientific literature. Tomato lycopene extraction was studied by Choudhari et al. [49] using cellulases and pectinases.

Using xylanase, cellulase, hemicellulase, and a ternary combination of these enzymes, Boulila et al. [50] found that the quantity of essential oil extracted from bay leaves could be increased. Using the enzymes amylase and amyloglucosidase, scientists were able to increase the quantity of curcumin extracted from turmeric by more than twofold. In terms of bioactive chemical extraction, EAE offers a number of advantages, but it also has a number of commercial and technical disadvantages [51]. The existing enzyme preparations cannot completely hydrolyze matrix cell walls, restricting the yields of phytochemical extraction. Great-scale or industrial-scale enzyme synthesis may cost more if the enzyme-to-substrate ratio is too large [52].

4.2.6.1 Important parameters

There are different factors like kinds of enzyme usage, enzymatic mixes, extraction duration, and temperature that impact the yield of the procedure. Enzymatic mixtures exhibit large impacts on hydrolytic capabilities through composition, enzymatic activity types of their elements, and their relative amounts. To accomplish complete cellular wall fragmentation, the chosen enzymes must have complementary activity. When the enzymatic concentration is raised twice, it can cut extraction time by up to half its initial value. Coinciding results can also be achieved by inverting the values of these parameters. A limiting issue may be the length of the extraction procedure since prolonged exposure to high temperatures or oxidation can lead to the degradation of bioactive compounds [53]. In addition to extraction temperature, enzymatic activity and the rheological characteristics of solubilized bioactive substances are influenced by EAE. Enzymatic activity tends to increase as the temperature rises.

Additionally, when temperatures rise, the viscosity of extraction media decreases, making it easier to dissolve bioactive chemicals. However, extremely high temperatures may disrupt three-dimensional enzyme structures, preventing hydrolysis and breaking down bioactive substances. Because it influences plant cell walls and enzymatic effectiveness, pH is a significant EAE parameter. For example, an acidic extraction medium causes hydrogen bonds to destabilize, resulting in enhanced cellular wall flexibility. In addition, because enzymes require acidic pH values, an acidic pH affects catalytic activity by changing protein structures and increasing substrate binding capacity [54].

4.2.7 Infrared-assisted extraction

Infrared radiation (IR) is a kind of electromagnetic radiation that covers near-, mid-, and far-infrared radiation and has a wavelength range of 0.78−1000 m. Its penetration diminishes with increasing wavelength (higher energy). Since the absorption wavelengths of water and most organic compounds are >2.5 m, the far-infrared extraction approach is often used [55]. Depending on the composition and incident infrared light absorption wavelengths, plants may absorb and convert energy. Vibrational excitation of the atoms or molecules of the plant material (for example, twisting, shaking, stretching) is induced by IR, which can create surplus thermal energy. This raises the temperature inside the cell, causing the liquid within to vaporize and the tissues to burst. Solvent characteristics are altered by IR. For instance, after using IR, water's dielectric characteristics, viscosity, surface tension, and polarity all diminish. As a result, as the temperature rises, the solubility of certain polar compounds in water increases, improving the mass transfer of target chemicals [43]. Higher temperatures promote internal and external diffusion of target substances by allowing them to exit the matrix and accelerating chemical reactions and molecular diffusion. Compared with typical convective extraction methods, infrared-assisted extraction's (IAE's) radiation heating improves efficiency of heat transfer and minimizes energy consumption. In the conventional heating procedure, a thermal solvent is convected onto a cell or tissue surface, promoting the outward diffusion of the target component. The poor heat transfer rate of this method may result in sample surface hardening and limited mass transfer. Infrared heating, on the other hand, may penetrate the sample's surface and operate on the internal matrix, allowing the cell and its surrounds to be heated at the same time. As a result, the sample experiences a transitory temperature gradient with homogeneous heating and a high heat transfer rate.

Components such as a round-bottom flask and an infrared lamp are prevalent in IAE systems. High-resistance metal filaments are encased in quartz glass bulbs or tubes, which can be vacuum sealed or filled with an inert gas to construct an infrared lamp. At 2200 K, the filament is resistively heated and emits IR. A rheostat is often used to manage the IAE system's output power since different bioactive phytochemicals and plant materials need varying degrees of infrared power for the extraction process. Although, the rheostat was unable to control the effectiveness of the radiative heating, and a sudden rise in solution temperature might cause thermally sensitive chemicals like polyphenols and flavonoids to degrade [56]. In the work of Wang et al. [57], it was found that a proportional-integral-derivative controller may be utilized to automatically regulate the power of an IR source. In this case, a cooling agent was used to dissipate heat from the reaction chamber to maintain a stable temperature within the chamber. IAE may be used in a wider range of applications now that this technology can effectively manage the temperature. As a starting point for future IAE systems, the authors feel these enhancements should be included.

4.2.7.1 Important parameters

The extraction efficiency is directly related to the type of solvent used. In order for a solution to form, a solute must overcome a certain amount of activation energy or the energies required for the solute to enter the solution. Bioactive chemicals such as polyphenols and flavonoids, which have low polarity, are difficult to extract from water because of their low solubility. The solubility of bioactive compounds has been improved by using organic solvents such as the bioactive component; however, extraction procedures have been deemed inefficient because of their long durations and high liquid-to-solid ratios. Studies on the usage of green solvents have been conducted in recent years as well. For the IAE of polyphenols from pomegranate peels, Mhanna et al. [58] examined the extraction yield by using three different solvents, i.e., water, deep-eutectic solvent, and 50% ethanol-water. The results revealed that water and the deep-eutectic solvent had the lowest and maximum extraction efficiencies, respectively. When compared to 50% aqueous ethanol and water, the deep-eutectic solvent enhanced polyphenol yields by 1.8 and 2.4 times, respectively.

Another important aspect of the IAE process is the liquid-to-solid ratio. Bioactive chemicals are dispersed in the region of the cell matrix at low ratios, increasing mass transfer resistance. Huang et al. [8] discovered that raising the liquid-to-solid ratio (100 mL/g) might enhance the yields of liquiritin and glycyrrhizic acid, while Cai et al. [59] observed that there was an increase in the production of phenolic acids, but the recovery of diterpenoids was not considerably influenced by this increase. Nevertheless, the scientists came to the conclusion that the high liquid-to-solid ratio, which did not appear to be taken into consideration, may explain for the slight shift in diterpenoids. If the amount of extra solvent exceeds an optimal ratio, it might result in waste and upset the balance of mass transfer of the target molecule.

Solute elimination from the sample matrix and solvent diffusion are influenced by the extraction temperature, which has a positive relationship with infrared power. Excessive extraction temperatures can cause thermally sensitive chemicals to degrade and increase impurity solubility, both of which impact the mass transfer process. As a result, infrared power is an important aspect in the IAE method and must be sensibly tuned. Several studies have examined the influence of infrared on phytochemicals extraction. Infrared has a substantial influence on the extraction of the flavonoid rutin from Flos Sophorae (*Sophora japonica*), according to Li et al. [60], with 200 W being the best value. Other researchers observed similar results, as well as an optimal infrared power of 200 W. Increasing or decreasing the infrared power from 60 to 250 W has minimal influence on the production of bioactive chemicals, according to Huang et al. [61]. However, damage to the delicate cellular material, which did not appear to be considered, might have led to the lower infrared power optimum.

4.2.8 Flash extraction

Designed for smashing up plants quickly, the flash extractor is ideal for this purpose. The analytical, experimental, pilot, and industrial flash extractors are among the four categories of extractors that may be found in the literature. The extraction pot is filled with the correct solvent, and the correct operating parameters are established in the control system, including rotation speed and extraction time, before the process begins. Once you have turned on the electric motor to drive the cutter, the extraction will come to an automated halt once the system setup time has expired. Raw materials must be pretreated to avoid plant fragments being too large to reach the crushing region; in other words, the diameter of the cutter head must be less than the raw plant fragments. Furthermore, the initial load on the motor is most significant when the extractor is turned on since plant tissue bits that have not been treated are more extensive and more compact. According to practical experience, inadequate motor power at the start can cause the plant bits to clog between the inner and outer edges, preventing the inner edge from rotating and damaging the motor. It is best to start the flash extractor in high gear and then lower it to the right level after a good run. Finally, the plant's serous fluid is filtered, and the filtrate is collected for further analysis [62].

The ultra-rapid spinning of the specifically designed cutter head, as well as various secondary effects including elevated shearing, extremely fast dynamic molecular permeation, dramatic agitation, and intense vibration, are responsible for flash extraction's great efficiency. The cutter's spinning speed can reach up to 15,000–30,000 rpm while working, resulting in a strong mechanical shear force that instantly breaks the plant tissue into small particles (approximately 50–80 m) [63]. The impediments to mass transmissions, for instance thick tissue and a strong cell wall, are reduced, and the mass transfer area increases due to smaller plant particles. As previously stated, the inner edge of the cutter head spins and the outside edge remains stationary. A negative pressure vacuum area forms between the inner and outer edges, causing a severe disturbance. Under negative pressure, ultra-dynamic molecular permeation accelerates phytochemical desorption and dissolution from the plant matrix. The target chemical molecules are promptly transported and penetrated into the bulk solvent after they are released from plant cells. The four effects work together to speed up and finish the extraction process [64].

Some key parameters and their linear, quadratic, and interdependent impacts must be taken into account to get satisfactory extraction results. It is vital to consider elements such as solvents, extraction duration, and rotation speed of the cutter head in the extraction process [62].

4.2.9 Membrane-assisted extraction process

As an alternative to conventional separation methods, membrane technologies including pervaporation, reverse osmosis, and nanofiltration provide the possibility for highly selective separation with low energy consumption, a compact design, and ease of scaling up [65,66]. As a result of its gentle operation conditions, liquid–liquid extraction is one of the most established and widely utilized unit operations in bio-based processes, making it particularly ideal for delicate phytochemical extraction. Furthermore, the process consumes a small amount of energy and is straightforward to regulate. The selection of the solvent and the recovery of the solvent are also critical considerations. Dhadge et al. [67] reported a novel technique for the purification and concentration of catechins from *Camellia sinensis*. Plant materials were filtered and processed through a membrane technology, which separated catechins from other phytochemicals after being extracted with hot water. Despite the fact that this approach has several advantages, only a small amount of study has been conducted on its application for the extraction of bioactive chemicals from plant sources.

4.3 Future perspectives

Bioactive compounds extracted from plant sources utilizing improved extraction methods have risen in recent years. However, each approach has its own set of obstacles. A few drawbacks include nonuniform sound wave dispersion, free radicals forming, and metal contamination if an ultrasonic probe is used in UAE, for example. In EAE, moderate processing parameters in aqueous solutions are one of the most critical difficulties. Other drawbacks include the high cost of enzymes required for large-scale extraction. Scaling up a process might be hampered if enzyme behavior changes under diverse environmental variables such as temperatures or the availability of nutrients. MAE has drawbacks, such as the recovery of nonpolar molecules and the change of the chemical structure of target compounds, which might affect bioactivity and restrict future applications. Other techniques, such as membrane-assisted extraction, SC-CO_2, and SWE, need scale-up procedures to assess yield, process parameters, and cost-benefit analysis for industrial settings. Standardized research and development facilities will be required for these operations. For the optimization of these extraction techniques, knowledge of the nature of the plant matrix as well as the chemistry of the target bioactive compound is also required. Modeling these technologies is necessary for continuous process monitoring, management, and forecasting.

4.4 Summary

The constant quest for effective extraction technologies is fueled by the ever-increasing demand for bioactive plant components. In the previous several decades, there has been a lot of progress in terms of extraction processes. The aforementioned nontraditional extraction techniques were primarily focused on boosting the yield of the desired chemicals. However, knowing every parameters of the advance extraction process is critical, as the majority of these approaches are based on distinct mechanisms, and extraction improvement is the outcome of several parameters. Some of the available approaches still require sufficient experimental data. The use of standard procedures also effects the assessment of extraction efficiency. On the other hand, the growing economic importance of bioactive compounds and bioactive compound-rich commodities may lead to more complex extraction technologies in the future.

References

[1] M. Cvjetko Bubalo, et al., Green solvents for green technologies, Journal of Chemical Technology & Biotechnology 90 (9) (2015) 1631–1639.
[2] S.O. Essien, B. Young, S. Baroutian, Recent advances in subcritical water and supercritical carbon dioxide extraction of bioactive compounds from plant materials, Trends in Food Science & Technology 97 (2020) 156–169.
[3] D. Haldar, M.K. Purkait, A review on the environment-friendly emerging techniques for pretreatment of lignocellulosic biomass: mechanistic insight and advancements, Chemosphere 264 (2021) 128523.
[4] A. Mouahid, et al., Supercritical CO_2 extraction of oil from Jatropha curcas: an experimental and modelling study, The Journal of Supercritical Fluids 141 (2018) 2–11.
[5] P. Arapitsas, C. Turner, Pressurized solvent extraction and monolithic column-HPLC/DAD analysis of anthocyanins in red cabbage, Talanta 74 (5) (2008) 1218–1223.
[6] S. Hemwimon, P. Pavasant, A. Shotipruk, Microwave-assisted extraction of antioxidative anthraquinones from roots of *Morinda citrifolia*, Separation and Purification Technology 54 (1) (2007) 44–50.
[7] M. Herrera, M. Luque de Castro, Ultrasound-assisted extraction for the analysis of phenolic compounds in strawberries, Analytical and Bioanalytical Chemistry 379 (7) (2004) 1106–1112.
[8] T. Huang, et al., Infrared-assisted extraction coupled with high performance liquid chromatography (HPLC) for determination of liquiritin and glycyrrhizic acid in licorice root, Analytical Methods 6 (15) (2014) 5986–5991.
[9] A. Alupului, I. Calinescu, V. Lavric, Microwave extraction of active principles from medicinal plants, UPB Science Bulletin, Series B 74 (2) (2012) 129–142.
[10] G. Cravotto, et al., Improved extraction of vegetable oils under high-intensity ultrasound and/or microwaves, Ultrasonics Sonochemistry 15 (5) (2008) 898–902.
[11] M. Dhobi, V. Mandal, S. Hemalatha, Optimization of microwave assisted extraction of bioactive flavonolignan-silybinin, Journal of Chemical Metrology 3 (1) (2009).

[12] J. Asghari, B. Ondruschka, M. Mazaheritehrani, Extraction of bioactive chemical compounds from the medicinal Asian plants by microwave irradiation, Journal of Medicinal Plants Research 5 (4) (2011) 495–506.
[13] C. Chiremba, L.W. Rooney, T. Beta, Microwave-assisted extraction of bound phenolic acids in bran and flour fractions from sorghum and maize cultivars varying in hardness, Journal of Agricultural and Food Chemistry 60 (18) (2012) 4735–4742.
[14] H. Teng, K. Ghafoor, Y.H. Choi, Optimization of microwave-assisted extraction of active components from Chinese quince using response surface methodology, Journal of the Korean Society for Applied Biological Chemistry 52 (6) (2009) 694–701.
[15] M. Desai, J. Parikh, P.A. Parikh, Extraction of natural products using microwaves as a heat source, Separation and Purification Reviews 39 (1–2) (2010) 1–32.
[16] C. Sparr Eskilsson, E. Björklund, Analytical-scale microwave-assisted extraction, Journal of Chromatography A 902 (1) (2000) 227–250.
[17] M. Vinatoru, T.J. Mason, I. Calinescu, Ultrasonically assisted extraction (UAE) and microwave assisted extraction (MAE) of functional compounds from plant materials, TrAC, Trends in Analytical Chemistry 97 (2017) 159–178.
[18] M.A. Rostagno, M. Palma, C.G. Barroso, Ultrasound-assisted extraction of soy isoflavones, Journal of Chromatography A 1012 (2) (2003) 119–128.
[19] H. Li, B. Chen, S. Yao, Application of ultrasonic technique for extracting chlorogenic acid from Eucommia ulmodies Oliv.(*E. ulmodies*), Ultrasonics Sonochemistry 12 (4) (2005) 295–300.
[20] Y. Yang, F. Zhang, Ultrasound-assisted extraction of rutin and quercetin from *Euonymus alatus* (Thunb.) Sieb, Ultrasonics Sonochemistry 15 (4) (2008) 308–313.
[21] L. Yang, et al., Ultrasound-assisted extraction of the three terpenoid indole alkaloids vindoline, catharanthine and vinblastine from *Catharanthus roseus* using ionic liquid aqueous solutions, Chemical Engineering Journal 172 (2–3) (2011) 705–712.
[22] D. Pingret, A.-S. Fabiano-Tixier, F. Chemat, Ultrasound-assisted extraction, Natural product extraction: Principles and Applications 21 (2013) 89.
[23] K. Ameer, H.M. Shahbaz, J.-H. Kwon, Green extraction methods for polyphenols from plant matrices and their byproducts: a review, Comprehensive Reviews in Food Science and Food Safety 16 (2) (2017) 295–315.
[24] A. Mustafa, C. Turner, Pressurized liquid extraction as a green approach in food and herbal plants extraction: a review, Analytica Chimica Acta 703 (1) (2011) 8–18.
[25] H. Wijngaard, et al., Techniques to extract bioactive compounds from food by-products of plant origin, Food Research International 46 (2) (2012) 505–513.
[26] J.O. Chaves, et al., Extraction of flavonoids from natural sources using modern techniques, Frontiers of Chemistry 8 (2020).
[27] A. Liazid, et al., Stability of anthocyanins from red grape skins under pressurized liquid extraction and ultrasound-assisted extraction conditions, Molecules 19 (12) (2014) 21034–21043.
[28] R.M. Alonso-Salces, et al., Pressurized liquid extraction for the determination of polyphenols in apple, Journal of Chromatography A 933 (1) (2001) 37–43.
[29] B.R. Sumere, et al., Combining pressurized liquids with ultrasound to improve the extraction of phenolic compounds from pomegranate peel (*Punica granatum* L.), Ultrasonics Sonochemistry 48 (2018) 151–162.
[30] J. Viganó, et al., Extraction of bioactive compounds from defatted passion fruit bagasse (*Passiflora edulis* sp.) applying pressurized liquids assisted by ultrasound, Ultrasonics Sonochemistry 64 (2020) 104999.
[31] N. Nastić, et al., New technological approaches for recovering bioactive food constituents from sweet cherry (*Prunus avium* L.) stems, Phytochemical Analysis 31 (1) (2020) 119–130.

[32] J. Ndayishimiye, B.S. Chun, Optimization of carotenoids and antioxidant activity of oils obtained from a co-extraction of citrus (*Yuzu ichandrin*) by-products using supercritical carbon dioxide, Biomass and Bioenergy 106 (2017) 1–7.

[33] S.G. Özkal, M.E. Yener, Supercritical carbon dioxide extraction of flaxseed oil: effect of extraction parameters and mass transfer modeling, The Journal of Supercritical Fluids 112 (2016) 76–80.

[34] T.C. Confortin, et al., Extraction and composition of extracts obtained from Lupinus albescens using supercritical carbon dioxide and compressed liquefied petroleum gas, The Journal of Supercritical Fluids 128 (2017) 395–403.

[35] R.N. Lima, et al., Extraction from leaves of piper klotzschianum using supercritical carbon dioxide and Co-solvents, The Journal of Supercritical Fluids 147 (2019) 205–212.

[36] K. Srinivas, J.W. King, Supercritical Carbon Dioxide and Subcritical Water: Complementary Agents in the Processing of Functional Foods, Functional food product development, 2010, pp. 39–78.

[37] M. Pillot, et al., High pressure intrusion of water and LiCl aqueous solutions in hydrophobic KIT-6 mesoporous silica: influence of the grafted group nature, Microporous and Mesoporous Materials 280 (2019) 248–255.

[38] H.R. Holgate, J. Tester, Oxidation of hydrogen and carbon monoxide in sub-and supercritical water: reaction kinetics, pathways, and water-density effects. 2. Elementary reaction modeling, The Journal of Physical Chemistry 98 (3) (1994) 810–822.

[39] E.S. Ong, J.S.H. Cheong, D. Goh, Pressurized hot water extraction of bioactive or marker compounds in botanicals and medicinal plant materials, Journal of Chromatography A 1112 (1–2) (2006) 92–102.

[40] P. Budrat, A. Shotipruk, Enhanced recovery of phenolic compounds from bitter melon (*Momordica charantia*) by subcritical water extraction, Separation and Purification Technology 66 (1) (2009) 125–129.

[41] Y. Yang, et al., Terpene degradation and extraction from basil and oregano leaves using subcritical water, Journal of Chromatography A 1152 (1–2) (2007) 262–267.

[42] J. Kronholm, et al., Comparison of gas chromatography–mass spectrometry and capillary electrophoresis in analysis of phenolic compounds extracted from solid matrices with pressurized hot water, Journal of Chromatography A 1022 (1–2) (2004) 9–16.

[43] J. Zhang, et al., Recent advances in the extraction of bioactive compounds with subcritical water: a review, Trends in Food Science & Technology 95 (2020) 183–195.

[44] M.S. Krieger, J.L. Wynn, R.N. Yoder, Extraction of cloransulam-methyl from soil with subcritical water and supercritical CO_2, Journal of Chromatography A 897 (1–2) (2000) 405–413.

[45] M.H. Eikani, F. Golmohammad, S. Rowshanzamir, Subcritical water extraction of essential oils from coriander seeds (*Coriandrum sativum* L.), Journal of Food Engineering 80 (2) (2007) 735–740.

[46] J. Wiboonsirikul, S. Adachi, Extraction of functional substances from agricultural products or by-products by subcritical water treatment, Food Science and Technology Research 14 (4) (2008), pp. 319–319.

[47] S. Latif, F. Anwar, Effect of aqueous enzymatic processes on sunflower oil quality, Journal of the American Oil Chemists' Society 86 (4) (2009) 393–400.

[48] P. Hanmoungjai, D. Pyle, K. Niranjan, Enzymatic process for extracting oil and protein from rice bran, Journal of the American Oil Chemists' Society 78 (8) (2001) 817–821.

[49] S.M. Choudhari, L. Ananthanarayan, Enzyme aided extraction of lycopene from tomato tissues, Food Chemistry 102 (1) (2007) 77–81.

[50] A. Boulila, et al., Enzyme-assisted extraction of bioactive compounds from bay leaves (*Laurus nobilis* L.), Industrial Crops and Products 74 (2015) 485–493.
[51] M. Marić, et al., An overview of the traditional and innovative approaches for pectin extraction from plant food wastes and by-products: ultrasound-, microwaves-, and enzyme-assisted extraction, Trends in Food Science & Technology 76 (2018) 28–37.
[52] C. Wen, et al., Advances in ultrasound assisted extraction of bioactive compounds from cash crops—A review, Ultrasonics Sonochemistry 48 (2018) 538–549.
[53] O. Gligor, et al., Enzyme-assisted extractions of polyphenols – a comprehensive review, Trends in Food Science & Technology 88 (2019) 302–315.
[54] L. Muniglia, et al., Enzymatic aqueous extraction (EAE), in: Alternative Solvents for Natural Products Extraction, Springer, 2014, pp. 167–204.
[55] S.A. Aboud, et al., A comprehensive review on infrared heating applications in food processing, Molecules 24 (22) (2019) 4125.
[56] B. Xiang, et al., Infrared assisted extraction of bioactive compounds from plant materials: current research and future prospect, Food Chemistry 371 (2022) 131192.
[57] L. Wang, et al., A simple and rapid infrared-assisted self enzymolysis extraction method for total flavonoid aglycones extraction from Scutellariae Radix and mechanism exploration, Analytical and Bioanalytical Chemistry 409 (23) (2017) 5593–5602.
[58] H.N. Rajha, et al., Innovative process of polyphenol recovery from pomegranate peels by combining green deep eutectic solvents and a new infrared technology, Lebensmittel-Wissenschaft & Technologie 111 (2019) 138–146.
[59] Y. Cai, et al., Study on infrared-assisted extraction coupled with high performance liquid chromatography (HPLC) for determination of catechin, epicatechin, and procyanidin B2 in grape seeds, Food Chemistry 127 (4) (2011) 1872–1877.
[60] F.j. Li, et al., Optimisation of infrared-assisted extraction of rutin from crude flos sophorae immaturus using response surface methodology and HPLC analysis, Phytochemical Analysis 23 (4) (2012) 292–298.
[61] G. Huang, et al., Determination of flavonoids in magnolia officinalis leaves based on response surface optimization of infrared assisted extraction followed by high-performance liquid chromatography (HPLC), Analytical Letters 53 (13) (2020) 2145–2159.
[62] D. Qin, J. Xi, Flash extraction: an ultra-rapid technique for acquiring bioactive compounds from plant materials, Trends in Food Science & Technology 112 (2021) 581–591.
[63] Y. Fan, et al., Tissue-smashing based ultra-rapid extraction of chemical constituents in herbal medicines, Journal of Pharmaceutical and Biomedical Analysis 95 (2014) 213–219.
[64] X.-s. Yin, et al., Ultra-rapid, enhanced and eco-friendly extraction of four main flavonoids from the seeds of *Oroxylum indicum* by deep eutectic solvents combined with tissue-smashing extraction, Food Chemistry 319 (2020) 126555.
[65] R. Singh, M.K. Sinha, M.K. Purkait, Stimuli responsive mixed matrix polysulfone ultrafiltration membrane for humic acid and photocatalytic dye removal applications, Separation and Purification Technology 250 (2020) 117247.
[66] U.B. Deepti, M.K. Purkait, Promising integrated technique for the treatment of highly saline nanofiltration rejected stream of steel industry, Journal of Environmental Management 300 (2021) 113781.
[67] V.L. Dhadge, M. Changmai, M.K. Purkait, Purification of catechins from *Camellia sinensis* using membrane cell, Food and Bioproducts Processing 117 (2019) 203–212.

CHAPTER 5

Neoteric solvents for extraction of bioactive phytochemicals

5.1 Introduction

Solvents are essential in synthesizing pharmaceutical solutions and suspensions and for the extraction of bioactive compounds from plant tissues or whole plants. Solution and suspension can be achieved by using a solvent, often a liquid, to dissolve or disperse one or more other substances. There has been an explosion of research into the extraction and recovery of bioactive phytochemicals like phenolic compounds, alkaloids, steroids, and pigments from plants and their diverse components because of growing knowledge of the health benefits of phytochemicals. While the extraction of phytochemicals from solid matrices has been extensively researched, new advances in hydrophobic neoteric solvents have increased interest in extraction from liquid matrices. Soxhlet extraction, maceration, and liquid—liquid extraction are all examples of distinct procedures that may be grouped within solid—liquid extraction, in which phytochemicals are removed from plant tissues by employing liquid solvents [1,2]. The best extraction process is typically determined by the kind of matrix (liquid or solid) and the type of molecule being extracted, including the intended use of the extracted extracts. Microwave-aided extraction and ultrasonic-assisted extraction represent substantial advances in decreasing solvent quantities, reducing extraction time, and enhancing extraction efficiency. These techniques are worth highlighting. Solvent selection based on properties, such as polarity, thermal properties, solvation power, toxicity, and physicochemical parameters, including boiling temperature, viscosity, and density, are critical to the extraction process's effectiveness [3].

A supercritical fluid, gas, or solid can serve as solvent in practical applications. Besides being able to remove active pharmaceutical ingredients (APIs) from a solution and break down their solid structure, solvents have a fluid structure that makes them useful as a delivery vehicle for a variety of different

Advances in Extraction and Applications of Bioactive Phytochemicals
ISBN 978-0-443-18535-9
https://doi.org/10.1016/B978-0-443-18535-9.00003-X

formulations, including emulsions and implants as well as injectable liquids, nanoparticles, oral liquids, and suspensions. In the pharmaceutical sector, water is the most widely utilized solvent. Both practical and financial considerations justify its use. Because of its low cost and ease of purification, as well as its nontoxicity and inertness, it is a popular choice for economic reasons.

Additionally, to develop procedures like crystallization and filtration, it might be advantageous to use water since it can be quickly transferred from one receptacle to another, producing little or no residue. At room temperature, the evaporation of the solvent is low since water has a boiling point of 100°C. Using water instead of alternative solvents in the development of pharmaceuticals saves money for the pharmaceutical industry, which helps keep prices for products lower. Some places of the globe, however, have a limited supply of water. Additionally, it demands a significant amount of energy to raise the boiling point of water in various temperature-based extraction processes. Distillation, for instance, needs a substantial amount of energy to get a high boiling point of water. Water-repellent properties of bioactive compounds have also prompted researchers to explore alternative solvent options, including typical organic liquids commonly used in the pharmaceutical sector [4].

The majority of conventional and traditional organic solvents are classified as volatile organic compounds (VOCs). The International Council for Harmonization (ICH) Q3C rules classify conventional solvents into one of three groups (Class 1, Class 2, or Class 3), as illustrated in Fig. 5.1. There are several ways in which conventional/traditional VOCs may be used to catalyze processes such as cleaning and disinfection as well as cryoprotection and degreasing of APIs and other compounds [5]. VOCs, on the other hand, can evaporate at ambient temperature since they are highly flammable and unstable. Anyone inhaling the resultant mist may be at risk. In addition, CO_2 elution from the oxidation of several traditional/conventional VOCs is a primary source of global climate change.

The environmental impact of VOCs, such as polluting water supplies is also substantial. Over the last decades, the pharmaceutical industry has been attempting to develop an alternative solvent to counteract the adverse effects of conventional solvents. The current focus of research, according to green chemistry, is on substituting more environmentally friendly solvents for unpredictable and dangerous VOCs. Fig. 5.2 and Table 5.1 illustrate the REACH (Registration, Evaluation, Authorization, and Restriction of Chemicals) regulation's suggested 12 green chemistry principles for developing green solvents.

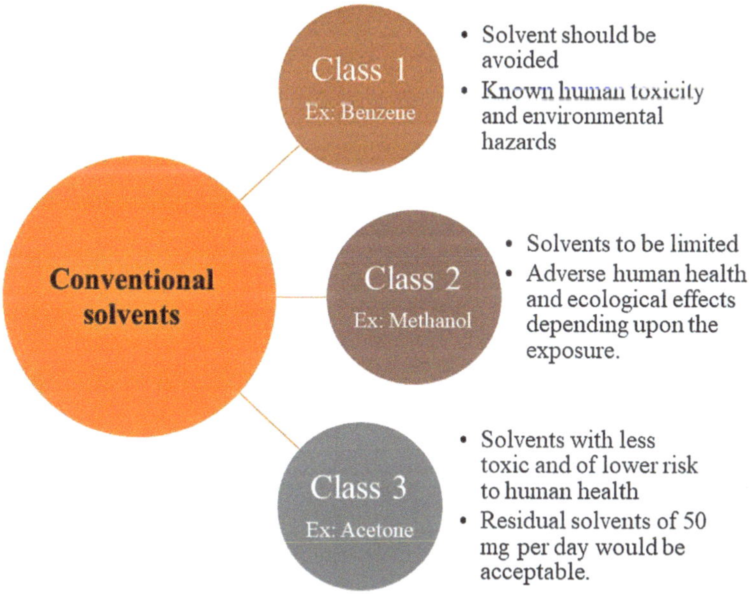

Figure 5.1 Categorization of conventional solvents in accordance with ICH Q3C recommendations.

It is desirable for a green solvent to have minimal toxicity, non-combustibility, long-term stability, no mutation potential, and wide availability. They also need to be cost effective, easy to handle, and reusable. Because of this, pharmaceutical companies are working hard to produce "neoteric" or unconventional solvents. As a result, these solvents will be more ecologically sound to meet chemical reaction demands and comply with environmental pollution regulations. Current neoteric solvents are classified and described here, along with their applicability in the pharmaceutical sector.

5.2 Classification of different synthetic solvents

5.2.1 Supercritical fluids

Supercritical fluids are compounds (H_2O, CO_2, and NH_3) that display characteristics of both liquids and gases at pressures and temperatures over their critical point. In general, a supercritical fluid is a mixture of both gas and liquid qualities. When compressed, it becomes a liquid, which means it has a similar density (0.1−1 g/mL) and solvent power to gas. It is only when the temperature and pressure of the substance exceed its critical point

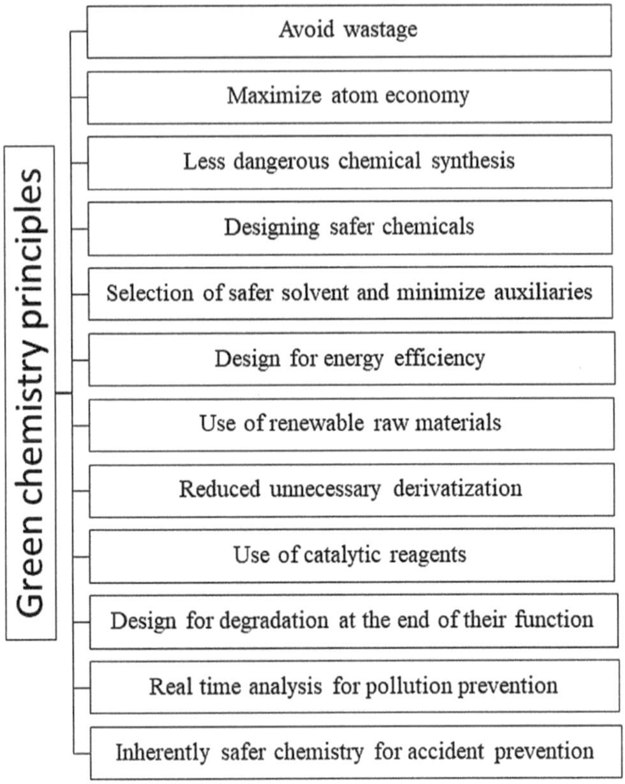

Figure 5.2 Green chemistry concepts that are applied in the formulation of green solvents in a systematic manner.

Table 5.1 The twelve principles of green chemistry.

S. no.	Principle	Brief description
1	Prevention	It is imperative to minimize waste rather than to manage or clean it up after it has occurred.
2	Atom economy	All components employed in the process should be included in the final product when using synthetic methods.
3	More environmentally friendly chemical synthesizes	Human health and the environment should be the primary considerations in developing synthetic procedures.
4	Designing safer chemicals	Toxicology and efficacy of chemical products should be considered in their development.

Table 5.1 The twelve principles of green chemistry.—cont'd

S. no.	Principle	Brief description
5	Safer solvents and auxiliaries	It is preferable to avoid using auxiliary chemicals (such as separation agents and solvents) if feasible, although their usage should never be considered harmful.
6	Energy-efficient design	For the sake of both the environment and the economy, chemical processes should have their energy requirements lowered. Chemical procedures should be executed at room temperature and pressure wherever possible.
7	Utilization of renewable feedstock	Wherever possible, raw resources and feedstocks should be replenished rather than depleted.
8	Reduce derivatives	Because needless derivatization necessitates the use of extra chemicals and may result in waste, it should be restricted or avoided whenever possible.
9	Catalysis	Stoichiometric reagents are substandard to catalytic reagents in terms of performance.
10	Design for degradation	When a chemical product has served its purpose, it should be designed to break down into nonhazardous degradation products with minimal ecologic impact.
11	Analysis in real time to aid in pollution prevention	For real-time, in-process operation and assessment before the formation of toxic compounds, additional improvements are needed in analytical methods.
12	Safer chemistry to avoid accidents	Hazardous processes should employ substances and forms of substances that limit the risk of chemical leaks, explosions, and fires.

that supercritical behavior begins. Conversely, pressures and temperatures above the critical values may not necessarily lead to a supercritical fluid, as previously stated. A supercritical fluid can exist at high pressures (for instance, >108 Pa) because the freezing curve can ascend into the supercritical fluid area. Conditions above and close to the critical temperature and pressure are commonly referred to as "supercritical" in the context of analytical scale extraction. When it comes to extraction medium and mobile phases, liquids typically have a better solvating capacity than supercritical fluids. However, there are many key potential advantages to using supercritical fluids in chromatography: the ease with which the solvating power of the fluid can be controlled. Solubility in a supercritical fluid is a function of pressure and temperature as well as density. To put it another way: if you increase the temperature while keeping the pressure the same, you will decrease the density and hence the solvent strength. Density, pressure, and temperature are the most important factors to consider [6]. A variety of equations of state have been constructed to characterize the connection between pressure, temperature, and density. Using Pitzer and coworkers' state equations, supercritical fluid properties may now be calculated numerically in several computer systems. Solvent strength calculations in binary systems were also established by various researchers. Moreover, the supercritical fluid's solvating strength diffusion coefficient, with reduced viscosity, among other benefits, considerably favors more effective component extraction than the subcritical process [7].

Table 5.2 highlights the critical pressure and temperature of various solvents used for the extraction of phytochemicals. CO_2 is the most often utilized supercritical fluid owing to it being a nontoxic, nonflammable, recyclable, and inexpensive substance with low critical pressure and temperature (73.6 atm and 31.1°C, respectively). CO_2 acts as a gas and a liquid in this supercritical state. It has the density of a liquid, the diffusivity of gas, and the viscosity of a gas. Unique properties of supercritical CO_2 have sparked interest in using it as a solvent for isolating necessary bioactive phytochemicals from plant biomass matrices [8,9]. When determining the solvating power of solvents, density is usually taken into account. CO_2 diffuses through the whole plant matrix during the extraction process,

Table 5.2 Critical temperature and pressure of various solvents used to extract phytochemicals.

Supercritical fluids	Temperature (°C)	Pressure (bar)
Water	373.85	220.889
Ammonia	132.85	113.484
Carbon dioxide	31.10	73.866
Ethane	31.85	48.839
Methane	−82.15	46.407
Argon	−122.15	49.143
Nitrogen	−147.15	33.944
Neon	−228.75	26.648
Hydrogen	−239.85	12.970

exploiting its solvent density qualities to dissolve essential phytochemicals. For the separation of phytochemicals without losing their valuable qualities, the supercritical CO_2 extraction technique requires moderate pressure and temperature. Also, after the extraction stage, a straightforward depressurizing setup ensures that the finished product is solvent-free. As a result, several valuable bioactive chemicals have been extracted from plant materials using supercritical CO_2 extraction methods [10].

The delignification procedure is also an essential part of the extraction process. Delignification of lignocellulosic materials is generally caused by pretreatment with supercritical CO_2. Furthermore, CO_2 generates carbonic acid in an aqueous solution, which helps hydrolysis of biomass carbohydrates. A rapid depressurization stage (explosion) can also be included in supercritical fluid pretreatment to encourage disruption of hemicellulose and cellulose structure, enhancing the cellulose surface area accessible for enzyme adsorption. Supercritical fluids often result in poorer enzymatic hydrolysis yields compared with ammonia fiber explosion and steam explosion pretreatments. Nonetheless, this approach is economical for biomass pretreatment and produces low amounts of biomass breakdown chemicals [11].

5.2.2 Fluorous solvents

Fluorocarbons, also known as perfluorocarbons or PFCs, are organofluorine compounds having the formula CxFy, indicating that they solely contain carbon and fluorine. Their nonpolar nature and weak intermolecular interactions make fluorocarbons, particularly perfluorinated alkanes, tertiary amines, and ethers, uncommon. Fluorocarbons can be employed as the nonaqueous phase since they are insoluble in water. Fluorocarbons have been effectively utilized as a transport medium of oxygen to aqueous biochemical systems due to their extraordinarily high oxygen solubility. Surprisingly, most common organic solvents, including toluene, tetrahydrofuran, acetone, and alcohols, have limited miscibility of perfluorinated alkanes, tertiary amines, and ethers, and these materials form biphase systems at the right circumstances [12]. As an analog to the term aqueous, fluorous is used to stress that the chemical transformation is predominantly controlled by a catalyst or reagent that dissolves favorably in the fluorous phase. The fluorous phase of a biphase system is described as the fluorocarbon-rich phase (mainly perfluorinated alkanes, ethers, and tertiary amines): hydroformylation catalyst with a fluorine biphase. The hydroformylation (or oxo) reaction, which typically takes place in the presence of homogeneous cobalt or rhodium catalysts, is a primary industrial process for the production of terminal aldehydes using olefins (where R is an alkyl group), CO, and H_2. Perfluorinated alkanes with functional groups, providing there are minimum favorable interactions between those groups, are the most effective fluorous solvents. Due to the fact that perfluoroaryl groups exhibit dipole—dipole interactions, they are less compatible with the fluorous biphase system (FBS) than perfluoralkyl groups. Tertiary amines and perfluoroalkyl ethers are also attractive fluorous phase options. Although having a substantial fluorous phase partition may be sufficient for some purposes, an FBS reagent or catalyst is intended to dissolve preferably in the fluorous phase. A fluorocarbon or fluoro hydrocarbon, with or without functional groups, might be used as an FBS compatible reagent or catalyst. Solubility in fluorocarbons may be limited by the presence of structural elements that interact favorably with one another, which should be avoided. These structural properties may also be attractive to the components of an opposing phase, resulting in fluorous phase leaching. Fluorohydrocarbons improve the chances of favorable interactions between the nonfluorinated parts of the molecule and the contents of the other phase. Fluorocarbon moieties should be used to reduce the attractive interactions in all of these circumstances. Linear or branching perfluoroalkyl chains with a large carbon number that may hold several heteroatoms are the most efficient fluorocarbon moieties (the fluorocarbon tethers or fluorous ponytails). To reduce the high electron-withdrawing properties of the fluorous ponytails, two or three ($-CH_2-$) groups must be inserted before the fluorous ponytail. This is a critical factor if the reactivity of the catalyst or reagent is to be approximated to that of the unmodified species in typical single-phase hydrocarbon solvents. Fluorination, functionalization with fluorocarbon compounds (for example, fluorocarbon groups can be added to reagents or catalysts), or complete synthesis can all be used to make ligands and reagents compatible with FBS (for transition-metal catalysts). Biphase extraction using fluorous soluble ligands to extract rhodium from a hydrocarbon phase is a unique technique to heavy-metal recovery, a required field of environmental chemistry. The chemistry of rhodium phosphine complexes is well documented, and it is one of the costliest transition metals employed in many homogeneous catalytic processes [12].

As a result of their lack of ability to combine with water and the organic phase at ambient temperature, fluorous solvents are referred to as the "third liquid phase." Perfluorohexane, perfluorooctane, perfluoropolyether perfluorodecalin, methylcyclohexane, and perfluorotributylamine are only a few of the high-fluorinated solvents [13]. The use of fluorous solvents in organic chemicals and metals extraction has been extensively studied, but the extraction of phytochemicals has received less attention. Fluorous solvents, according to the literature, can be employed as a unique extraction and cleaning procedure for food matrices such as cheese [14]. Nevertheless, there are various drawbacks to using these solvents, notably expensive costs, minimal application on strongly nonpolar solutes, and environmental problems [15].

5.2.3 Ionic liquids

An increasing number of green solvents for the fractionation of biomass have recently emerged, including ionic liquids (ILs) and IL-based solvent systems. However, this processing technology's commercial scalability is still hampered by various technologic, economic, and environmental constraints [16]. Inorganic anions and significant organic cations make up IL salts, which are liquid at temperatures below 100°C, have strong thermal and chemical stability, are nonflammable, and have excellent solvating capabilities for various materials [17]. Since Swatloski et al. [18] showed the capacity of several imidazolium-based ILs to dissolve substantial quantities of cellulose, the scientific interest in ILs for lignocellulose pretreatment has expanded significantly (over 15%). Because their hydrogen-bonding network is effectively disrupted, the ILs can solubilize carbohydrates. It is possible to employ ILs to deconstruct lignocellulose, boosting the separation of lignin, cellulose, and other components while reducing the creation of biomass degradation chemicals [19]. Lignocellulose feedstock and pure crystalline cellulose have been used to demonstrate the efficacy of ILs. Lignulosic materials have been treated with 1-ethyl-3-methyl-imidazolium chloride and 1-allyl-3-methylimidazolium chloride, two of the several ILs. In comparison to untreated biomass, pretreatment of barley straw with 1-ethyl-3-methyl-imidazolium acetate increased cellulose conversion by a factor of 10 and xylan conversion by a factor of 13. Another method that reduced sugars by 54.8% in wheat straw after 12 h of enzymatic hydrolysis was the use of 1-ethyl-3-methylimidazolium diethylphosphate. Economically viable chemical production costs, acceptable ecotoxicity profiles, and improved biodegradability make protic ILs like 2-hydroxy-ethyl-ammonium acetate attractive chemicals [20]. [FurEt$_2$NH][H$_2$PO$_4$] and [p-AnisEt$_2$NH][H$_2$PO$_4$] are two examples of ILs that have been produced recently and exhibit good hydrolysis potentials. Implementing energy-efficient recovery systems is necessary for large-scale use of ILs, just as it is for organosolv processes. In addition, the inhibitory capability of ILs to enzymes and fermentative bacteria must be explored thoroughly. While fermenting wheat straw hydrolysates pretreated with IL, Li et al. [21] found that *Saccharomyces cerevisiae* growth was unaffected by IL's deleterious effects (washed twice with the antisolvent). Even at 0.5% IL concentration, imidazolium-based ILs can suppress *S. cerevisiae* growth [22]. Finally, at a 10% (v/v) IL concentration, imidazolium-based ILs have been demonstrated to suppress cellulase activity by 70%–85% [23].

Most of the physical qualities of ILs may be modified and fine-tuned for a specific application, just as their chemical properties can be. The density of ILs is an essential consideration. There are two main reasons why ILs are denser than traditional solvents: their density is in the range of 0.9–1.7 g/cm^3 and viscosity. There are a number of factors that impact density, including temperature, pressure, molecular mass, and interactions. Viscosity is a key consideration when using ILs in transdermal drug delivery systems. The viscosity of a particular IL can range from 10 to 1000 cP at room temperature, making it a critical feature [24]. Because ILs do not exhibit Arrhenius behavior, viscosity is given as a viscosity coefficient rather than a stated value. The Vogel–Tammann–Fulcher equation, on the other hand, takes into consideration another element, namely, the transition to glass. Although ILs are naturally ionic, the lower melting points of ILs are one of their most intriguing features. As a result of their unique properties, including excellent thermal stability, low vapor pressures, and high conductivity, ILs are viable alternatives to conventional organic solvents [25]. Charge distribution, H-bonding capability, and symmetry all play a role in defining room temperature ILs, which have melting points at or below room temperature. Since ILs endure varying rates of supercooling, freezing point estimations are generally experimental and incorrect. The molecule structure, symmetry, rotational freedom, and electrostatic interactions were found experimentally by Katritzky et al. [26] to impact these characteristics. Solvent–solvate interactions depend heavily on polarity. There are no unifying principles for ILs. Instead, structure-related alterations may be tweaked and optimized for a particular purpose, as mentioned for each of the aforementioned qualities. Polarity studies have used solvatochromic dyes, which exhibit unique absorption and emission bands depending on the solvents in which they are dissolved. The hydrophobicity of long and branching chains is increased by chain length variation, a significant factor in IL polarity.

In spite of being considered environmentally friendly, there are several downsides to using ILs that have been recently identified. Although their substantially low vapor pressure and nonflammability make ILs "environmentally benign," research has shown that their usage pollutes the air and may affect aquatic and terrestrial ecosystems. For each creature, the toxicity varies according to the trophic level. The degradation rate and toxicity of ILs both rise with increasing bulk of organic moiety, according to a number of studies [27]. IL's biodegradability cannot be sacrificed in an effort to lessen its toxicity. When it comes to inadvertent discharge or pollution of waterways, the majority of ILs are water soluble. Toxicologic research on ILs revealed that they have significant impacts on enzymes, as well as on bacteria, algae, other cells, aquatic plants, invertebrates, and vertebrates of all kinds [28].

5.2.3.1 Preparation of ionic liquid

Many ILs are available in the market or maybe made easily by reacting the proper cation and anion bodies. Metathesis of a halide salt with, for example, silver, a group 1 metal, or the ammonium salt of the desired anion and acid-based neutralization reactions are the two fundamental procedures utilized in synthesizing ILs.

A reaction of the right halogenoalkane with amine produces several alkylammonium halides. In a similar way, pyridinium and imidazolium halides can be made. The low boiling points of halogenoalkanes necessitate either a sealed tube or an elaborate process, as in the production of 1-ethyl-3-methylimidazolium chloride ([EMIM][Cl], wherein [EMIM] is the 1-ethyl-3-methylimidazolium cation). As a result, salts with longer chain substituents, such as 1-butyl-3-methylimidazolium chloride ([BMIM][Cl], where [BMIM] is the 1-butyl-3-methylimidazolium cation), have become popular. Wilkes and Zaworotko synthesized 1-butyl-3-methylimidazolium tetrafluoroborate ([EMIM][BF_4]) from 1-ethyl-3-methylimidazolium iodide ([EMIM][I]) and Ag[BF_4] in methanol in 1992 [29]. This salt has a low melting point and could be made cheaply using acetone and ammonium tetrafluoroborate ([NH_4][BF_4]) [30]. 1-Ethyl-3-methylimidazolium hexafluorophosphate ([EMIM][PF_6]) was produced via the reaction of [EMIM][Cl] with fluorophosphoric acid. It is less desirable than tetrafluoroborate because of its greater melting point, which creates difficulties for room temperature activities ([BF_4]) [31]. Metathesis processes have yielded tris((trifluoromethyl)sulfonyl)methide ([$(CF_3SO_2)_3C]^-$), nonafluorobutanesulfonate ($[NfO]^-$), bis((trifluoromethyl)sulfonyl) imide ($[Tf_2N]^-$), trifluoroacetate ($[CF_3CO_2]^-$), heptafluorobutanoate, and thiocyanate ($[SCN]^-$). Although the foregoing metathesis processes are promising for creating new ILs, a minor amount of halide ions from the ILs may react with the solute materials. Tetraalkylammonium tetraalkylborides are usually made by combining tetraalkylammonium bromide and lithium tetraalkylboride in a metathesis synthesis. In the metathesis procedure, reactions to manufacture suitable quaternary amines were used to formulate a number of 1-alkyl-3-methylimidazolium trifluoromethanesulfonate ([EMIM][TfO]) ILs. The best way to make monoalkylammonium nitrate ILs is to neutralize aqueous amine solutions with nitric acid [32].

5.2.4 Eutectic solvents

When two or more compounds are combined, the resulting eutectic mixture (EM) inhibits each other's crystallization process, leading to a lower melting point than any of the components alone. The term eutectic is derived from the Greek word eutektos, which signifies "effortlessly dissolved or quickly melted." Since EMs have similar bioactivity, are eco-friendly, have poor volatility and instability, and fire-resistant properties to water, they are often utilized in water treatment. Urea (proline: urea), sugar and organic acids (citric acid, glucose), organic acid and amino acids (malic acid, glutamate, lactic acid, etc.), as well as choline chloride can be used to make EMs; these polymers include synthetic and natural ones [33]. Significant characteristics of EMs include the capacity to boost API bloodstream absorption by increasing API solubility and then enhancing intestinal permeability. In their liquid state at ambient temperature, EMs are referred to as deep eutectic solvents (DESs). Hybrid DESs are synthesized by reacting a hydrogen bond acceptor (HBA) with a hydrogen bond donor (HBD). For instance, quaternary ammonium halide salts (which is an HBA) and HBD (for example, carboxylic acid, alcohol, amides, carbohydrates, metal chloride) are connected by hydrogen bonds communication. When HBA and HBD are mixed, charge delocalization occurs, resulting in DESs with massive nonsymmetric ions that have low lattice energy and low melting temperatures [34]. DESs offer many of the same advantages as ESs, such as being less hazardous, affordable, environmentally benign, and noncombustible. Depending on HBA and HBD, DESs may be categorized into four categories [35] described in Table 5.3.

5.2.4.1 Deep eutectic solvent preparation

A DES is an ambient-temperature liquid created by combining two solid compounds at their eutectic composition, which includes a quaternary ammonium salt (for example, choline chloride) and an HBD. Near the eutectic composition, a variety of room temperature liquids can frequently

Table 5.3 Classification of DES with general formulas.

Types	General formula	Components	Term
Type I	$Cat^{+}X^{-}zMCl_x$	Organic salt (HBA) + metal salt (HBD)	M = Zn, Sn, Al, Fe, Ga, In
Type II	$Cat^{+}X^{-}zMCl_x \cdot yH_2O$	Organic salt (HBA) + metal salt hydrate (HBD)	M = Cr, Co, Ni, Cu, Fe
Type III	$Cat^{+}X^{-}zRZ$	Organic salt (HBA) + any HBD	Z = COOH, $CONH_2$, OH
Type IV	$MCl_x + RZ = MCl_{x-1}^{+} \cdot RZ + MCl_{x+1}^{-}$	Metal salt (HBA) + any HBD	Z = OH, $CONH_2$ and M = Al, Zn

be produced. As a result, a broader word, DES derivatives (DESDs), is easier to use to represent a broad range of DES-like derivatives, together with those formed from ternary mixes. Because hydrogen bonding between DESD components lowers the lattice energy of eutectic system components, the melting point of the combination is decreased. This correlation between melting point depression as well as the disparity between the hydrogen bonding contribution and the polar contribution to the solubility parameter of an HBD component have been shown by the study by Li et al. [33] using data from 22 choline chloride-based DES pairings. The association was confirmed using a novel DESD prepared by choline chloride and glycolic acid, which generate DESDs with DES-like characteristics when molar ratios of 1:1 to 1:4 are used. This particular DESD displays an extensive range of solubility increase on various mildly basic, inadequately water-soluble pharmaceuticals as a room temperature liquid. When compared with their aqueous solubility at room temperature, the solubility of itraconazole, lidocaine, posaconazole, and piroxicam increased by 6700, 430, 28, and 6400 times, respectively. This is in addition to an entirely new ternary DESD that has been revealed to enhance the solubility of itraconazole to a notable 5.36 mg/mL based on a molar ratio of 1:1.6:0.4. The possible usefulness of appropriate DESDs to drug delivery, particularly in improving drug solubility for topical formulations, might be highly appealing owing to the components of such DESDs that can include biodegradable ones that have already been utilized in prepared human products [33].

In most cases, DESs are made by first grinding the ingredients in a mortar and pestle. It is possible to create a clear liquid by placing the blended mixture in a magnetic stirrer and allowing it to whirl for a few minutes without applying heat [36]. To produce a liquid product after combining equal amounts of each component, heat is required. Mixing without heating over lengthy periods will not produce a distinct DES, even if the ratio of one component remains constant and the other component's ratio increases. DESs can also be made by freezing the component combination, which is then thawed to provide a clear liquid for use in the DES. Vacuum evaporation can be used to make DESs, then evaporate at 323 K in a rotatory flash evaporator with the component combinations dissolved in water. A natural deep eutectic solvent (NADES) can be created by mixing two naturally existing excipients to create a DES. Therapeutic deep eutectic solvents (THEDES) may also be created by combining APIs with excipients or two APIs. Polymeric deep eutectic solvents may be made similarly by mixing EM with any polymer. This is because the main problem of native DESs is their high viscosity at room temperature, which limits their usefulness as extraction solvents.

For the extraction of bioactive chemicals from plant tissues, foods, and other naturally occurring substances, NADES were explicitly developed. In contrast, THEDES were used as excipients to make any pharmaceutical product; they were used to enhance solubility, promote permeation, and raise absorption levels. There were several NADES with primary metabolites such as sugars and formed by choline chloride. Numerous NADESs containing a sweetener such as fructose or sucrose have been discovered, as well as those containing acids or bases such as malic acid, sorbitol, and choline chloride; these are all sugar-based NADESs [37]. Biosynthesis of NADESs might be facilitated by these components, which are commonly accessible in plants. It was proven by NMR spectroscopy that these mixes had a high degree of hydrogen bonding between their components, a characteristic of NADESs. DNA, proteins, and polysaccharides may all be dissolved by NADESs. This means that NADESs stimulate the biosynthesis of water-insoluble natural products, and they dissolve both the substrates and enzymes, which is not feasible on taking water into account [36].

5.3 The emergence of solvent-free reactions in pharmaceutical industries

Pharma has recently grown to be one of the most sophisticated industries. One reason for this sector's expansion has been the steady progression of science and technology as a whole. Other industrial sectors have progressed toward more sustainable manufacturing methods, goods, and processes in the pharmaceutical business. Every pharmaceutical industry's ultimate objective has always been to offer new pharmaceuticals to improve people's lives worldwide. This objective can only be achieved by moving away from old synthetic techniques to a more modern, environmentally friendly mechanism. Solvent-free extraction methods for biochemicals are presently being developed by pharmaceutical companies in tandem with advancements in other domains. However, even though the neoteric solvents covered here were primarily employed to extract phytochemicals or produce API-loaded drugs, many pharma firms are interested in minimizing excipient consumption and eliminating conventional or traditional neoteric solvents from their operations. Pharmaceutics has begun looking at the idea of "solvent-less or solvent-free reactions" to that aim. Products in the pharmaceutical business can also be made without using VOCs by employing thermal procedures, irradiation with ultraviolet, ultrasound, microwaves, and so on. Reduced contamination and handling costs, avoidance of solvent toxicity, simplified synthesis and separation, reduced waste, low energy consumption, reduced costs, rapid reactions, and no requirement for special apparatus are some of the potential benefits of exploring solvent free reactions in both chemical reactions and formulation development.

5.4 Summary

Aqueous or traditional VOC-based extraction procedures are often used to separate phytochemicals. Of them, water is by far the most commonly utilized solvent. However, the usage of water as an extractant is limited when the lead molecules have inadequate solubility in aqueous solutions. Neoteric solvents, on the other hand, were created and employed to extract bioactive components from entire plants or plant tissues or to produce API-loaded pharmaceutical products due to the evaporation of conventional VOCs at ambient temperature. DESs and SCFs offer the most significant potential for creating extracted or formulated APIs among the four neoteric solvents mentioned here (SCFs, ILs, FSs, and DESs). In the pharmaceutical business, DESs, particularly, exhibit potential in producing hydrophilic polymer-based microcapsules and oil-free emulsions. As we all know, few things in this world do not have two sides, and neoteric solvents are no exception. The effects and toxicity of these solvents on the environment and humans are currently poorly understood. As a result, many pharmaceutical companies are interested in reducing excipient usage and removing traditional and neoteric solvents from their processes. Solvent-free reactions or solvent-less ones are a significant addition to the reaction spectrum for API synthesis and product development in this situation since they allow for a substantial decrease in solvent consumption.

References

[1] N.P. Kelly, A.L. Kelly, J.A. O'Mahony, Strategies for enrichment and purification of polyphenols from fruit-based materials, Trends in Food Science & Technology 83 (2019) 248–258.
[2] M. Sharma, P. Kaushik, Vegetable phytochemicals: an update on extraction and analysis techniques, Biocatalysis and Agricultural Biotechnology 36 (2021) 102149.
[3] W. Routray, V. Orsat, Microwave-assisted extraction of flavonoids: a review, Food and Bioprocess Technology 5 (2) (2012) 409–424.
[4] T.R. Sekharan, et al., Neoteric solvents for the pharmaceutical industry: an update, Drug Discovery Today 26 (7) (2021) 1702–1711.
[5] K. Miazek, et al., Effect of organic solvents on microalgae growth, metabolism and industrial bioproduct extraction: a review, International Journal of Molecular Sciences 18 (7) (2017) 1429.
[6] J.R. Dean, Applications of Supercritical Fluids in Industrial Analysis, Springer Science & Business Media, 2012.
[7] T. Arumugham, et al., Supercritical carbon dioxide extraction of plant phytochemicals for biological and environmental applications – a review, Chemosphere 271 (2021) 129525.
[8] E. Naziri, et al., Advantages of supercritical fluid extraction for recovery of squalene from wine lees, The Journal of Supercritical Fluids 107 (2016) 560–565.
[9] A.P. Sánchez-Camargo, et al., Supercritical CO_2 extraction of lipids and astaxanthin from Brazilian redspotted shrimp waste (*Farfantepenaeus paulensis*), The Journal of Supercritical Fluids 56 (2) (2011) 164–173.
[10] L. Baldino, M. Scognamiglio, E. Reverchon, Supercritical fluid technologies applied to the extraction of compounds of industrial interest from *Cannabis sativa* L. and to their pharmaceutical formulations: a review, The Journal of Supercritical Fluids 165 (2020) 104960.
[11] V. Balan, et al., Lignocellulosic biomass pretreatment using AFEX, Biofuels (2009) 61–77.
[12] I.T. Horváth, J. Rábai, Facile catalyst separation without water: fluorous biphase hydroformylation of olefins, Science 266 (5182) (1994) 72–75.
[13] A. Saini, P.S. Panesar, Beneficiation of food processing by-products through extraction of bioactive compounds using neoteric solvents, LWT 134 (2020) 110263.
[14] V.A. Bailey, D. Clarke, A. Routledge, Extraction of perfluorinated compounds from food matrices using fluorous solvent partitioning, Journal of Fluorine Chemistry 131 (6) (2010) 691–697.
[15] H. Matsuda, et al., Liquid–liquid equilibria containing fluorous solvents as environmentally benign solvent, Fluid Phase Equilibria 357 (2013) 71–75.
[16] P. Reddy, A critical review of ionic liquids for the pretreatment of lignocellulosic biomass, South African Journal of Science 111 (11–12) (2015) 1–9.
[17] A. Pinkert, et al., Ionic liquids and their interaction with cellulose, Chemical Reviews 109 (12) (2009) 6712–6728.
[18] R.P. Swatloski, et al., Dissolution of cellose with ionic liquids, Journal of the American Chemical Society 124 (18) (2002) 4974–4975.

[19] N. Sathitsuksanoh, A. George, Y.-H.P. Zhang, New lignocellulose pretreatments using cellulose solvents: a review, Journal of Chemical Technology & Biotechnology 88 (2) (2013) 169−180.
[20] E.G.A. Rocha, et al., Evaluation of the use of protic ionic liquids on biomass fractionation, Fuel 206 (2017) 145−154.
[21] Q. Li, et al., Improving enzymatic hydrolysis of wheat straw using ionic liquid 1-ethyl-3-methyl imidazolium diethyl phosphate pretreatment, Bioresource Technology 100 (14) (2009) 3570−3575.
[22] M. Ouellet, et al., Impact of ionic liquid pretreated plant biomass on *Saccharomyces cerevisiae* growth and biofuel production, Green Chemistry 13 (10) (2011) 2743−2749.
[23] P. Engel, et al., Point by point analysis: how ionic Liquid affects the enzymatic hydrolysis of native and modified cellulose, Green Chemistry 12 (11) (2010) 1959−1966.
[24] Z. Sidat, et al., Ionic liquids as potential and synergistic permeation enhancers for transdermal drug delivery, Pharmaceutics 11 (2) (2019) 96.
[25] Y.H. Choi, R. Verpoorte, Green solvents for the extraction of bioactive compounds from natural products using ionic liquids and deep eutectic solvents, Current Opinion in Food Science 26 (2019) 87−93.
[26] A.R. Katritzky, et al., QSPR correlation of the melting point for pyridinium bromides, potential ionic liquids, Journal of Chemical Information and Computer Sciences 42 (1) (2002) 71−74.
[27] R. Cañadas, et al., Overview of neoteric solvents as extractants in food industry: a focus on phenolic compounds separation from liquid streams, Food Research International 136 (2020) 109558.
[28] T.P. Thuy Pham, C.-W. Cho, Y.-S. Yun, Environmental fate and toxicity of ionic liquids: a review, Water Research 44 (2) (2010) 352−372.
[29] J.S. Wilkes, M.J. Zaworotko, Air and water stable 1-ethyl-3-methylimidazolium based ionic liquids, Journal of the Chemical Society, Chemical Communications (13) (1992) 965−967.
[30] J. Fuller, R.T. Carlin, R.A. Osteryoung, The room temperature ionic liquid 1-Ethyl-3-methylimidazolium tetrafluoroborate: electrochemical couples and physical properties, Journal of the Electrochemical Society 144 (11) (1997) 3881−3886.
[31] J. Fuller, et al., Structure of 1-ethyl-3-methylimidazolium hexafluorophosphate: model for room temperature molten salts, Journal of the Chemical Society, Chemical Communications (3) (1994) 299−300.
[32] B. Tang, et al., Application of ionic Liquid for extraction and separation of bioactive compounds from plants, Journal of Chromatography B 904 (2012) 1−21.
[33] Z. Li, P.I. Lee, Investigation on drug solubility enhancement using deep eutectic solvents and their derivatives, International Journal of Pharmaceutics 505 (1) (2016) 283−288.
[34] F.M. Perna, P. Vitale, V. Capriati, Deep eutectic solvents and their applications as green solvents, Current Opinion in Green and Sustainable Chemistry 21 (2020) 27−33.
[35] E.L. Smith, A.P. Abbott, K.S. Ryder, Deep eutectic solvents (DESs) and their applications, Chemical Reviews 114 (21) (2014) 11060−11082.
[36] M.B. Singh, et al., A mini review on synthesis, properties and applications of deep eutectic solvents, Journal of the Indian Chemical Society 98 (11) (2021) 100210.
[37] A. Hayyan, et al., Fruit sugar-based deep eutectic solvents and their physical properties, Thermochimica Acta 541 (2012) 70−75.

CHAPTER 6

Application and effectiveness of computational methods in improving the production of bioactive phytochemicals

6.1 Introduction

There has been an increasing interest in phytochemicals over the past 3 decades due to their numerous health advantages. In addition to treating common illnesses like diabetes and liver disease, phytochemicals are used to treat a wide range of other diseases, including digestive, pulmonary, cardiac, neurological, and reproductive problems. In recent decades, there has been a considerable surge in the study of medicinal plants because of secondary metabolites, which play a significant role in drug design, medicine, food, and other fields. Secondary metabolites, essential to human well-being, are produced in small amounts in plants. Various circumstances like biotic and abiotic environments significantly impact their production [1]. As the concentration of secondary metabolites is reliant on so many various natural circumstances, the occurrence of it does not have a set process.

The search for novel medication elements necessitates the creation of accurate screening procedures for natural products' bioactive components. Over the years, various screening methodology has been developed. However, pharmacologic screening of bioactive phytochemicals demands more time, work, money, and other resources. In silico, technologies including molecular dynamic (MD) simulation, molecular docking, and artificial intelligence (AI) are some of the most promising new alternatives for the screening and optimization process. From drug design to culture optimization, AI has been used in a variety of fields in pharmacology in recent years. Morishige and Scoog Media, Driver and Kuniyuki wood plant medium, Gamborg's B5 Woody Plant medium, etc., are used as basal mediums in plant

Advances in Extraction and Applications of Bioactive Phytochemicals
ISBN 978-0-443-18535-9
https://doi.org/10.1016/B978-0-443-18535-9.00007-7

biotechnology. In in vitro research, altering the medium helps to improve the desired outcome [2]. To be fair, though, the change is a challenge because so many macro- and microelements are added to the medium at the same time. It becomes increasingly difficult to estimate the effects of various culture components on plant growth. When it comes to plant development and phytohormones, AI has a critical function to play in the selection of optimum culture mediums along with their components [3]. AI can be used to improve phytohormones by modeling the results of in vitro research to account for the effects of various confounding circumstances. In *Centella Asiatica* cultures, artificial neural network-based modeling was used to predict growth conditions and biomass production [4]. An artificial neural network (ANN) predicts interactions between the elements and provides a nutritional imbalance report for the plant, focusing on the parameters that affect plant growth. Utilizing cutting-edge technology like AI and microfluidics has accelerated the design and development of new pharmaceuticals [5]. ANNs are designed to handle noisy, incomplete, and nonlinear data. A modest amount of experimental data may be used to swiftly create mathematical models using ANNs to discover and approximate any complicated nonlinear systems. In addition, ANNs are more precise than other commonly used fitting approaches. The hidden layer's number of neurons and the training function both have a direct impact on neural network performance. Tenfold cross-validation may be used to estimate errors in neural network training functions and the number of neurons in the hidden layer of neural networks, based on previous research. When it comes to solving optimization computational problems mathematics, genetic algorithms (GAs) have been widely employed. It is common to practice to employ GAs in conjunction with ANNs to solve optimization issues based on the evolutionary principles of natural selection and genetic mutation. The genetic algorithm is a type of metaheuristic algorithm.

Machine learning (ML) is also becoming increasingly popular in the study of pharmacology. For instance, in plant tissue culture, ML has improved the production of secondary metabolites in *Bryophyllum* [6]. Phytochemicals from different medicinal plants can now be mass produced considerably from in silico work. In addition, AI forecasts which medicinal plant species are in danger of extinction and aids in their preservation. The identification of medicinal plant leaves can also be aided by image processing. Herbal interactions are predicted by AI as well. Secondary metabolites in medicinal plants that have therapeutic potential are enhanced by ML methods, making them more suitable for industrial usage. An ANN uses leaf size, color, and dimensions to classify medicinal plants [6]. Nutrition is a crucial aspect of tissue culture plant growth in plant biotechnology. Photochemistry and its nutritional activity can be studied holistically using ML methods such as ANN and support vector machines (SVMs).

In bioinformatics, docking is an essential method for determining the binding pose and binding score. From identifying phytochemicals to developing a pharmacologic lead, docking has taken the lead. It is easier to sift through the best candidate complexes if the two compounds bind precisely, reducing time and money spent on experiments. The docking technique assists in resolving a number of critical difficulties in pharmacology research. As one of the most difficult challenges in research, dengue serotype antigenic diversity has been bridged by introducing a novel plant scaffold against dengue targets [7]. Dasatinib and imatinib have been developed as a result of advances in computational technology [8]. The pharmacology network approach has improved the binding relationships between ligands and various targets. Aside from approximately 100 docking software products, the rising number of protein structures in the protein database (PDB) is one of the sophisticated aspects that aid in docking. The PDB now has 148,827 nuclear magnetic resonance (NMR)-based protein structures, up from 45,651 in 2008 [9]. Because of the enormous development of 3D X-ray and NMR structures, as well as their higher resolution reported in the PDB, molecular docking has become one of the most widely used virtual screening approaches, and it has proven to be quite effective throughout the course of time.

MD simulations are another common approach in drug development and discovery. They give enough dynamic information about proteins, as well as an understanding of how protein–ligand interactions operate energetically. Understanding the dynamic connection between protein and ligand is more accessible by this information. MD also helps with detailed studies of specific binding sites to improve docking accuracy. For example, computational techniques have successfully designed and developed anticancer medications derived from nature-based plant phytochemicals for prostate and lung cancers. Binding energy is generated during 50 ns using the molecular mechanics generalized Born surface area technique [10]. MD simulations can also find the root-mean-square deviation (RMSD) of particles and dynamic stability, as well as determining the radius of gyration. RMS improves the effectiveness of the virtual screening procedure for ligand and target stability in a body-like environment before recommending it for use in clinical uses [11]. This chapter discusses the advancements in computational techniques, ranging from static molecular docking to dynamic modeling and sophisticated AI techniques such as ML, ANN, and deep learning.

6.2 Insight into the progress of different computational tools

6.2.1 Artificial intelligence

In the field of pharmaceutical research and development, AI has made significant advances. It has served as a catalyst in the advancement of technology to design lead candidates or phytochemicals that are more accurate and precise. It is becoming increasingly common in this industry to use ML, a sort of AI that allows software programs to get more accurate at predicting events without being specifically designed to do so. Cutting-edge new technology in the pharmaceutical industry is deep learning, a subset of ML. It was recently reported that Iktos and Servier researchers used deep learning models to successfully optimize compounds that were wholly ligand-built, even for targets that remained concealed until later in the optimization procedure. Beyond these, there are a variety of other AI computing tools, including linear regression, SVM, and other ML models, that have been utilized successfully in drug discovery.

6.2.2 Artificial intelligence in improving the production of secondary metabolites from plants

Several examples of successful applications of AI in enhancing phytochemical production may be found in recent decades. An advanced computational effort in detecting phylogenic similarity in plants is a grouping strategy to surround plants based on their region-based secondary metabolites content generation. Total polysaccharides and flavonoids in *Chrysanthemum morifolium* were calculated using an SVM and multivariate analysis [12]. By combining in vitro and in silico methods, researchers were able to maximize the synthesis of phenolic compounds. AI predicts promising phytochemicals in underutilized medicinal plants.

Combining in vitro plant characteristics with ML to increase phenolic compound synthesis has been very successful. It employed an ANN to represent the influence of various factors on a specific variable and the effects of different nutrients in the medium responsible for the same effects. A nonlinear optimization approach was used to extract the phytonutrients crocin, geniposide, and total phenolic compounds (TPC) from the plant gardenia. Based on the preceding data, the GA projected the optimal parameters for TPC extraction from gardenia [13]. Farhadi et al. [14] used an ML-GA to forecast the optimization of secondary metabolites in *Corylus avellane* using paclitaxel as input. AI is capable of analyzing large amounts of data and pinpointing the parameters that maximize the generation of secondary metabolites and drug development.

6.2.3 Artificial intelligence in plant tissue culture

One of the most extensively used methods in the field of plant research and agricultural production is the employment of plant tissue culture techniques to investigate plant development, differentiation, gene function, as well as genetic recombination. Tissue culture is a typical method for growing plants since it does not need the use of precise tools. A few drawbacks remain in plant tissue cultures, such as extended cycle times and laborious experiments. Modeling and optimizing all stages of in vitro culture for optimal development is a time-consuming and challenging undertaking. It is also difficult to do studies in plant tissue culture. In the last few decades, AI-based modeling has advanced in plant tissue culture. These tools are becoming increasingly important in the improvement of plant tissue culture. By gathering in vitro data and developing models from it, AI modeling has a significant influence on overcoming these obstacles and assisting in making the best optimization decisions [15]. Tissue culture optimization has a considerable influence on reducing experimental time and even resources in statistical optimization. When maximizing more than two parameters at the same time in plant tissue culture, a conflict emerges [16]. The consequences of one function conflicts with the impacts of other functions. A multiobjective method can be used to address this. Plant tissue culture is a nonlinear process in which various variables influence numerous processes, such as the medium's environment and the combinations and concentrations of plant hormones. Tissue culture procedures employ ML-based models to improve the efficiency of each stage. Explant sterilization in vitro is influenced by a number of variables, including the type of explants used, the age of the explants, and even the size of the explants used for the inoculation process itself. Tissue culture optimization is made more difficult by the several stages involved. According to published reports, extended exposure times to the sterilant have a positive effect on sterilization but a detrimental effect on the explant's viability. This needs to be balanced to benefit the explant's health [17].

Surface sterilization has been optimized using multilayer perception to report the highest possible outcome without damaging the explant. Using hormones, vitamins, and other nutrients as learning data, neuro-fuzzy logic has predicted the number of *Prunus armeniaca* shoot multiplications [18]. ML was used to forecast the shoot's characteristics by using image processing as an input tool. Naphthalene acetic acid (NAA) has a significant impact on rhizogenesis in the laboratory. Charcoal may also be used for rooting; however, the interactions between the two factors must be tuned to produce the greatest possible output. In vitro rooting has been improved by using AI-based modeling, which has reduced the incidence of caulogenesis by reporting charcoal as an essential variable [19]. As a result, ML approaches may be used to monitor and adjust medium conditions.

Callogenesis is a crucial aspect of plant micropropagation. A variety of variables drive the production of calluses, resulting in a variety of textures and colors. The callogenesis of many plants has been studied using image-based modeling. *Cuminum cyminum* callus generation has been predicted using the backpropagation approach in neural networks [20]. For the prediction of shoot development in bioreactors, *Chlorophytum borivilianum* was used to apply three different models of neural networks [21]. A backpropagation neural network was shown to be the best tool for predicting the fresh weight of plantlets compared to the other two methods, which used pH, density, and energy concentration as feedback data. Nutrients in strawberry cultivation have been studied using MARS (multivariate adaptive regression splines)-based modeling. Using ML, Barone et al. [22] predicted the nitrogen supply influence on shoot organogenesis in *Pinus taeda*. They compared two approaches, namely multiple analysis and multilayer perception.

The process of in vitro rooting is a critical component of tissue culture. Gago et al. [23] have used ML-based modeling to improve the rooting of grapevines by optimizing many parameters. The media used in tissue culture is another important component of the process. To a significant extent, the growth of shoot propagation is influenced by mineral elements. For better micropropagation of *Actinidia arguta*, another group of researchers has developed three ML algorithms to reduce mineral and salt content in the culture medium [24].

ML was used to develop *Grynops walla*'s chemical composition for callus generation, as well as to forecast the excellent composition of callus weight and callus induction. Tissue culture development of *Prunus* rootstock by micropropagation is best accomplished using a medium recommended by

AI-based research [25]. Pear rootstock macronutrients may be predicted using regression analysis—based modeling. The relationship between macronutrients and several growth characteristics, including explant growth rate, shoot length, shoot tip necrosis, chlorosis, and vitrification, was predicted using ANN models and a GA. For example, the melon cultivation conditions have been improved by using neural networks and GA-based modeling [26].

6.2.4 Artificial intelligence in drug design and discovery

AI algorithms in drug discovery must be used sequentially, and the issue domain should be well defined. This often entails defining the problem, preparing the data, designing the AI architecture, training and evaluating the model, and interpreting and explaining the findings. The process flow for developing an AI prediction model is illustrated in Fig. 6.1. Prior to making any architectural decisions, one should be clear about the problem at hand since the ML approach chosen should be suited for the challenge at hand. One must first determine if the problem is a discriminative or generative one. The next stage is to create a model architecture suited for AI modeling. The selection of an appropriate algorithm and the setting of reasonable hyperparameter values are part of this stage. SVM, random forest (RF), and ANNs have been the most often utilized algorithms for discriminative tasks to date. Deep Boltzmann machine (DBM), deep belief network (DBN), variational autoencoder (VAE), generative adversarial network (GAN), and adversarial autoencoder (AAE) are a few models

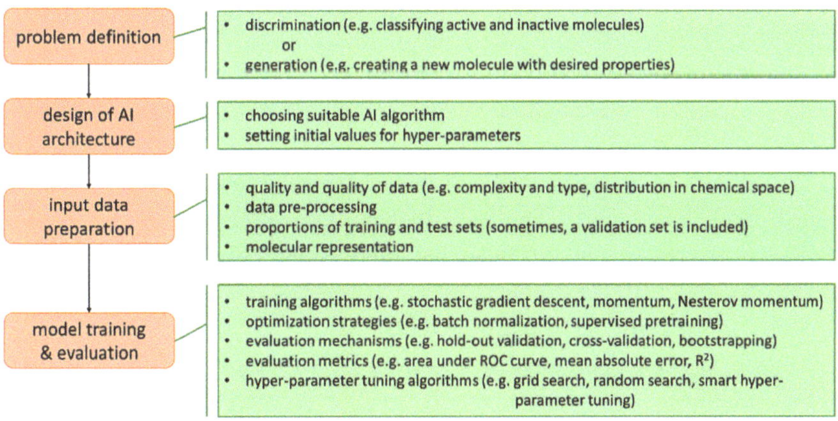

Figure 6.1 Process flow for developing an AI prediction model. *(Reproduced with permission from Yang et al. [27].)*

available for generative jobs. Because of their generalizability and theoretical capacity to simulate any input-output connection function, ANNs are often the go-to component of the field for these tasks. AI algorithms use different hyperparameters. The error penalty and the kernel parameters are two examples from the world of SVM algorithms. In addition to the number of neurons and layers (and their kind), learning rate and decay, regularization parameters, and connections between neurons or neighboring layers, the architectural characteristics of a neural network include but are not limited to those parameters.

ML can predict the increase or decrease in the effectiveness of numerous pharmacologic interactions occurring simultaneously, as well as the pace at which one drug inhibits another. Using a prediction accuracy of 91%, Islam et al. (2018) employed ML to predict the association between medication and symptoms, and this prediction was used as input [28]. The use of vector machines for medication repositioning in the field of schizophrenia illness is also reported in the literature. For predicting medication interactions, Ning et al. [29] used an SVM supervised learning approach.

Drug design and other biomedical fields rely heavily on neural networks. A convolutional neural network trained on two separate protein datasets yielded impressive accuracy at the ATP site of the corresponding protein. Knowing a protein's ATP site is critical in drug design because it allows the ligand and protein to create a protein–ligand complex, which aids in drug discovery. A crucial development in the field of drug design has been the use of deep neural networks for the identification of novel medication–disease pairings. To address the problems that emerge in traditional drug design, AI is used at all phases of drug design, such as the validation of drugs, identification of pharmaceuticals, and repurposing of medications. Integrated drug use is becoming more and more frequent. Drug compatibility has been calculated using Traditional Chinese medicine (TCM) prescriptions as the database [30].

There are many aspects of the pharmacologic arena covered by Chinese herbal medicines, which are multiherbal. The effectiveness of AI was proved in a case study of TCM that used AI to develop three separate models to anticipate side effects of prescriptions. To improve traditional Chinese remedies, integrating science and AI is becoming more commonplace. It is being used as a basis for TCM recipes based on a variety of herbs. Chinese medications, which are also classified as the meridian, are based on the practice from TCM. Meridian categorization is uncertain even with extensive knowledge of Chinese medicines [31]. The AI-based model was created with the goal of better understanding the categorization system. To forecast the relationships with TCM, a convolutional neural network was used to progress this categorization. Drug repurposing is a new method for the pharmaceutical industry that saves money and time. Kim et al. [32] proposed an ML technique to exploit undiscovered therapeutic characteristics of herbal bioactive compounds, which might improve medication repurposing.

Regulated least square is a semisupervised novel modeling approach that may be used to leverage the new pharmacologic significance of current medications. Numerous therapeutic plants have yet to be recognized for their phytochemicals' function. The therapeutic efficacy of the Xiaoxuming decoction as a neuroprotective ingredient has been discovered using an ML technique [27].

6.3 Insight into the advancement of molecular docking

Docking is a computer tool used extensively in designing and discovering new pharmaceuticals. Binding two molecules and analyzing their capacity to bind together is the primary goal of this tool. As a result, it provides a platform to identify the optimal therapeutic ligand chemical from a broader pool of compounds. Lamarckian GA-based AutoDock tools calculate the energy of a ligand at protein active sites by computing the multiple ligand conformations utilizing grid design [33]. An AutoDock-calculated Phytoligand from TCM has been successfully tested and proven to be a therapeutic target protein cruzain from *Trypanosoma cruzi* preferred by the FDA [34]. The semiempirical version of AutoDock4, AutoDock Vina, and other versions are available for free download and installation. GLIDE is another docking tool that lists compounds based on two scoring systems, SP and XP, used to rank compounds. The OPLS-AA force field (Optimized Potentials for Liquid Simulations) uses GLIDE to convey an orientation and positional browsing of docked ligand complexes. GOLD, in addition to docking ligands to their targets, is a tool that does postdocking processing. There are three types of software that make up the GOLD Suite, and they are GOLD, Hermes, and GOLDMINE. The flexibility of docking is the prime advantage of this software [35].

In 2004, docking of 100 wt ligands using a variety of tools, including DOCK, FLEXX, FRED, GLIDE, GOLD, SLIDE, SURFLEX, and QXP were compared to determine which compounds were enzyme inhibitors and which were drug-like compounds using X-ray images [36]. Identifying and distinguishing between binding and nonbinding sites in ligand–target interactions is the fundamental goal of scoring functions. The use of molecular mechanics, which administers molecules in conjunction with the law of classical mechanics, can reduce the cost of quantum mechanical calculation. For the most part, atoms are thought of as an electrically charged sphere connected by a spring, with no consideration given to the existence of electrons on the perimeter. In mechanics, potential energy, or force field, is the sum of all bound and unbounded energy values. The torsional potential is a trigonometric function, whereas harmonic potential is a function of bond stretching and bending together. AutoDock, GBVI/WSA, and GoldScore are some examples of scoring functions. Hydrogen bonds, van der Waals, hydrophobicity, and electrostatic are all considered when calculating the empirical scoring function. A few examples of empirical scoring functions include LUDI, ChemScore, GlideScore, and PLANTSCHEMP. The statistical measurement of ligand–target binding provides the foundation for knowledge-based scoring functions. For instance, GOLD/ASP and DrugScore are two examples of knowledge-based scoring functions. Unknown active sites can be found using a variety of tools and web servers, including POCKET (Putative Active Sites with Pockets), GRID, PASS (Putative Active Site with Spheres), SURFNET, and MMC (Mapping Macromolecular Topography) [37].

There are two phases to docking: the production of a conformational posture and the evaluation of the stability of a complex based on its scoring functions. The scoring functions connect the structural pose to the minimal energy score to offer the best-docked structure. The sampling typically discovers the conformational spaces of ligand at the catalytic site of protein by free energy. GLIDE and GOLD, two programs that generate 90% correct conformational poses, have enhanced docking performance. Table 6.1 lists the docking data for ligands and their therapeutic targets for action against certain diseases.

6.3.1 Molecular docking in drug design

In the realm of drug discovery, molecular docking techniques are commonly employed. When medications interact with targets, they are frequently mixed noncovalently, limiting ability to conduct research and development. Researchers created covalent docking is a novel molecular docking approach that now allows modeling the covalent force between

Table 6.1 Detail list of proteins and phytochemicals for computational docking along with therapeutic potential.

Phytochemicals	Medicinal plants	Protein	Therapeutic significance	Docking software
9-Octadecenoic acid,3-dodecanol	*Aloe castellorum* and *Aloe pseudorubroviolacea*	Musashi −1	Anticancer activity	AutoDock vin
Artesunic acid, homogenol	*Withania somnifera, Bacopa monnieri*, and *Morus alba*	Monoamine oxidase (MAOB), beta-secretase 1 (BACE1), and phosphodiesterase 4D	Alzheimer disease	Autodock vina
3,4-Di-*o*-caffeoylquinic acid, apigenin, and 7-*o*-methylwogonin	*Andrographis paniculata* and *Spilanthespaniculata*	B protease	Antiamyloid	GLIDE
Lycorine	*Pancratium foetidum*	LpxC	Antibacterial properties	MOE version
Juniperuschinensis, artoflavanocoumarin 3	*Juniperuschinensis*	BACE 1	Neurological disease	Autodock 4.2
Physostigimine and tacrine	*Tetrapterysmucronata*	Acetylcholinesterase	Parkinson disease	Autodock vina
Glycerol, magnesium ions	*Cornus capitata*	Alpha glucosidase	Postprandial hypoglycemia	Autodock 4
Floribundiquinone B	*Berchemia*	Acetylcholinesterase	Alzheimer disease	SYBYL-X2.0
Vitexin, isovetxin, betulin, llanasterol	*Grewia tiliaefolia*	Acetylcholinesterase	Alzheimer disease	Ligand fit from discovery studio

Continued

Table 6.1 Detail list of proteins and phytochemicals for computational docking along with therapeutic potential.—cont'd

Phytochemicals	Medicinal plants	Protein	Therapeutic significance	Docking software
Ganoderic acid J	*Ganoderma lucidum* karst	P2Y1R protein	Anti-thrombotic drug	Dockscore
Gallic acid, glucogallic acid, and citric acid	*Eucalyptus globulus*	Glutathione s-transferase	Antioxidant, hyperglycemia	Discovery studio
3-Hydroxyhericenone F	*Hericium erinaceus*	β-Secretase	Alzheimer disease	LibDock
Cyclovirobuxine D	*Buxux microphylla*	Human serum albumin	Arrhythmias, angina pectoris	Sybyl 6.9
Puerarin, mirificin, genistinc	*Puerariae lobatae*	Tyrosinase	Skin disease	GLIDE, gOLD, libdock, and cdocker
Punicalagin and chebulagic acid	Triphala (*terminalia bellirica*, *terminalia chebula*, and *embelica officinalis*)		Angiogenesis	AutoDock vina 1.0.2

Reprinted with permission from Singh et al. [37].

drug molecules and their targets, considerably expanding our study possibilities. However, there are a number of difficulties with molecular docking that still need to be addressed. For instance, in the docking procedure, the shape of protein molecules during actual binding may not be appropriately depicted. In the market, molecular docking software with improved computation accuracy and more accurate prediction outcomes is continually appearing. The integrated services can be utilized for computing to increase the speed of operations. Other technologies, including MD, network pharmacology, and ML, can be integrated with molecular docking to increase theoretical accuracy and offer advice for experimentation.

Phytochemicals from *Allophytus serratus* plants were shown to have greater binding energy than the control medication diclofenac when docked against the target cyclooxygenase 2 enzymes. This was used as a lead phytochemical for drug discovery. Antifilarial lead chemical is a combination of phytochemicals docked to protein B-tubulin. Snake venom is neutralized by docking and simulating plant phytochemicals crepside E beta glucopuyranoside against the target PLA2 [37].

Natural phytochemicals from the mangrove plant, such as taraxasterol, heritonin, stigmasterol, tretinoin, tricin, and ascochitin, have been shown to be antidiabetic drugs in docking studies. Persian shallot phytochemicals have the property to be employed as a future study for antidiabetic medicine, according to another report on docking for antidiabetics. If subsequent simulations show that the phytochemical sitosterol is stable, it has a strong chance of being used as a therapeutic candidate for diabetes therapy. Ahmed et al. [38] revealed docking results for 10 distinct phytochemicals, as well as molecular docking modeling and drug-like characteristics against the target compound pancreatic lipase. Alam et al. [39] performed a docking investigation using 45 distinct natural ligands against 13 different targets, indicating that it is a good candidate for Alzheimer disease by destroying brain nerve cells.

6.3.2 Application of molecular docking in the treatment of various diseases

For a variety of ailments, this in silico procedure has been elevated by improvements in science and technology in the current period. To combat osteoarthritis, researchers used medication repurposing against the target MMP-13 (matrix metalloproteinase 13) and osteoarthritic inhibitors as a starting point for their docking [37]. An estimated two million people die each year from malaria across the world. Docking analysis is the primary method used by scientists nowadays to reduce the number of instances of this. To identify the pharmacologic potential of herbal phytochemicals against malaria, Sahayarayan et al. used docking methods [40]. Studies on multicentric Castleman illness have used an herbal ingredient to treat lymph node growth and other inflammatory issues related to lymph [41].

Antiwrinkling properties of lupeol and botulin from triterpenoids have been demonstrated in a docking study using the protein matrix metalloproteinase as the target [42]. Protozoa sickness can be treated with the use of bioactive compounds from Nigerian medicinal plants, according to computational research. Antimyocardial activities of 13 herbal components from *Panax notoginseng* are described in another paper from China [43]. Many individuals have died as a result of respiratory sickness caused by the recent pandemic outbreak of COVID 19. With regard to COVID-19 and its ligands, a lot of research has been done on docking and the use of herbal substances as potential treatments [37].

6.4 Insight on molecular dynamics simulation for diseases and drug design

All the chemicals in the simulation box are handled as flexible in this in silico program, which simulates the changing behavior of a system as a result of parameters such as time and space. It is based on the physics theory of interatomic interactions and regulates the movement of every atom in every entity in the system across time. The docked complex's structural properties must be known before designing a drug. MD simulations shed information on the complex's dynamic functions as well as their stability. Experiments like as X-ray crystallography, electron paramagnetic resonance, cryo-electron microscopy, NMR, and Förster resonance energy transfer can also be used in conjunction with MD modeling.

Due to the rapid development of supercomputers and the ability to deliver findings in a short period of time, this type of simulation has grown in relevance during the last 2–3 decades. Fig. 6.2 describes the various applications of MD. Many fields, like drug discovery and development involving the nervous system and neuronal signaling, have benefited from its extensive usage in locating protein information. MD simulation is used to determine the binding energy and stability of the docking molecule that yielded the best results in terms of scoring functions. The docked compound's high-quality structure is exploited through simulation. There are a variety of MD simulation tools available, including AMBER, NAMD,

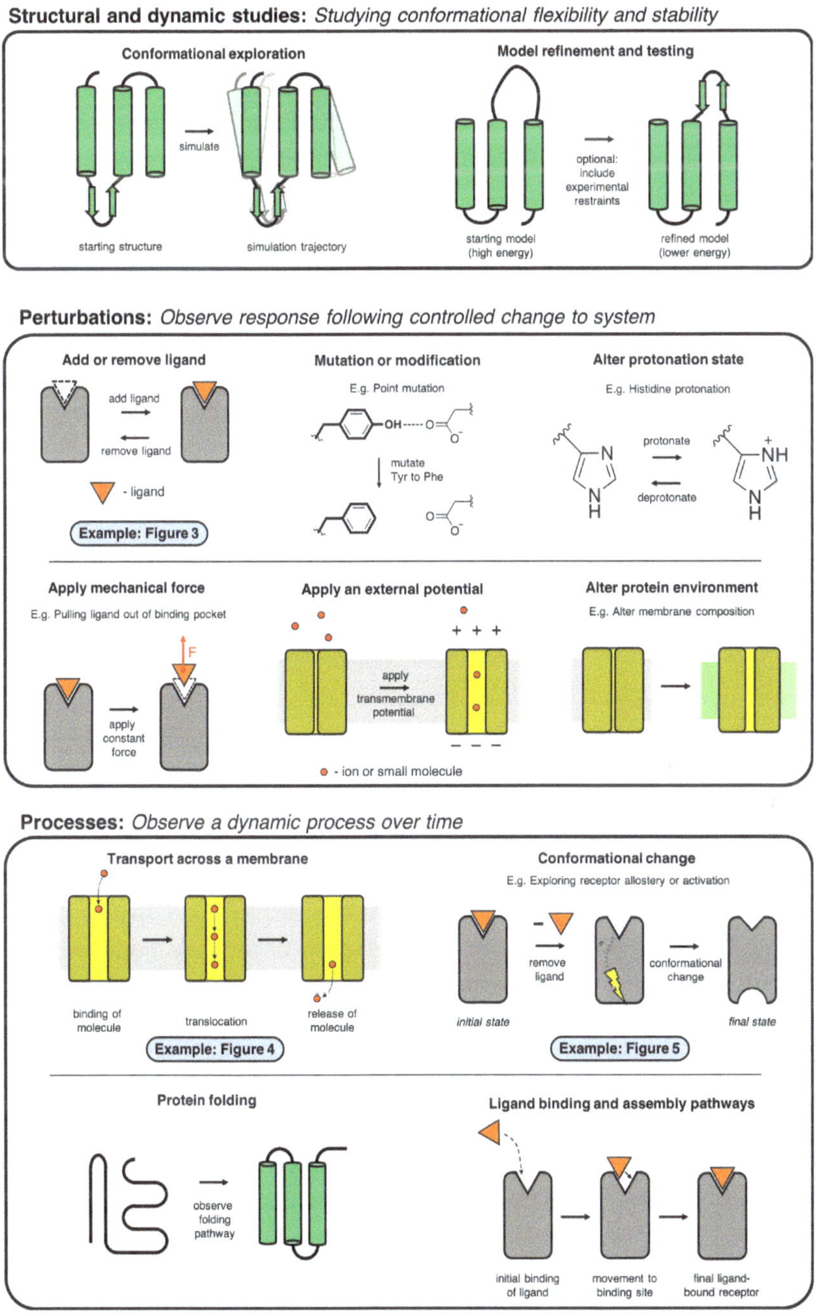

Figure 6.2 Applications of molecular dynamic simulation. *(Reproduced with permission from Hollingsworth et al. [44].)*

GROMACS, Desmond, AMBER, and OpenMM [45]. On a supercomputer, these programs produce quick results. The ligand and target PSF files are generated mostly using VMD (visual dynamics). MD simulation has been upgraded thanks to improvements in computer hardware that allow it to run at millisecond speeds [46].

MD simulation is based on Newton's principles of motion, and this simulation mimics the system's behavior as it changes through time. It aids in the comprehension and prediction of the biologic system. The counter ions counteract the protein simulations in the solvent. Simulation results are expressed in terms of RMSD. Ligand and target structures are compared to each other using the RMSD.

Ligand–protein interaction, folding, and membrane transport are all processes that may be studied using simulations. Developing a new drug can take as long as 40 years and cost as much as 800 million dollars. MD simulation was able to go forward in its experiment cost-effectively and rapidly because of the high costs associated with traditional drug design. Lead optimization, in which a ligand is improved to boost its effectiveness and other qualities, is aided by MD simulations. Simulating ligand optimization helps by providing a variety of data. Simulating ligand binding helps increase the number of binding sites by discovering various locations for ligand binding. Through the use of molecular modeling, the drug aliskiren was created [47].

In addition to optimizing the dissociation mechanism of the medicinal molecule, the MD simulation also highlighted the link between structure and kinetics. Even though high-resolution structures of each component are available, MD simulation uses low-resolution maps to construct atomic-level structures. The combination of MD simulation and spatial autoregressive (SAR) models resulted in the discovery of DPP-IV inhibitors. The bonding mechanism and, by extension, the stability have been improved under the guidance of modeling [47].

6.4.1 Adaptation of MD simulation for various diseases

For the treatment of neurodegenerative diseases like Alzheimer disease, MD simulation is commonly employed because of its ability to minimize the increase in free radical production. As more and more disorders emerge on a daily basis, there is a lot of study being done in the neurological portions of the body. A potent therapy for neurological illnesses may be derived from its characteristics, which are based on MD simulation's insights into the chemical world.

There are several additional examples of the application of this high-tech tool that may be found in the literature. The neutralizing action of ligand ikshusterol3-O-glucoside on snake venom was demonstrated in a molecular dynamic simulation of docked complex PLA2 (phospholipase 2) [48]. Researchers found that the optimal time interval for simulated stability of eight docked ligand—target pairs was at 80 ns, which they characterized as "candidates" against bacterial leaf blight (BLB)illness [49]. Irritable conditions can be treated by targeting JAKa (Janus kinases 3). Su et al. [50] found that three substances from TCM, cryptotanshinone, icaritin, and indurubin, exhibited the best potential inhibition.

In Alzheimer disease therapy, a ML-based MD is a revolutionary approach. Caspase 8 inhibitor ligands were predicted by ML using MD simulation data. Potential natural antifungal agents have reduced the pathogenicity of the fungal infection protein mrlip through molecular mechanics [51] using the surface area of the Poisson Boltzmann equation. Sclerostin, an osteoporosis target protein, promotes bone growth. Researchers Yooin et al. [52] evaluated the effects of baicalin on sclerostin loop two within a 50-ns time frame to establish that baicalin is a new chemical for the treatment of osteoporosis.

6.4.2 Adaptation of MD simulation for drug designing

A key new tool for drug design is funnel metadynamics, an improved form of dynamics that depicts the surface-bound binding energy in absolute terms. MD modeling plays a critical role in improving enzyme-mediated prodrug activation over the course of drug development. Pharma core modeling has been widely utilized to determine the conformational space of ligands in the active site of proteins, such as vitamin D inhibitors, for example. Using docking and simulation, GSK-3β, an essential Alzheimer disease target, has been bound to beta-amyloid plaque compounds [53].

Using data from MD simulation trajectories for screening libraries and identifying the top drug candidates has proven to be a crucial and influential part of the drug discovery process. Phytochemicals including curcumin, rosmarinic acid, and capsaicin have been shown to have pharmacologic activity against breast cancer, according to Rampogu et al. [54]. Additionally, these molecules reveal a scaffold characteristic that may be employed in the design and development of new medicines. Granzyme B has lately been linked to reports of host cell damage and an uptick in infection levels throughout the body. Potential inhibitors such as tannic acid and xenaxoic acid have been shown to be most effective against granzyme B by reducing its activity by drug repurposing and MD modeling. As a result of MD simulations and docking scores, pharmacologic studies can be improved. Compound LHB 8 and a phosphodiesterase 2 inhibitor were discovered by Zhang et al. [55] using MD modeling techniques, combined with a structural alteration in the compound.

6.5 Summary

Phytochemicals are being studied using in silico technologies to better understand the pharmacologic relevance of such compounds. Computational potentials in today's period have been expanded by an approach that uses two chemicals, such as target and phytochemicals, as docking partners and then simulates their binding affinity. The dynamic behavior of a stable docking complex may then be modeled. For the docking approach, this proves the dynamic stability of binding complex poses. The latter verifies this claim. AI-based techniques for building models from a massive dataset to speed up plant science research and the development of new drugs have offered great potential for computer science, as well. By offering a better alternative, this strategy helps to save both money and resources when it comes to the manufacturing of pharmaceuticals.

More databases and pharmacologic information about plants will be generated as a result of in silico study on medicinal plants, which will aid in the search for a treatment option for a certain ailment. In computational research, the proliferation of biomolecule databases continues to be a problem since each one serves a distinct purpose. As a result, new and improved software is needed to detect diverse plant databases and deliver the best possible results. As a result, there will be more research, more software upgrades, and more pharmacologic knowledge, which will lead to more drug candidates for further study and discovery. The pharmacologic qualities of medicinal plants can be used for human health using in silico approaches. They help bridge the gap between plants of therapeutic significance and various ailments. More study using computational methods will improve our understanding of medicinal plants' pharmacologic value. As a result, we will be able to produce drugs that are quick, inexpensive, and herbal.

References

[1] A.M.L. Seca, D.C.G.A. Pinto, Biological potential and medical use of secondary metabolites, Medicines 6 (2) (2019) 66.

[2] G.C. Phillips, M. Garda, Plant tissue culture media and practices: an overview, In Vitro Cellular and Developmental Biology—Plant 55 (3) (2019) 242–257.

[3] M.M. Arab, et al., Modeling and optimizing a new culture medium for in vitro rooting of G×N15 Prunus rootstock using artificial neural network-genetic algorithm, Scientific Reports 8 (1) (2018) 9977.

[4] A. Prasad, et al., Artificial neural network-based model for the prediction of optimal growth and culture conditions for maximum biomass accumulation in multiple shoot cultures of *Centella asiatica*, Protoplasma 254 (1) (2017) 335–341.

[5] L. Jiang, et al., A method to predict different mechanisms for blood–brain barrier permeability of CNS activity compounds in Chinese herbs using support vector machine, Journal of Bioinformatics and Computational Biology 14 (01) (2016) 1650005.

[6] P. García-Pérez, et al., From ethnomedicine to plant biotechnology and machine learning: the valorization of the medicinal plant Bryophyllum sp, Pharmaceuticals 13 (12) (2020) 444.

[7] M. Tahir ul Qamar, et al., Computational screening of medicinal plant phytochemicals to discover potent pan-serotype inhibitors against dengue virus, Scientific Reports 9 (1) (2019) 1–16.

[8] A.K. Ghosh, S. Gemma, Structure-Based Design of Drugs and Other Bioactive Molecules: Tools and Strategies, John Wiley & Sons, 2014.

[9] P.A. Onguéné, et al., The potential of anti-malarial compounds derived from African medicinal plants, part III: an in silico evaluation of drug metabolism and pharmacokinetics profiling, Organic and medicinal chemistry letters 4 (1) (2014) 1–9.

[10] G. Singh, et al., Cadmium-induced conformational changes in type 2 metallothionein of medicinal plant C optis japonica: insights from molecular dynamics studies of apo, partially and fully metalated forms, Journal of Biomolecular Structure and Dynamics 37 (6) (2019) 1520–1533.

[11] P. Parida, et al., Insight into the screening of potential beta-lactamase inhibitors as antibacterial chemical agents through pharmacoinformatics study, Journal of Biomolecular Structure and Dynamics 39 (3) (2021) 923–942.

[12] J. He, et al., Determination of total polysaccharides and total flavonoids in Chrysanthemum morifolium using near-infrared hyperspectral imaging and multivariate analysis, Molecules 23 (9) (2018) 2395.

[13] K. Deep, V. Katiyar, Multi objective extraction optimization of bioactive compounds from gardenia using real coded genetic algorithm, in: 6th World Congress of Biomechanics (WCB 2010). August 1-6, 2010 Singapore, Springer, 2010.

[14] S. Farhadi, et al., Modeling of paclitaxel biosynthesis elicitation in Corylus avellana cell culture using adaptive neuro-fuzzy inference system-genetic algorithm (ANFIS-GA) and multiple regression methods, PLoS One 15 (8) (2020) e0237478.

[15] M. Hesami, et al., Development of support vector machine-based model and comparative analysis with artificial neural network for modeling the plant tissue culture procedures: effect of plant growth regulators on somatic embryogenesis of chrysanthemum, as a case study, Plant Methods 16 (1) (2020) 1–15.

[16] T. George, T. Amudha, Genetic algorithm based multi-objective optimization framework to solve traveling salesman problem, in: Advances in Computing and Intelligent Systems, Springer, 2020, pp. 141–151.

[17] M. Cuba-Díaz, et al., Advances of native and non-native Antarctic species to in vitro conservation: improvement of disinfection protocols, Scientific Reports 10 (1) (2020) 1–10.

[18] J. Gago, et al., Improving knowledge of plant tissue culture and media formulation by neurofuzzy logic: a practical case of data mining using apricot databases, Journal of Plant Physiology 168 (15) (2011) 1858–1865.
[19] M.R. Mridula, A.S. Nair, K.S. Kumar, Genetic programming based models in plant tissue culture: an addendum to traditional statistical approach, PLoS Computational Biology 14 (2) (2018) e1005976.
[20] A. Mansouri, A. Fadavi, S.M.M. Mortazavian, An artificial intelligence approach for modeling volume and fresh weight of callus—A case study of cumin (Cuminum cyminum L.), Journal of Theoretical Biology 397 (2016) 199–205.
[21] M. Rizvi, A.K. Kukreja, N.S. Bisht, Retracted article: plant regeneration in Chlorophytum borivilianum Sant. et Fernand. from embryogenic callus and cell suspension culture and assessment of genetic fidelity of plants derived through somatic embryogenesis, Physiology and Molecular Biology of Plants 18 (3) (2012) 253–263.
[22] J.O. Barone, Use of multiple regression analysis and artificial neural networks to model the effect of nitrogen in the organogenesis of Pinus taeda L, Plant Cell, Tissue and Organ Culture 137 (3) (2019) 455–464.
[23] J. Gago, M. Landín, P.P. Gallego, A neurofuzzy logic approach for modeling plant processes: a practical case of in vitro direct rooting and acclimatization of Vitis vinifera L, Plant science 179 (3) (2010) 241–249.
[24] P. García-Pérez, et al., Machine learning unmasked nutritional imbalances on the medicinal plant Bryophyllum sp. cultured in vitro, Frontiers of Plant Science 11 (2020).
[25] S.P. Munasinghe, et al., Prediction of chemical composition for callus production in Gyrinops walla Gaetner through machine learning, Information Processing in Agriculture 7 (4) (2020) 511–522.
[26] Q. Zhang, et al., Optimization of culture conditions for differentiation of melon based on artificial neural network and genetic algorithm, Scientific Reports 10 (1) (2020) 1–8.
[27] X. Yang, et al., Concepts of artificial intelligence for computer-assisted drug discovery, Chemical Reviews 119 (18) (2019) 10520–10594.
[28] T. Islam, et al., Detecting adverse drug reaction with data mining and predicting its severity with machine learning, in: 2018 IEEE Region 10 Humanitarian Technology Conference (R10-HTC), IEEE, 2018.
[29] A. Ning, et al., Fulfillment of retailer demand by using the MDL-optimal neural network prediction and decision policy, IEEE Transactions on Industrial Informatics 5 (4) (2009) 495–506.
[30] W. Wan-Ying, et al., TCM-based new drug discovery and development in China, Chinese Journal of Natural Medicines 12 (4) (2014) 241–250.
[31] H.-Y. Yeh, et al., Predicting the associations between meridians and Chinese traditional medicine using a cost-sensitive graph convolutional neural network, International Journal of Environmental Research and Public Health 17 (3) (2020) 740.
[32] E. Kim, A.-s. Choi, H. Nam, Drug repositioning of herbal compounds via a machine-learning approach, BMC Bioinformatics 20 (10) (2019) 33–43.
[33] S. Forli, et al., Computational protein–ligand docking and virtual drug screening with the AutoDock suite, Nature Protocols 11 (5) (2016) 905–919.
[34] I. Palos, et al., Repositioning FDA drugs as potential cruzain inhibitors from Trypanosoma cruzi: virtual screening, in vitro and in vivo studies, Molecules 22 (6) (2017) 1015.
[35] P.G. Jamkhande, M.H. Ghante, B.R. Ajgunde, Software based approaches for drug designing and development: a systematic review on commonly used software and its applications, Bulletin of the Faculty of Pharmacy Cairo University 55 (2) (2017) 203–210.

[36] N. Paul, et al., Recovering the true targets of specific ligands by virtual screening of the protein data bank, Proteins: Structure, Function, and Bioinformatics 54 (4) (2004) 671–680.
[37] H. Singh, N. Bharadvaja, Treasuring the computational approach in medicinal plant research, Progress in Biophysics and Molecular Biology 164 (2021) 19–32.
[38] B. Ahmed, U. Ali Ashfaq, M. Usman Mirza, Medicinal plant phytochemicals and their inhibitory activities against pancreatic lipase: molecular docking combined with molecular dynamics simulation approach, Natural Product Research 32 (10) (2018) 1123–1129.
[39] A. Alam, et al., Pharmacokinetic and molecular docking studies of plant-derived natural compounds to exploring potential anti-alzheimer activity, in: D.K. Choudhary, et al. (Eds.), In Silico Approach for Sustainable Agriculture, Springer Singapore, Singapore, 2018, pp. 217–238.
[40] J.J. Sahayarayan, et al., Identification of potential drug target in malarial disease using molecular docking analysis, Saudi Journal of Biological Sciences 27 (12) (2020) 3327–3333.
[41] A. Aher, et al., In silico insights on IL-6: a potential target for multicentric castleman disease, Current Computer-Aided Drug Design 16 (5) (2020) 641–653.
[42] S. Yasmeen, P. Gupta, Interaction of selected terpenoids from Dalbergia sissoo with catalytic domain of matrix metalloproteinase-1: an in silico assessment of their anti-wrinkling potential, Bioinformatics and Biology Insights 13 (2019), p. 1177932219896538.
[43] C.-Y. Lin, et al., Screening of active anti-myocardial ischemia components of Panax notoginseng based on molecular docking technology, Zhongguo Zhong yao za zhi = Zhongguo Zhongyao Zazhi = China Journal of Chinese Materia Medica 45 (11) (2020) 2560–2567.
[44] S.A. Hollingsworth, R.O. Dror, Molecular dynamics simulation for all, Neuron 99 (6) (2018) 1129–1143.
[45] D.A. Case, T.A. Darden, T.E. Cheatham III, C.L. Simmerling, J. Wang, R.E. Duke, P.A. Kollman. AMBER 9, University of California, San Francisco, 2006, p. 45.
[46] D.E. Shaw, et al., Anton 2: raising the bar for performance and programmability in a special-purpose molecular dynamics supercomputer, in: SC'14: Proceedings of the International Conference for High Performance Computing, Networking, Storage and Analysis, IEEE, 2014.
[47] T. Altarejo Marin, et al., The use of aliskiren as an antifibrotic drug in experimental models: a systematic review, Drug Development Research 81 (1) (2020) 114–126.
[48] N.A. Morris, B.M. Czeisler, A. Sarwal, Simulation in neurocritical care: past, present, and future, Neurocritical Care 30 (3) (2019) 522–533.
[49] T. Joshi, et al., Molecular docking and molecular dynamics simulation approach to screen natural compounds for inhibition of Xanthomonas oryzae pv. Oryzae by targeting peptide deformylase, Journal of Biomolecular Structure and Dynamics 39 (3) (2021) 823–840.
[50] D. Su, et al., Identification of Chinese herbal compounds with potential as JAK3 inhibitors, Evidence-based Complementary and Alternative Medicine 2019 (2019).
[51] S. Ali, et al., Identification and evaluation of inhibitors of lipase from Malassezia restricta using virtual high-throughput screening and molecular dynamics studies, International Journal of Molecular Sciences 20 (4) (2019) 884.
[52] W. Yooin, et al., Discovery of potential sclerostin inhibitors from plants with loop2 region of sclerostin inhibition by interacting with residues outside Pro-Asn-Ala-Ile-Gly motif, Journal of Biomolecular Structure and Dynamics 38 (5) (2020) 1272–1282.
[53] N.D. Elangovan, et al., Screening of potential drug for Alzheimer's disease: a computational study with GSK-3 β inhibition through virtual screening, docking, and

molecular dynamics simulation, Journal of Biomolecular Structure and Dynamics 39 (18) (2021) 7065–7079.
[54] S. Rampogu, et al., Natural compounds as potential Hsp90 inhibitors for breast cancer-Pharmacophore guided molecular modelling studies, Computational Biology and Chemistry 83 (2019) 107113.
[55] C. Zhang, et al., Discovery of novel phosphodiesterase-2A inhibitors by structure-based virtual screening, structural optimization, and bioassay, Journal of Chemical Information and Modeling 57 (2) (2017) 355–364.

CHAPTER 7

Advances in encapsulation strategies for bioactive phytochemicals

7.1 Introduction

Natural resources have been utilized by humans from the beginning of time in the search for sustenance and bioactive compounds to employ as poisons and to treat a variety of maladies. Together with natural light and water, photosynthetic organisms on land and at sea have the potential to gather carbon dioxide and employ their multiple complex processes to produce bioactive chemicals, which can be used to treat diseases [1,2]. Historically, plants have been the most significant source of these chemicals for humans. Bioactive compounds derived from plant species are used in the commercial manufacturing of functional meals to enhance color, flavor, texture, and health benefits such as antioxidant capabilities. It is challenging to prepare functional components in the industrial setting since many of these chemicals are unstable even under standard processing conditions like heat or pH changes [3].

The functional potential of bioactive constituents is preserved while its stability is improved through the use of encapsulation methods. In terms of particle size, microencapsulation and nanoencapsulation may be divided into two major groups. When it comes to capsule particle size, nano-encapsulation and microencapsulation fall into two distinct categories: 10−1000 nm (nano) and 3−800 nm (micro), respectively [4,5]. These approaches allow bioactive core chemicals to be coated with wall materials to make capsules that provide an effective barrier against environmental and chemical interactions. Encapsulation permits functional chemicals to be delivered to the target location in a regulated manner, boosting their bioavailability and water solubility while also increasing their stability. An effective bioactive chemical encapsulation system must be able to achieve

Advances in Extraction and Applications of Bioactive Phytochemicals
ISBN 978-0-443-18535-9
https://doi.org/10.1016/B978-0-443-18535-9.00005-3

the following: (1) make things that are fit for human consumption; (2) use food matrices with high physical-chemical stability and minimum influence on the product's sensory characteristics to integrate bioactive constituents; (3) protect encapsulated chemicals against temperature, light, and pH degradation; (4) enhance encapsulated compound absorption after intake for controlled release; and (5) be ready to be mass produced at a rapid rate [6–8].

Spray drying, freeze-drying, electro spraying, electrospinning, and layer-by-layer (LbL) disposition are some of the popular encapsulating techniques used in the food and pharmaceutical sectors [9,10]. Other techniques include extrusion and polyelectrolyte layer-by-layer assemblies [11–13]. Several research studies have successfully produced unique encapsulate systems that improve the efficiency and long-term stability of bioactive compounds in a variety of fields of study. As a result, the purpose of this chapter is to give an extensive collection of information about advancements in the encapsulating process of bioactive compounds.

7.2 Different encapsulation processes for bioactive compounds

7.2.1 Spray drying

The concept of spray drying, which involves spraying feed into a gaseous drying medium to turn it from a liquid to a dry powder, has been around for a long time. It was not until 1872 that the first patent for spray drying was obtained, although this drying process was first mentioned in print in 1860. It was a challenge to use the spray drying method at that time because of issues with the continuous process performance, process efficiency, and process safety, all of which impeded its use. Until the 1920s, research into this approach was hampered by these disadvantages. Spray dryers were possible to be used in milk powder manufacturing at that time because of their progress. Spray drying had its first use in the manufacturing industry, and it continues to hold an essential place in the industry today [14].

Schematic illustration of spray drying process is depicted in Fig. 7.1. Spray drying can be broken down into three distinct stages. The first stage uses an appropriate instrument to atomize the liquid stream. Following that, the feed is exposed to a drying gas at a temperature that is just suitable for the small droplets to interact with one another. Drying takes place during this phase because the solvent in the dispersion droplets has evaporated. Particles of solid products start to form. The dried particles must be

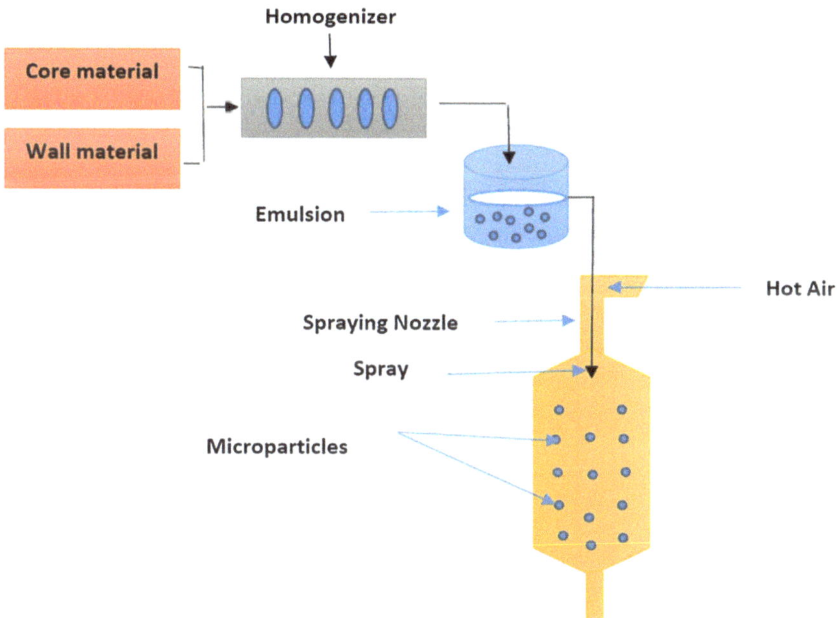

Figure 7.1 Schematic illustration of spray drying process. *(Reproduced with permission from Mohammed et al. [15].)*

separated from the drying gas and collected in a receptacle tank during the final stage. The effectiveness of the drying process and the qualities of the final product are greatly influenced by each of the preceding stages and the conditions in which they are carried out.

Atomization is forming a gaseous suspension of a powder or liquid while also reducing the particle size of the liquid. Spray drying uses a drying gas to disperse the dispersion. As a result, the drying gas is forced to interact with a far larger surface area than possible. Drying gas transfers heat to fluid atomized particles over a broad surface area, which speeds up the process of solvent evaporation and mass transfer back into the gas phase. Consequently, the drying material never becomes hot enough to enter the drying gas. When the atomization phase is included in the spray drying process, it becomes not just a drying technique for heat-sensitive substances but also the one and the only way of drying that may provide the appropriate morphologic and physicochemical qualities. The atomization effect is possible using a wide variety of tools. Hydraulic (pressure) nozzles, rotary atomizers, pneumatic nozzles, and ultrasonic nozzles are the most common [16]. Peristaltic pumps are the most common method of transporting feed to the atomization equipment. A constraint on feed viscosity comes about due to pumps, which necessitate uniform and reproducible feeding. Clogging the tubes might be a concern if the feed is overly viscous.

The feed droplets are immediately exposed to the drying gas following atomization. Air is the most common type of drying gas. Preheated air is obtained straight from the atmosphere and passed through filters. The expense of the gas itself and the cost of the installation necessitates the usage of a closed circulation system for nitrogen and other inert gases. However, in other cases, inert gas is required because the material is unstable. Throughout the chamber, the dispersion droplets are exposed to a variety of air temperatures and humidity levels as they move through the various airflows. This is because of the chamber's nonlaminar gas flow. Because each droplet loses its solvent, it is plausible to assume that each dried particle is unique. The elimination of liquid from the dispersion is greatly influenced by the drying air's initial temperature. This temperature is set so that the process may run as efficiently as possible without risking the product's destruction. The ultimate solvent content in the product is affected by both the drying air temperature and the air humidity; however, the temperature is the only variable that can be modified at any moment.

The humidity of the incoming air has a considerable impact on the drying process' effectiveness and efficiency. Depending on the humidity of the ambient air, the drying conditions alter with the seasons. On a small scale, Goula and Adamopoulos were able to test this idea. The researchers used a Buchi-191 spray drier that had been modified and had a high-performance mechanism for absorbing humidity from the drying air that was brought in from the environment. The investigation unequivocally proved a favorable influence of humidity absorption on process efficacy and product drying, as well as the potential of decreasing the drying temperature. Furthermore, it has been demonstrated that drying with dried air enhances product qualities greatly. There has never been any research done on the impact of moisture in the air used for atomization in pneumatic nozzles on the drying process [9].

7.2.2 Freeze-drying

To preserve heat-sensitive foods and biologic materials, freeze-drying dehydrates them at low pressures and temperatures. As a result of this method, water in the material is able to immediately transition from solid to gas phase. Freeze-drying is used to encapsulate bioactive phytochemicals, and the process takes four phases. Freeze-dryers are usually made with four fundamental components: a drying chamber, a vacuum pump, a heat source, and a condenser, as shown in Fig. 7.2. First, a liquid dispersion medium must be prepared; next, it must be frozen; then, it must be sublimated (primary drying); and last, it must be evaporated (secondary drying) [4]. At this stage, extracts are mixed with a wall material or carrier agent to create the liquid dispersion medium that will be used in subsequent steps of the process. González-Ortega et al. [17] synthesized the solution by mixing olive leaf powder extract in an aqueous solution comprising wall material, maltodextrin, at 350 rpm for 30 min at room temperature. The solution was then homogenized for 30 min in a centrifuge at 4000 rpm before being filtered to eliminate any leftover solids and get clear solutions. This step is identical to the ones included in the spray drying procedure.

For the second phase, known as freezing, liquid solutions are cooled to a low temperature so that they can harden. Pressure and temperature must be less than 0.006 atm for water to transition from liquid to solid and eventually to vapor. Amorphous or glassy bioactive chemicals are left behind as the water molecules in the materials crystallize into ice. As a result, the operating costs for this stage are rather substantial. At this point, the pressure is decreased to less than ice's vapor pressure, and sublimation begins to remove most of its water content. Once the product temperature reaches

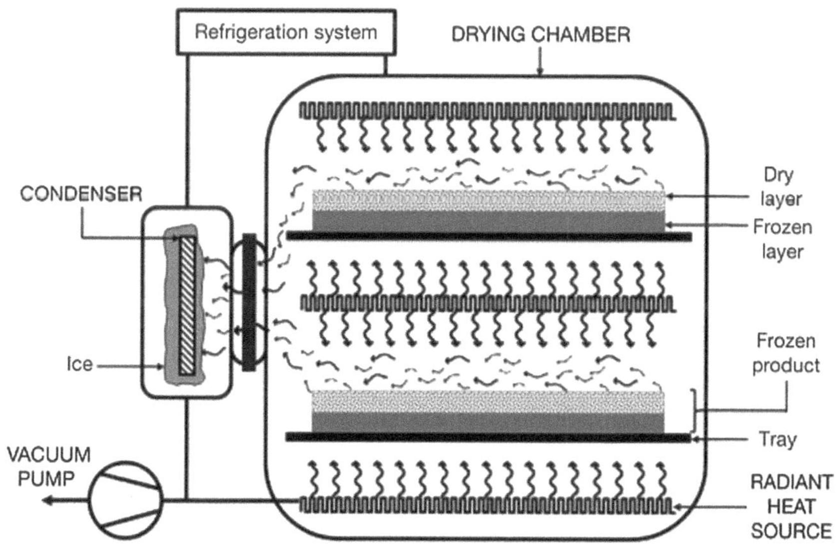

Figure 7.2 Schematic representation of the freeze-drying process. *(Reproduced with permission from Amezquita et al. [18].)*

the desired shelf temperature, the process repeats itself until it does. The fourth phase, evaporation, will remove the remaining liquid water from the mixture. In comparison to the sublimation step, the evaporation stage is shorter and uses less energy. Temperatures of −20 to −40°C for 6 h during the freezing phase, for example, are operated by Malik et al. [19], followed by primary drying at −40°C for 12 h and second drying at −20°C for 6 h with Arabic gum as an encapsulating agent in the subsequent drying stages.

Encapsulated fish oil was created with the use of β-cyclodextrin (β-CD), an emulsion diffusion technique, and a freeze-drying procedure by Choi et al. [20]. In comparison to polycaprolactone (PCL)/fish oil particles, the average particle size of β-CD fish oil was observed to be between 250 and 700 nm. One hundred percent of the fish oil was loaded and encapsulated with more efficiency in PCL/fish oil than in β-CD, resulting in less fish oil leakage (84%−87%). Bejrapha et al. [10] examined the stability of fish oil-loaded nanocapsules encapsulated in a PCL to the impacts of vacuum freeze-drying and standard freeze-drying procedures. Fish oil nanocapsules were discovered to have a particle size below 360 nm and to be aggregated, according to their research. Vacuum freeze-drying had a higher encapsulation efficiency than traditional freeze-drying, except at temperatures below −30°C. PCL membrane fragility may be impacted by the vacuum freezing method, which has a poorer encapsulation effectiveness and more aggregation of particles. Fish oil−loaded nanocapsules were also shown to be more stable when conventional freeze-drying was used rather than vacuum freeze-drying.

The ionic gelation and freeze-drying procedures of Dube et al. [21] were used to encapsulate catechin and epigallocatechin gallate (EGCG). Researchers tested the efficiency of nanoencapsulation with the addition of reducing agents such dithiothreitol, ascorbic acid, and (tris 2-carboxyethyl) phosphine (TCEP) for their ability to protect catechins and EGCG against degradation and found that nanoencapsulation was superior. Average particle size of less than 200 nm was found in the nanocapsules used in the research. Catechin and EGCG nanoencapsulation showed superior protection against TCEP and ascorbic acid reductases. Using the emulsion diffusion method, Surassmo et al. [22] encapsulated capsicum oleoresin in PCL using a water-miscible solvent that contained the drug and a polymer aqueous phase; adding water to the system causes the solvent to diffuse to the external phase, resulting in nanospheres that were then frozen to preserve their properties. Pluronic F68 was used as a surfactant to adjust the process conditions. The resulting nanoemulsions were between 320 and

460 nm in diameter. Increased emulsifier content led to smaller nanocapsule particles. The particle size reduced as the surfactant concentration was increased. Recent research by Nakagawa et al. [23] evaluated the dispersibility of capsicum oleoresin that was encapsulated in PCL, stabilized with gelatin, and dried using an emulsion diffusion process and a freeze-drying methodology. The nanocapsules had a mean diameter of less than 200 nm, which is extremely small. The freeze-dried capsules were also found to have variable dispersion qualities in the dried bulk sample at various locations. Heterogeneity was influenced by the cooling technique used during processing. A gel network in nanocapsule gelatin might help generate better dispersion qualities after drying, according to the researchers. Bejrapha et al. [24] employed a modified emulsion diffusion technique in conjunction with freeze-drying to produce capsicum oleoresin—loaded nanocapsules containing PCL in capsicum. Capsicum oleoresin—loaded nanocapsules were tested at −40, −20, and −15°C to determine the effects of chilling temperature on their properties. The freeze-thawing and freeze-drying durability of capsicum-loaded nanocapsules was tested using a variety of excipients, including gelatin and k-carrageenan. A relatively high freezing temperature (15°C) had an influence on the nanocapsule size maintenance after freeze-thawing and freezing drying, according to their results. According to Abdelwahed et al. [25], freeze-drying of PCL nanocapsules containing Miglyol 829 oil, which was generated via emulsion diffusion and stabilized by polyvinyl alcohol (PVA), was examined. In the freeze—thaw study, PVA and PCL concentrations, cooling rate, cryoprotectant concentrations (polyvinyl pyrrolidone and sucrose), type of encapsulated oil, and nanocapsule purity were all examined. Nanocapsule stability and sublimation rate were both studied in relation to annealing. A sufficient concentration of PVA stabilizer in PCL nanocapsules, they found, allowed them to be freeze-dried without adding any cryoprotectant (5%). When freeze-drying nanocapsules, the choice of cryoprotectant had no influence on their size or rehydration, and the annealing technique expedited the sublimation process while preserving nanocapsule size. The microemulsion method and freeze-drying were used by Tiyaboonchai et al. [26] to load curcuminoids into solid lipid nanoparticles. An integration efficiency of up to 70% was observed in lyophilized curcuminoid-loaded nanoparticles when the process parameters were improved. It was discovered that the amount of components such as fat and emulsifier had a substantial influence on curcuminoid loading capacity and size distribution. When stored for 6 months, the physical and chemical

stability of curcuminoids was maintained in in vitro release studies for up to 12 h. The freeze-drying approach was used by Zhang et al. [27] to encapsulate trehalose in a thermally sensitive pluronic nanocapsule. Nanocapsules that contain trehalose are able to physically retain the trehalose and release it with little release in hours for cellular absorption at 37°C, and their cytotoxicity is low.

Tocopherol was encapsulated in zein and zein/chitosan complexes by Luo et al. [28] via freeze-drying. The particle size ranged from 200 to 800 nm. The encapsulation efficiency was between 77% and 87%. Tocopherol demonstrated a burst effect followed by a delayed release in terms of kinetic release profile. Chitosan coatings on the zein/chitosan complex outperformed zein in terms of tocopherol release protection from gastrointestinal disorders. Using thin-film ultrasonic dispersion and lyophilization, Zhao et al. [29] created conventional liposomes and polyethylene glycol (PEG)-coated vitamin E lyophilized proliposomal (PLP) forms. PLPs coated with PEG had a mean diameter of 164 nm and an encapsulation efficiency of 84%. Compared to other liposomes, PLP's vitamin E exhibited a 90% retention rate at 4°C after 15 days. Using freeze-drying to stabilize nanocapsules appears to be an effective method of drying. Although it dried to a particle size below 400 nm, it retained the nanometric range of particle size, enhancing the durability of the core component against degradation and demonstrating superior encapsulation effectiveness of around 70%. Drying heat-sensitive foods and bioactive components may benefit greatly from this method as well. There are a few different encapsulation processes and methods for breaking down droplets into nano sizes that can affect the final features of freeze-dried nanoparticles. Cryoprotectants, such as sucrose, trehalose, and mannitol, are required to maintain particle size and prevent aggregation during freeze-drying. They are also necessary. The size of the nanocapsules was found to vary with the freezing temperatures. Polymers like PCL and chitosan were commonly employed as wall materials in this research [4].

7.2.3 Electrospraying

Electrospraying is based on Rayleigh's 1882 discovery that an electric field may operate on a liquid drop, which was later confirmed by Zeleny in 1914 and Taylor in 1964 as a fundamental concept. Microparticles can be created by using voltage to atomize a substance by electrical atomization pioneered by Vonnegut and Neubauer in 1952 [30]. By delivering 5−10 kV (DC) to liquids in microscopic capillaries, they were able to create a stream with uniform droplets of roughly 0.1 mm in diameter. Electrospraying has been researched extensively by researchers. High-voltage electrostatic forces atomize the liquid into tiny droplets, and the solvent is evaporated as the droplets fall toward a ground electrode in this method. Electric spinning and electrospraying have different degrees of molecular interaction, and this is what makes the difference between the two processes Fig. 7.3 illustrates a basic setup and mechanism of the electrospraying process. A fiber is formed when there is a high degree of contact, but a particulate stream is formed when there is a lower degree. Spinneret with needle-like form, ring electrode, collector, feed pump, and power supply source make up the apparatus. It is common practice to use a blunt hypodermic needle as the needle (or spinneret), while the ring electrode and collector are grounded. It is not uncommon for the collector or ring to be at high voltage when the needle is grounded. There are certain molecules that are better at transporting a positive charge than a negative charge, and vice versa. This can be due to differences in molecular polarity in the electric field. When a strong

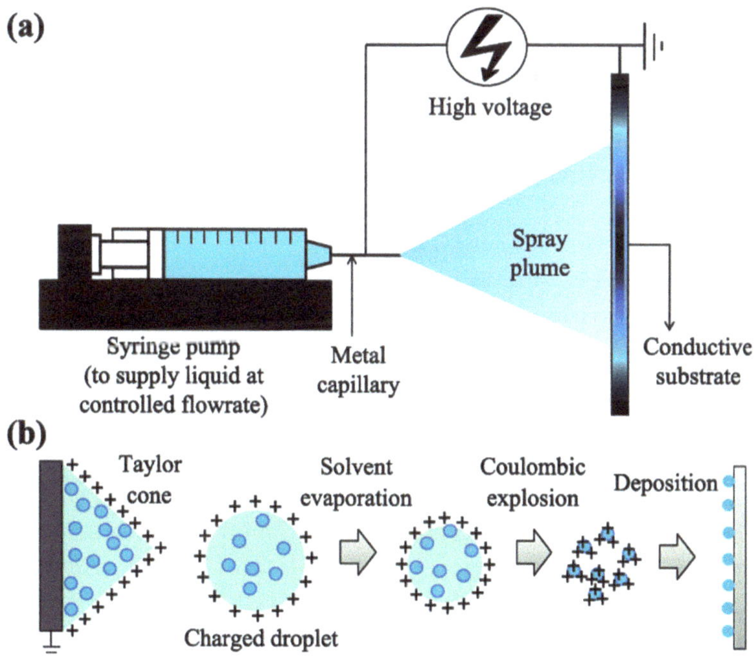

Figure 7.3 Schematic representation of electrospraying (A) setup and (B) mechanism. *(Reproduced with permission from Saallah et al. [35].)*

electric field is needed at the needle's tip to keep the spinning process going across a wide range of flow rates, a protective circular electrode may be employed [31]. For low conductivity solutions, this circular shielding electrode may steady the liquid meniscus ejected by the needle [32]. An extra ring electrode is said to stabilize the homogeneity of microencapsulation size. For example, in the electrospraying method, Xie and Wang (2007) investigated droplet formation and development of mono-dispersed microencapsulation of live cells with adjustable size [33]. Both the nozzle and the ring electrode received two positive volts. They noticed that raising the voltage given to the ring electrode reduced the dripping frequency and caused somewhat bigger droplets to form [34].

A substantial role is played by chain entanglements of polymer solutions in fiber or capsule creation during the electrospinning/spraying process. Varicose instability causes a jet to destabilize, resulting in tiny spherical bodies—microparticles—being generated as a result [37]. Due to electrostatic repulsion, these highly charged droplets self-disperse in space, avoiding droplet aggregation and coagulation [32]. Because of their tiny size, droplets are typically smaller than those produced by traditional mechanical atomizers, maybe down to less than 1 μm in diameter. To begin with, Rayleigh was the first to notice and quantify the electrostatic force's ability to break up charged droplets into smaller ones. With Coulombic fission of the droplets, this results in numerous smaller, more stable droplets from the initial scattered droplet. The charged droplet is subject to a variety of bulk forces, including electrodynamics, inertia, gravity, and drag.

Definition of materials that can be electrosprayed is the first stage in converting this technology for culinary applications. Polymers come in a wide variety of forms and can be used to enclose, cover, or encapsulate various things. If the materials are to be used to encapsulate food components, they should be food-grade chemicals that are generally considered safe [38]. It is also important to consider elements like the cost of raw materials, the simplicity with which the distribution system can be constructed, and regulatory status when deciding on wall material. The size, shape, charge, permeability, bioadhesion, and environmental stability of nanocarriers should also be taken into consideration. They are also crucial. The biocompatibility, biodegradability, and lack of toxicity requirements are generally met more readily by materials derived from nature, so they are frequently favored [39]. Functioning matrices derived from biologic sources, such as proteins and carbohydrates, are being developed to counteract the potential environmental or health hazards posed by the use of nonbiodegradable materials [40]. Bioactive delivery systems made from food-grade polymers and biopolymers have been studied for application in food.

7.2.4 Electrospinning

An emerging technique for improving the performance of functional materials in the food industry is the incorporation of bioactive compounds within electrospun fibers. Innovative functional foods are now easier to develop thanks to this new approach, which has revolutionized the entire food supply chain, from production all the way through to processing. Thorough knowledge of the electrospinning mechanism is necessary for optimizing production conditions and maximizing throughput, hence expanding the range of industrial applications in food science and beyond.

Electrospinning is a good way to make submicron or nanoscale fibers from polymers. Fig. 7.4 provides a schematic representation of an electrospinning process. To deposit a droplet of polymer solution on a grounded collector, an electrical field draws the droplet into a fine fiber. Electrically spun yarn is fed into an electrospinning machine by injecting it into a metal needle—equipped injection pump that is connected to a grounded collector. Syringe pumps are used to expel a solution or molten polymer at the needle tip in electrospinning, which creates a droplet at the needle tip. The droplet's hemispherical surface is twisted into a conical form

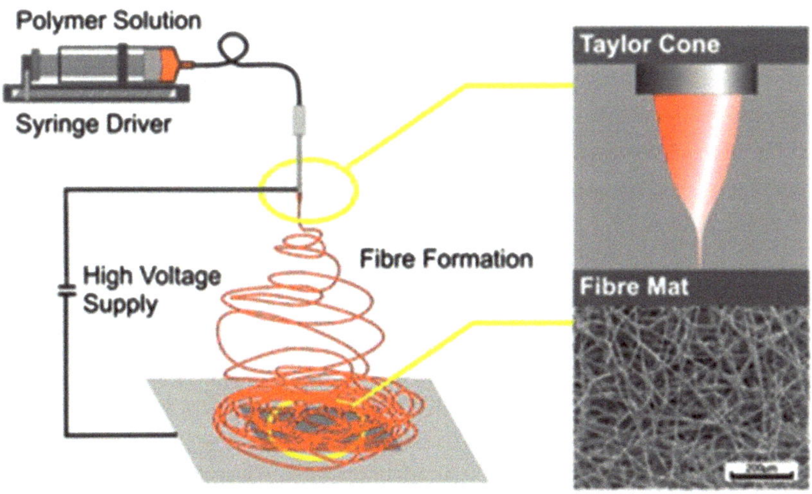

Figure 7.4 Schematic illustration of an electrospinning process. *(Reproduced with permission from Nieuwland et al. [36].)*

as a result of the operation of two primary electrostatic forces, the internal electrostatic repulsion and the external Coulombic force.

The electrically charged jet of polymer is expelled from the tip of the Taylor cone and directed toward the collector with opposing charges. Due to the jet's whipping or bending action as it is propelled toward the collection, polymer nanofibers are deposition on the grounded collector as a randomly arranged nonwoven mat as a result of fast evaporation of solvent and jet elongation.

Spinnability, fiber shape, and diameter distribution may all be influenced by electrospinning process parameters as well as environmental factors [12,41]. Because of the aforesaid factors, the electrospinning technology is highly customizable, allowing for the alteration of fiber shape, targeted collection, and fiber orientation through the use of setup modifications. It is possible to incorporate bioactive compounds into nanofibers with relative ease, making electrospinning an attractive alternative to other production methods.

Another advantage of electrospinning is that it does not generate heat during the electrospinning process, making it an attractive option for food applications. Furthermore, electrospun nanofibers have submicron to nanoscale diameters, a high surface-to-volume ratio, acceptable porosity, variable fiber diameters, and good encapsulation effectiveness for bioactive chemicals, among other structural and functional advantages. The bioactive chemicals enclosed in electrospun fibers have improved stability and bioavailability as a result of these structural benefits and can accomplish the targeted distribution and sustained release [42].

Compounds known as bioactive molecules have a variety of health-promoting properties, such as anticancer, antioxidant, antiinflammatory, and so on. Many types of bioactive chemicals exist, including small hydrophilic substances, small hydrophobic substances, and macromolecular active substances (e.g., enzymes, probiotics, active proteins). Because they are very prone to oxidation, light, temperature, or other severe circumstances, their use in the food sector is limited. Using encapsulation might be an excellent way to deal with this. Electrospinning's benefits and prospective uses in the nanoencapsulation of bioactive substances have been studied in depth. When it comes to the creation of new functional foods like probiotics and other microorganisms, this technology can make a huge difference in the stability and bioavailability of bioactive compounds. The ability to disguise unpleasant scents and tastes is another major advantage. Nanofibers have also been employed as delivery methods for nutraceuticals and gastrointestinal (GIT) medications, with the regulated or sustained release [43]. The fabrication of active packaging materials or the production of food packaging nanostructured layers using electrospinning is also a promising technique with applications ranging from the control of microbial growth to the inhibition of chemical degradation reactions, as well as the achievement of specific biocatalysis. Additionally, electrospun fibers might be used as filtering membranes in the food and beverage processing industry. Food-grade polymers (polysaccharides and proteins) hold considerable promise as matrices for the encapsulation of bioactive chemicals in the food sector since they are nontoxic, biocompatible and biodegradable, renewable, and sustainable.

7.2.5 Extrusion

It is possible to describe extrusion technology as a process in which a material is forced to flow through an orifice of varying diameters at a specified rate under a range of circumstances (various temperatures and speeds, different concentrations of moisture). Extrusion can manufacture a broad range of goods that are difficult to produce using other methods. The extrusion technique requires high temperatures (80–150°C) to be applied for a short period of time (less than 1 min), which is one of the technology's disadvantages because most bioactive chemicals are thermolabile.

With its high productivity and cheap production costs, the extrusion processing of food products has become an increasingly important manufacturing technology. Due to the low-moisture procedure, extrusion is a more ecologically friendly approach than other methods. As a result, the cost of water treatment and the level of environmental contamination can be reduced [44]. Extruders are machines that aid in extrusion procedures. They are made up of one or two rotating screws that are securely fitted within a barrel, with the die at the end [45]. All extruders operate on the same principle, which includes loading the barrel with raw materials through a feeder and then pushing the barrel toward the die and cutter using a screw. Preconditioning systems, feeding systems, screws, barrels, die, and cutting mechanisms can all be found on more specialized extruders. Additionally, the screw, barrel, and die configurations can all be altered according to the raw materials utilized and the ultimate output sought [45].

Based on the type of extruder (a machine used for extrusion) used, the state of extrusion, and other criteria such as the type of extrudate produced, there are several extrusion technologies. It is possible to divide extrusion technology into five distinct types, namely, hot-melt extrusion, melt injection, centrifugal/co-extrusion, electrostatic/electrospinning, and particle from gas saturated solution).

Single or double screws are used in the first kind of extrusion, depending on the desired final result. When it comes to temperature control, it features an extrusion barrel and a thermostat linked to it. Using multiple types of forces and dies is required for the screwless extrusions (centrifugal, melt injection, and electrostatic). Melt injection extrusion is a low-temperature extrusion technique that uses encapsulation of bioactive compounds in molten wall materials as a mechanism of encapsulation. Centrifugal extrusion makes use of centrifugal force to drive the bioactive component loaded within the concentric orifices into the revolving cylinder's outer circumferential wall material [46]. Electrostatic extrusion is a needle-based technique that utilizes electrostatic charges to extrude material. When the bioactive chemicals are electrostatically forced into a hardening solution, they are encapsulated by the electrostatic charges that pass through the extrusion needle.

7.2.5.1 Hot-melt extrusion

Using a continuous screw-extrusion technique, hot-melt extrusion creates molten plastic. There are many similarities between this process and melt injection extrusion, but one important distinction is that whereas melt injection is a vertical screwless process with surface-cleaned particles, hot-melt extrusion is a horizontal screw process with particles that have not been surface washed [5]. Encapsulation is a primary goal of hot-melt extruders, which are cylinders containing thermomechanical mixers that have a single or double screw with self-wipe screws.

A variety of screw profiles, liquid and solid feed intake ports, and barrel temperatures may be adjusted based on the active ingredient and biopolymer matrix in the extruder. There are three stages to hot-melt extrusion [47].

The extruder is initially filled with the powder combination of the encapsulant. If required, a plasticizer or other additives can be added at this time before the active chemicals are introduced. When the wall material is plasticized, the bioactive ingredient may easily interact with the wall, which is how hot-melt extrusion encapsulates it. Plasticized carrier matrices are used to encapsulate bioactive compounds. In hot-melt extrusion, adding a plasticizer lowers the glass transition temperature by decreasing the attraction between polymer chains in the encapsulant (wall material) [5]. To preserve heat-sensitive bioactive chemicals, the encapsulation occurs at lower temperatures when the temperature of the glass is reduced [48].

A cold surface can be used to chill an extrudate, or the air might be used. It is important to note that semicrystalline polymers have a low melting point and a high solidification temperature. When extruding semicrystalline polymers, selecting the cooling rate is critical to achieving the desired crystallinity. To get more crystals and more overall crystallinity, annealing would be better than rapid cooling, which would produce smaller crystals and a lower overall crystalline density. In this case, the extrudate should be cooled at a rate that is defined by the throughput rate and the cooling medium's temperature [11].

Some bioactive substances have been enclosed via the hot-melt extrusion approach, which has been employed for encapsulation. In hot-melt extrusion, maltodextrin has been the most widely utilized wall material since it is inexpensive and easily accessible. Maltodextrin is a starch hydrolysate with essential matrix-forming capabilities that can tolerate high temperatures and serve as a wall material [49]. Microencapsulation of oil-soluble supplies such as flavors, vitamins, and oils is commonly done with starch hydrolysates. Due to their lack of emulsifying power, they (maltodextrin) can only be utilized to encapsulate water-soluble compounds. They are combined with additional emulsifying ingredients, including gums (such as gum Arabic) and water-soluble proteins.

Extrusion of hot melt is a solvent-free process that requires only a small amount of water. Continuous, rapid, and with fewer unit actions, the process is efficient. The extrusion channel is not exposed to oxygen, resulting in excellent mixing of components and a rapid rate of production. The residence period is minimal, and bioactive compounds can be added at various stages of the extrusion process while being monitored online. With hot melt extrusion, bioactive chemicals may be stabilized, allowing for regulated release, flavor masking, and uniform particle size (500−1000 μm) [48].

In comparison to spray drying, hot-melt extrusion is more costly since it necessitates many machines; the anticipated processing costs for this method are about twice as high. The substance to be extruded must also be temperature resistant [50]. Hot-melt extrusion requires a material with excellent flow properties. Cooking using hot-melt extrudates is problematic because of their large size (500−1000 μm), which may necessitate further processing, such as grinding, before use. Maltodextrin DE 17 was used to encapsulate orange turpentine at temperatures between 105 and 145°C. In addition, maltodextrin DE 12 was used to encapsulate tocopherol at the same temperature range of 105–145°C as well [51].

7.2.5.2 Melt injection extrusion process

Melt injection is a screwless, vertical extrusion method. Compounds distributed in carbohydrate melts (80–140°C) are extruded through one or more orifices into a bath of cold, dehydrating liquid in a melt injection extrusion method. The encapsulant or wall material solidifies with the liquid, generating an encapsulating matrix, which encapsulates or traps the bioactive molecule in the system. The dehydrating solvent causes the wall material to stiffen, encasing the bioactive ingredient [5]. The extruded strands are broken into little pieces by rapid swirling in the cold solvent, which reduces the strands' diameter. The dehydrating solvent will remove any active agent remains from the surface. From 200 to 2000 μm in particle size, melt injection encapsulates are water soluble [48].

Despite the fact that the researchers did not identify any disadvantages of the melt injection extrusion method, it was observed that melt extrusion generated large granule sizes (200–2000 μm), which limited its usage in food applications due to the tiny surface area and long diffusion route [51]. Because of this, melt extrusion may not be suitable for encapsulating bioactive substances that need to be released in a regulated manner in the human body. Melt injection extrusion is a batch method that uses a finite amount of water to produce the finished product. With fewer unit operations, the bioactive chemical has a shorter residence period. Encapsulated bioactive compounds are more stable in this small-scale equipment [52].

Isopropanol, a solvent not commonly used in food production operations, limits the usage of melt injection in food. The melt injection extrusion technology restricts the commercialization of encapsulated bioactive compounds since it is a batch procedure [47].

7.2.5.3 Centrifugal extrusion (co-extrusion)

The third type of extrusion mode employed in encapsulating bioactive compounds such as olive oil and caffeic acid is centrifugal extrusion, which is one of the varieties of co-extrusion. Co-extrusion is often employed in the manufacturing of core-shell particles, with a concentric feed tube through which the encapsulant (wall material) and bioactive substance are pushed separately through a number of nozzles located on the extruder's outer surface [53].

Centrifugal co-manner extrusion of encapsulation is based on the mechanism of interfacial polymerization. Another method of encapsulating bioactive compounds is co-extrusion technology, which is often not suited for food applications due to harmful reactions between the wall components and the bioactive molecule [54]. An organic solvent is used to emulsify an aqueous mixture containing the enzyme and hydrophilic monomer via interfacial polymerization. The bioactive chemical polymerizes with the encapsulant to generate microcapsules during interfacial polymerization. With the aid of centrifugal force acting on the extruder's surface, two soluble reactive monomers are brought together at the interface during co-extrusion. A polymer microsphere is formed when the bioactive chemical reacts with the wall material (microcapsule) [55]. Polymeric membrane—encased droplets of microcapsules may be gathered on moving beds, and they can be dissolved in water. The encapsulation of olive oil, caffeine acid, essential oils, and protein has all been accomplished through the technique of co-extrusion [7].

The benefits of co-extrusion over other encapsulation processes, such as spray drying, are that the encapsulated oil is more resistant to oxidation and that the shelf life of encapsulated ligands is extended by avoiding oxygen interaction during storage [56]. Co-extrusion uses more than one wall material and has a long residence time between the wall material and the bioactive compound (>1 min), in contrast to spray drying, which uses mononuclear wall materials and short contact times (less than 1 min) for the wall materials and bioactive compound. In addition, it reduces the rate of essential oil evaporation while it is stored [57]. Due to the high cost and huge particle size (150—8000 μm) produced by co-extrusion, it may not be suitable for many applications. Small surface area and longer diffusion route length lower the bioavailability, delivery characteristics, and solubility of the functional (nutraceutical) food in the target location [5].

A drawback to co-extrusion is the nonuniformity of the wall material (encapsulant), which means the combination of one or more wall materials with varying components and structures. Ineffective encapsulation and interfacial instability of bioactive compounds can be caused by wall material nonuniformity. In addition, improper wall material adhesion might cause separation during the extrusion process if it is not done correctly. As a result, bioactive chemicals encapsulated by co-extrusion become unstable in storage. Co-extrusion method also has the drawback of requiring a second process to obtain the powder. It is necessary to dry the encapsulated bioactive component in a mist chamber, flash volatilization chambers, powdered beds, or liquid hardening baths [54].

7.2.5.4 Electrostatic extrusion

Electrostatic extrusion, also known as electrospraying or electrostatic atomization, is a kind of electrostatic extrusion. Electrospinning and electrospraying are two easy one-step methods for producing dried micro and nano encapsulates. Because it is operated at ambient temperature and under atmospheric strain, this extrusion method is appropriate for encapsulating warm, labile substances. Biodegradable, biocompatible, food-grade conducting polymeric components are used as wall substances in electrospinning and electrospraying to encapsulate bioactive chemicals. Whey protein isolate, whey protein concentrate, soy protein isolate, collagen, zein, egg albumen, casein, and gelatin are common protein-based encapsulating compounds used in electrospinning and electrospraying [58].

Electrostatic extrusion is a technique that can be used to encapsulate certain bioactive substances. With the use of electrostatic extrusion, Prüsse et al. [59] were able to encapsulate ethyl vanillin in alginate gel microbeads. Alginate containing about 2% (wt/wt) alginate was used to encapsulate about 10% (wt/wt) of ethyl vanillin. Electrostatic extrusion was used to encapsulate *Thymus serpyllum* L. in calcium alginate beads. *T. serpyllum* L. encapsulation efficacy in calcium alginate ranged from 50% to 80%, according to Stojanovic et al. [60], who used calcium alginate beads with a diameter of 730 m for electrostatic extrusion. Six polyphenolic antioxidants from medicinal plants were electrostatically extruded by Belak-Cvitanovi et al. [6]. All of the extracts in alginate chitosan were encapsulated with an effectiveness of 80%−89%.

By changing the applied voltage, electrostatic extrusion may produce microbeads that are significantly smaller than traditional needles. High concentrations of bioactive chemicals can also be encapsulated via electrostatic extrusion. The encapsulating of bioactive compounds in high quantities is one of the drawbacks of electrostatic extrusion. There are also restrictions on the types of encapsulant (wall material) that may be utilized (alginates and gums).

Unlike other methods (such as co-extrusion and melt injection), electrostatic extrusion does not need heating or a second step to dry the enclosed product. It has a wide range of sizes, wall polymers, and long-term storage capabilities [58]. Low-energy electrostatic extrusion is able to provide bioactive chemicals with a unique property since it uses less energy.

Scale-up or poor throughput is one of the key downsides. Because of this, large-scale commercial exploitation of these products is out of the question [58].

Researchers have proposed employing a multineedle configuration for encapsulating bioactive substances to solve the setup's structural disadvantages. Continuous operation in a bioreactor using immobilized enzymes is also being studied.

7.2.6 Layer-by-layer disposition

The design and production of soft nano- or micro-sized assemblies for encapsulation and increased bioavailability of active compounds have been hot issues in recent decades. The field's rapid growth is owing to its significant implications in a wide range of scientific and technologic fields, from functional foods to pest management and cosmetics to medicine delivery. The increased interest in the use of supramolecular functional materials in the aforementioned applications has resulted in the rapid development of several strategies for controlling the self-assembly of materials. The building blocks can be selected to have the required qualities and structures to meet the needs of the many application domains. For creating materials with customizable composition, structure, and dimensionality, many approaches have been developed, with the LbL process being one of the most notable owing to its incredible simplicity and adaptability [61]. Iler established the LbL approach more than 50 years ago, and Decher et al. reviewed it in the early 1990s. Initially, the LbL approach relied on electrostatic interactions to alternately deposit oppositely charged components, mostly polyelectrolytes, onto a flat, macroscopic, solid, charged substrate. To put it another way, the LbL technique may be regarded as a template-assisted technology that requires a precursor structure to make the final supramolecular substance, whether that structure is sacrificial or not. Apart from macroscopically large, flat, solid substrates, a wide range of smaller, more complex substrates, such as colloidal particles, liposomes, and fluid interfaces, are also commonly used as templates for nanofabrication. In addition to the traditional LbL assembly mediated by electrostatic contacts, the LbL approach may also be used to construct materials via other types of interactions such as hydrogen bonds, chemical bonds, host–guest interactions, or acid–base reactions. There is now a wide range of materials that can be used as building blocks, from basic polyelectrolytes to carbon nanotubes or nano- or microparticles, and from synthetic polymers to various types of biomolecules. This has broadened the spectrum of materials that may be utilized as building blocks [62–64]. LbL materials can be used as platforms for the encapsulation and delivery of active chemicals in a variety of ways, ranging from onion-like particles to sponges, membranes, and nanotubes [65]. It is also possible to control a variety of physical and chemical characteristics of the manufactured materials using the LbL approach. In this way, it is possible to adjust the delivery procedure based on environmental cues [66]. Due to these groundbreaking studies, the creation of LbL materials for the encapsulation and controlled release of active compounds has evolved into a research challenge that has brought researchers from various fields of interfacial nanoengineering together to address a variety of issues critical to the advancement of modern society. These include chemistry, physics, materials science, and biology. Aside from the variables stated before, there is a slew of others such as charge density of the molecules, ionic strength and type of ions, solvent quality for the molecules, concentration, temperature, and pH that have a significant influence on the manufacturing of functional materials. Supramolecular materials with regulated and adjustable structural and physicochemical characteristics can only be synthesized with a thorough grasp of their role. These factors have a significant impact on the characteristics of any material. LbL films, on the other hand, need a far higher degree of control. Since the foundational efforts by Decher et al. [67], the assembly procedures utilized for the manufacture of LbL materials have not altered greatly, and only minor adjustments have been added owing to the specific properties of the templates. Alternating dips of flat macroscopic substrates into solutions include intermediate rinse cycles to remove material that is not highly adsorbent. For polyelectrolytes, this is especially important as undesired interpolyelectrode complex precipitates, altering the material's composition and structure [68]. The utilization of colloidal particles, vesicles, and liposomes or micelles as templates for LbL deposition is particularly intriguing from a practical standpoint for the construction of platforms for the encapsulation and controlled release of active chemicals. Because the substrate is dispersed or suspended in the solvent, the manufacturing procedure must be adjusted. Sukhorukov et al. used a unique way of making capsules using the LbL method. The process involved coating microparticles with two polyelectrolytes. Particles can be used as either a template for creating core-shelled or hollow capsules, depending on how they are treated with the appropriate chemicals. To avoid interpolyelectrolyte compounds from forming in the media when successive oppositely charged polyelectrolytes are added, conventional polyelectrolytes are alternatively deposited onto particle surfaces in aqueous medium and cleaned and centrifuged. Hollow capsules can be made by chemically dissolving the core after the requisite number of layers has been attained. The agent used should not impact the integrity of the shell but should be able to dissolve the core. Dissolved hydrochloride acid for melamine formaldehyde resin crystals, fluoride acid for silicon oxide crystals, or tetrahydrofuran for polystyrene latex crystals are all instances of this procedure [69].

The inclusion of intermediate centrifugation cycles, which are difficult to accomplish when microparticles are substituted by nanoparticles, complicates the process outlined for the manufacture of LbL films on colloidal templates. Other techniques of separation can be used to remove the excess polyelectrolyte from the dispersion of coated nanoparticles, thereby solving this issue. One of the best methods is serum replacement, which also allows for the manufacture of capsule dispersions. Voigt et al. demonstrated that the adoption of filtration-based technologies for capsule production might speed up the coating process and increase the recovery yield. This is especially essential because the LbL approach is one of the primary limitations for industrial use of capsule suspensions. The LbL approach, whether used with flat templates or colloidal particles, has a significant scaling problem at the industrial level. The spray-aided deposition has helped overcome this barrier for LbL materials on flat templates, but it is still challenging to fabricate materials on colloidal templates. Elizarova et al. [70] have partially overcome this problem by employing a tubular flow reactor that allows the continuous production of capsules with the necessary layers. A certain polyelectrolyte stays in solution after each deposition cycle, which causes some difficulties. Microfluidic chips might also be used to increase the production of LbL capsules. However, monitoring and optimizing the process for each specific case necessitate the use of costly equipment, which is a constraint [13].

7.3 Future perspectives

The stability and durability of bioactive compounds in unfavorable temperature, light, humidity, and oxygen circumstances, as well as during storage, are the primary purposes of the encapsulation approach. Although there is no encapsulation approach that is specific to a technology or suggested for each bioactive chemical, some research has employed two or three distinct technologies to encapsulate bioactive compounds and compared the results of these investigations. Depending on the technique utilized, there were considerable variances in encapsulation efficiency and core material loss throughout the encapsulation process. While we can still propose encapsulation technology in certain situations, the version chosen may not be the best option. The variations were not only due to the bioactive molecule. They have more to do with the wall materials and operational parameters utilized; i.e., if other process circumstances were employed, the technique chosen might not be the best. As a result, investigations frequently involve a second step to improve encapsulation technology. A large majority (almost all) of the research chose the encapsulation method on the basis of prior investigations on similar chemicals or the availability and affordability of equipment. The expense of conducting these investigations must be minimized if they are to be used on a large scale. Additionally, it is required to conduct certain research, such as toxicologic assessments of bioactive compounds for pharmaceutical applications. These analyses must be carried out to ensure the safety of novel additives.

7.4 Summary

This chapter gives an overview of recent advancements in encapsulation technologies, which are widely employed in a variety of industries, including pharmaceuticals. Bioactive compounds derived from plant species are used in the commercial manufacturing of functional meals to enhance color, flavor, and texture. The functional potential of bioactive constituents is preserved while their stability is improved through the use of encapsulation methods such as microencapsulation and nanoencapsulation. These approaches allow bioactive chemicals to be coated with wall materials to make capsules that provide an effective barrier against environmental and chemical interactions. Encapsulation of bioactive compounds allows functional chemicals to be delivered to the target location in a regulated manner, boosting their bioavailability and water solubility while also increasing their stability. Spray drying, freeze-drying, electrospinning, extrusion, and LbL disposition are all encapsulating procedures used in the food and pharmaceutical industries. Spray drying is the most common method used in industry. All of the encapsulating technology that is now available, however, has significant limits. The usage of expensive equipment, which significantly increases the overall cost of the operation, is one of the key challenges associated with all of the encapsulation technologies available today. For large-scale applications, minimizing the total cost of the process is a critical criterion. Additionally, to maximize the performance of today's encapsulation methods, retro-design flavor encapsulation is required, where knowledge of both core and wall carriers is critical. It is also critical to recognize and comprehend how bioactive compound encapsulates develop physical, mechanical, chemical, and microbiological qualities that ensure long-term quality for end users and consumers.

References

[1] B. Debnath, D. Haldar, M.K. Purkait, Potential and sustainable utilization of tea waste: a review on present status and future trends, Journal of Environmental Chemical Engineering 9 (5) (2021) 106179.

[2] T.N. Baite, B. Mandal, M.K. Purkait, Ultrasound assisted extraction of gallic acid from Ficus auriculata leaves using green solvent, Food and Bioproducts Processing 128 (2021) 1−11.

[3] V.L. Dhadge, M. Changmai, M.K. Purkait, Purification of catechins from Camellia sinensis using membrane cell, Food and Bioproducts Processing 117 (2019) 203−212.

[4] P.N. Ezhilarasi, et al., Nanoencapsulation techniques for food bioactive components: a review, Food and Bioprocess Technology 6 (3) (2013) 628−647.

[5] A.M. Bakry, et al., Microencapsulation of oils: a comprehensive review of benefits, techniques, and applications, Comprehensive Reviews in Food Science and Food Safety 15 (1) (2016) 143−182.

[6] A. Belščak-Cvitanović, et al., Encapsulation of polyphenolic antioxidants from medicinal plant extracts in alginate−chitosan system enhanced with ascorbic acid by electrostatic extrusion, Food Research International 44 (4) (2011) 1094−1101.

[7] C. Dolçà, et al., Microencapsulation of rosemary essential oil by co-extrusion/gelling using alginate as a wall material, Journal of Encapsulation and Adsorption Sciences 5 (03) (2015) 121.

[8] P. Duarah, D. Haldar, M.K. Purkait, Technological advancement in the synthesis and applications of lignin-based nanoparticles derived from agro-industrial waste residues: a review, International Journal of Biological Macromolecules 163 (2020) 1828−1843.

[9] K. Cal, K. Sollohub, Spray drying technique. I: hardware and process parameters, Journal of Pharmaceutical Sciences 99 (2) (2010) 575−586.

[10] P. Bejrapha, et al., Physicothermal properties of freeze-dried fish oil nanocapsules frozen under different conditions, Drying Technology 28 (4) (2010) 481−489.

[11] H.F. Giles Jr., E.M. Mount III, J.R. Wagner Jr., Extrusion: The Definitive Processing Guide and Handbook, William Andrew, 2004.

[12] B. Ghorani, N. Tucker, Fundamentals of electrospinning as a novel delivery vehicle for bioactive compounds in food nanotechnology, Food Hydrocolloids 51 (2015) 227−240.

[13] E. Guzmán, et al., Layer-by-Layer polyelectrolyte assemblies for encapsulation and release of active compounds, Advances in Colloid and Interface Science 249 (2017) 290−307.

[14] K.S.I. Masters, Spray Drying in Practice, Charlottenlund, 2002.

[15] N.K. Mohammed, et al., Spray drying for the encapsulation of oils—a review, Molecules 25 (17) (2020) 3873.

[16] R. Vehring, Pharmaceutical particle engineering via spray drying, Pharmaceutical Research 25 (5) (2008) 999−1022.

[17] R. González-Ortega, et al., Microencapsulation of olive leaf extract by freeze-drying: effect of carrier composition on process efficiency and technological properties of the powders, Journal of Food Engineering 285 (2020) 110089.
[18] L.E. Garcia-Amezquita, et al., Freeze-drying: the basic process, in: B. Caballero, P.M. Finglas, F. Toldrá (Eds.), Encyclopedia of Food and Health, Academic Press, Oxford, 2016, pp. 104–109.
[19] N. Malik, et al., Microstructure and reconstitution of freeze-dried gum Arabic at a range of concentrations and primary drying temperatures, Food Hydrocolloids 104 (2020) 105712.
[20] M.-J. Choi, et al., Physical characteristics of fish oil encapsulated by β-cyclodextrin using an aggregation method or polycaprolactone using an emulsion diffusion method, Food Chemistry 119 (4) (2010) 1694–1703.
[21] A. Dube, et al., Effective use of reducing agents and nanoparticle encapsulation in stabilizing catechins in alkaline solution, Food Chemistry 122 (3) (2010) 662–667.
[22] S. Surassmo, et al., Effects of surfactants on the physical properties of capsicum oleoresin-loaded nanocapsules formulated through the emulsion diffusion method, Food Research International 43 (1) (2010) 8–17.
[23] K. Nakagawa, et al., Dispersibility of freeze-dried poly (epsilon-caprolactone) nanocapsules stabilized by gelatin and the effect of freezing, Journal of Food Engineering 102 (2) (2011) 177–188.
[24] P. Bejrapha, et al., Studies on the role of gelatin as a cryo-and lyo-protectant in the stability of capsicum oleoresin nanocapsules in gelatin matrix, Journal of Food Engineering 105 (2) (2011) 320–331.
[25] W. Abdelwahed, G. Degobert, H. Fessi, A pilot study of freeze drying of poly (epsilon-caprolactone) nanocapsules stabilized by poly (vinyl alcohol): formulation and process optimization, International Journal of Pharmaceutics 309 (1–2) (2006) 178–188.
[26] W. Tiyaboonchai, W. Tungpradit, P. Plianbangchang, Formulation and characterization of curcuminoids loaded solid lipid nanoparticles, International Journal of Pharmaceutics 337 (1–2) (2007) 299–306.
[27] W. Zhang, et al., The encapsulation and intracellular delivery of trehalose using a thermally responsive nanocapsule, Nanotechnology 20 (27) (2009) 275101.
[28] Y. Luo, et al., Preparation and characterization of zein/chitosan complex for encapsulation of α-tocopherol, and its in vitro controlled release study, Colloids and Surfaces B: Biointerfaces 85 (2) (2011) 145–152.
[29] L. Zhao, et al., PEG-coated lyophilized proliposomes: preparation, characterizations and in vitro release evaluation of vitamin E, European Food Research and Technology 232 (4) (2011) 647–654.
[30] K. Wang, J.P. Stark, Voltage effects on the nanoelectrospray characteristics in fully voltage-controlled atomisation of gold nanocolloids, Analytica Chimica Acta 679 (1–2) (2010) 81–84.
[31] Q. Guo, et al., Fabrication of polymeric coatings with controlled microtopographies using an electrospraying technique, PLoS One 10 (6) (2015) e0129960.
[32] A. Jaworek, Micro-and nanoparticle production by electrospraying, Powder Technology 176 (1) (2007) 18–35.
[33] J. Xie, C.H. Wang, Electrospray in the dripping mode for cell microencapsulation, Journal of colloid and interface science 312 (2) (2007) 247–255. https://doi.org/10.1016/j.jcis.2007.04.023.
[34] X. Xu, et al., Preparation and properties of electrospun soy protein isolate/polyethylene oxide nanofiber membranes, ACS Applied Materials and Interfaces 4 (8) (2012) 4331–4337.
[35] S. Saallah, W. Lenggoro, Nanoparticles carrying biological molecules: recent advances and applications, KONA Powder and Particle Journal 2018 (2018).

[36] M. Nieuwland, et al., Reprint of "Food-grade electrospinning of proteins", Innovative Food Science & Emerging Technologies 24 (2014) 138–144.
[37] A. Jaworek, A.T. Sobczyk, Electrospraying route to nanotechnology: an overview, Journal of Electrostatics 66 (3–4) (2008) 197–219.
[38] S. Freiberg, X. Zhu, Polymer microspheres for controlled drug release, International Journal of Pharmaceutics 282 (1–2) (2004) 1–18.
[39] Z. Liu, et al., Polysaccharides-based nanoparticles as drug delivery systems, Advanced Drug Delivery Reviews 60 (15) (2008) 1650–1662.
[40] M. Aceituno-Medina, et al., Development of novel ultrathin structures based in amaranth (Amaranthus hypochondriacus) protein isolate through electrospinning, Food Hydrocolloids 31 (2) (2013) 289–298.
[41] A.C. Mendes, K. Stephansen, I.S. Chronakis, Electrospinning of food proteins and polysaccharides, Food Hydrocolloids 68 (2017) 53–68.
[42] R. Pérez-Masiá, J.M. Lagaron, A. López-Rubio, Development and optimization of novel encapsulation structures of interest in functional foods through electrospraying, Food and Bioprocess Technology 7 (11) (2014) 3236–3245.
[43] E. Mascheroni, et al., Encapsulation of volatiles in nanofibrous polysaccharide membranes for humidity-triggered release, Carbohydrate Polymers 98 (1) (2013) 17–25.
[44] George, M., Extrusion Cooking: Technologies and Applications edited by R Guy Woodhead Publishing, Cambridge, 2001 pp 206, price£ 115.00 ISBN 1-85573-559-8. Journal of the Science of Food and Agriculture, 2003. 83(4): pp. 361–361.
[45] H. Ramachandra, M. Thejaswini, Extrusion technology: a novel method of food processing, International Journal of Innovative Science, Engineering and Technology 2 (4) (2015) 358–369.
[46] D. Seth, H.N. Mishra, S.C. Deka, Effect of microencapsulation using extrusion technique on viability of bacterial cells during spray drying of sweetened yoghurt, International Journal of Biological Macromolecules 103 (2017) 802–807.
[47] M. Emin, H. Schuchmann, Droplet breakup and coalescence in a twin-screw extrusion processing of starch based matrix, Journal of Food Engineering 116 (1) (2013) 118–129.
[48] N.J. Zuidam, E. Shimoni, Overview of microencapsulates for use in food products or processes and methods to make them, in: Encapsulation Technologies for Active Food Ingredients and Food Processing, Springer, 2010, pp. 3–29.
[49] K. Ravichandran, et al., Effects of different encapsulation agents and drying process on stability of betalains extract, Journal of Food Science & Technology 51 (9) (2014) 2216–2221.
[50] N.M. Gately, J.E. Kennedy, Processing stability and the significance of variation in extrusion speeds and temperatures on SSB® 55 pharma grade shellac for oral drug delivery, Journal of Manufacturing and Materials Processing 1 (1) (2017) 9.
[51] J.M. Lakkis, Encapsulation and Controlled Release Technologies in Food Systems, John Wiley & Sons, 2016.
[52] M.R.I. Shishir, et al., Advances in micro and nano-encapsulation of bioactive compounds using biopolymer and lipid-based transporters, Trends in Food Science & Technology 78 (2018) 34–60.
[53] J. Oxley, Coextrusion for food ingredients and nutraceutical encapsulation: principles and technology, in: Encapsulation Technologies and Delivery Systems for Food Ingredients and Nutraceuticals, Elsevier, 2012, pp. 131–150.
[54] N. Garti, D.J. McClements, Encapsulation Technologies and Delivery Systems for Food Ingredients and Nutraceuticals, Elsevier, 2012.
[55] C. Perignon, et al., Microencapsulation by interfacial polymerisation: membrane formation and structure, Journal of Microencapsulation 32 (1) (2015) 1–15.

[56] S. Gouin, Microencapsulation: industrial appraisal of existing technologies and trends, Trends in Food Science and Technology 15 (7–8) (2004) 330–347.

[57] E.A. Soliman, A.Y. El-Moghazy, M.S. Mohy El-Din, M.A. Massoud, Microencapsulation of essential oils within alginate: formulation and in vitro evaluation of antifungal activity, Journal of Encapsulation and Adsorption Sciences 3 (1) (2013) 48–55.

[58] J.A. Bhushani, C. Anandharamakrishnan, Electrospinning and electrospraying techniques: potential food based applications, Trends in Food Science and Technology 38 (1) (2014) 21–33.

[59] U. Prüsse, et al., Comparison of different technologies for alginate beads production, Chemical Papers 62 (4) (2008) 364–374.

[60] R. Stojanovic, et al., Encapsulation of thyme (Thymus serpyllum L.) aqueous extract in calcium alginate beads, Journal of the Science of Food and Agriculture 92 (3) (2012) 685–696.

[61] G. Decher, J.B. Schlenoff, Multilayer Thin Films: Sequential Assembly of Nanocomposite Materials, John Wiley & Sons, 2006.

[62] E. Guzman, et al., Influence of the percentage of acetylation on the assembly of LbL multilayers of poly (acrylic acid) and chitosan, Physical Chemistry Chemical Physics 13 (40) (2011) 18200–18207.

[63] B.B. Hsu, S.R. Hagerman, P.T. Hammond, Rapid and efficient sprayed multilayer films for controlled drug delivery, Journal of Applied Polymer Science 133 (25) (2016).

[64] A. Zhuk, R. Mirza, S. Sukhishvili, Multiresponsive clay-containing layer-by-layer films, ACS Nano 5 (11) (2011) 8790–8799.

[65] W. Tong, X. Song, C. Gao, Layer-by-layer assembly of microcapsules and their biomedical applications, Chemical Society Reviews 41 (18) (2012) 6103–6124.

[66] F.-X. Xiao, et al., Layer-by-layer assembly of versatile nanoarchitectures with diverse dimensionality: a new perspective for rational construction of multilayer assemblies, Chemical Society Reviews 45 (11) (2016) 3088–3121.

[67] G. Decher, J. Schmitt, Fine-tuning of the film thickness of ultrathin multilayer films composed of consecutively alternating layers of anionic and cationic polyelectrolytes, Trends in Colloid and Interface Science VI (1992) 160–164.

[68] Y. Xiang, S. Lu, Layer-by-layer self-assembly in the development of electrochemical energy conversion and storage devices from fuel cells to supercapacitors, Chemical Society Reviews 41 (21) (2012) 7291–7321.

[69] H.G. Bagaria, M.S. Wong, Polyamine–salt aggregate assembly of capsules as responsive drug delivery vehicles, Journal of Materials Chemistry 21 (26) (2011) 9454–9466.

[70] I.S. Elizarova, P.F. Luckham, Fabrication of polyelectrolyte multilayered nano-capsules using a continuous layer-by-layer approach, Journal of Colloid and Interface Science 470 (2016) 92–99.

CHAPTER 8

Applications of herb-derived bioactive phytochemicals

8.1 Introduction

Since the beginning of human civilization, herbs have been employed for therapeutic applications. Herbs have a wide spectrum of phytochemical ingredients or secondary metabolites that contribute to their therapeutic effectiveness [1,2]. Medicinal herbs have been utilized for centuries to treat a variety of diseases. For instance, Ayurveda, or Ayurveda medicine, is a system of ancient Indian medicine that has been practiced for thousands of years. Ayush is a Sanskrit term for long life, and Veda is Sanskrit for wisdom or science. It was during the Vedic period in India in the second millennium when the oldest literature on Indian medical treatment appeared. The famous medical encyclopedias *Susruta Samhita* and *Charak Samhita* were created between BCE and CE 500. Ayurveda relies heavily on these writings as the foundation of its practice. In Ayurveda medicine, there are a number of plant-based medications that have been used to treat fractures. Evidence of the usage of medicinal plants in the middle Gangetic area dating back to the second millennium BC has been unearthed by archaeobotanical excavations. Science has been affecting intellectual life since Buddha's time, leading people to reexamine long-held beliefs and look for concrete evidence to support them. Throughout the lower Himalayas and Indo-Gangetic region, tribal and wandering healers were taught the physician ascetic and yogic traditions of Buddhism and Jainism and philosophical schools like Samkhya, Vaisheshika, and Nyay, all of which contributed to the emergence of Ayurveda [3].

In addition to traditional herbs, researchers have lately discovered hundreds of new innovative bio-derived sources for extracting phytochemicals and for preparing novel materials such as metal nanoparticles for biomedical uses [4,5]. During the last several years, it has been seen that traditional medicine is returning to the scene in a new and more effective

Advances in Extraction and Applications of Bioactive Phytochemicals
ISBN 978-0-443-18535-9
https://doi.org/10.1016/B978-0-443-18535-9.00009-0

form for the benefit of patients today. Traditional herbs such as *Azadirachta indica, Phyllanthus emblica, Picrorhiza kurroa, Ocimum tenuiflorum, Withania, somnifera, Piper nigrum, Zingiber officinale,* and *Curcuma longa* are extensively used plants in traditional remedies. They are known for their numerous biologic properties throughout the world [6—10]. They are still used today to treat a wide range of ailments, from the ordinary cold to life-threatening conditions like cancer. Even during the COVID-19 pandemic, these herbs were extensively researched to discover a remedy. The potential of these plants for the treatment of various diseases, as well as their diverse qualities, are discussed in this chapter. Recent research activity on these plants is highlighted. Furthermore, the usefulness of nanoformulation technology for efficient medication delivery is emphasized.

8.2 Treatment of orthopedic diseases using herbal extracts

An important aspect of bone healing is restoring the tissue to its preinjury state, which can be accomplished in three separate and intertwined stages. Proliferation and protection of fractured and dislocated bone regions are aided by a number of stages of bone healing. The amount of time it takes depends on the severity of the injury, but in general, upper-body fractures should be prepared within 2—3 weeks, and lower-body fractures should be ready by 4 weeks. Periosteum plays a major role in the healing process. In the periosteum, the progenitor cells for chondroblast and osteoblast, two cell types critical to bone repair, may be found. Precursor cells can also be found in the bone marrow, endosteum, tiny blood vessels, and fibroblast. Fracture repair is divided into two prime categories: primary/direct and secondary/indirect. There is limited callus development in the initial healing of the fracture. Because it is an immediate effort to repair bone integrity, the cells in the cortex must be directly connected to the bone. Secondary or indirect healing is the primary mode of healing for most fractures. A hematoma develops, which is followed by an early inflammatory phase, a healing phase, and a late remodeling phase [11]. Fig. 8.1 describes the various phases of healing.

In the initial few hours and days following a fracture, a hematoma forms at the site of the injury. This leads to granulation tissue creation, new blood vessels, and mesenchymal cell migration when prostaglandins are administered. This process is accompanied by inflammation and fibrosis of the bone. Cancellous bone and muscle are the key sources of nutrients and

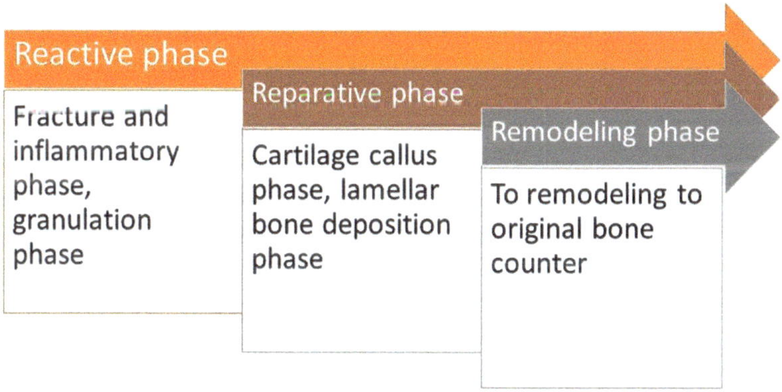

Figure 8.1 The phases of fracture healing.

oxygen during this early stage of the process. It is possible to change the inflammatory response and limit bone repair by using antiinflammatory or cytotoxic medicine during the first week of treatment. For example, at this stage of the healing process, the collagen matrix is laid down, and osteoid is released, which leads to the development of the soft callus around the repair site; this callus is then mineralized. A brace or internal fixation is necessary to provide enough protection during the first 4–6 weeks of the healing phase because the callus's resistance to movement is inadequate. The callus eventually ossifies, generating a bridge of braided bone across the fragmented pieces of bone. Another possibility is an unstable fibrous union to form instead of callus solidification if adequate immobilization is not applied. In the remodeling stage, the healed bone is returned to its previous form, structure, and mechanical stress. This is when fracture healing is completed. There are times when axial loading forces cause the bone to be deposited at the fracture site and reabsorbed at the place where it is not needed. It usually takes 3–6 months to reach a sufficient level of strength [12]. Fractures can cause a great deal of discomfort, functional impairment, and cosmetic disfigurement. If the patient's fracture does not heal, they may be permanently disabled. Implant development and bone quality enhancement are two approaches to speed up and improve callus formation during fracture healing. It is not enough to have surgery or any other gadget to help fracture healing; appropriate nutrition and general health are just as important. This is because damaged bones can mend on their own. Just to aid in the natural healing process, therapy is required. Capillaries, vascularization of the clot, and the creation of callus are the first steps in bone regeneration, according to Hunter (1779). These vessels arise from the periosteum, the outer layer of bone. According to John Goodsir, a 19th-century researcher, bone corpuscles, the live cells that reside underneath the periosteum, are responsible for bone formation. Biologic factors regulate the healing of fractures, and mechanical measures must be coordinated with them, according to Phemister (1951), who noted that mechanical methods are often required to decrease and stabilize shattered bones [3]. It has been shown that protein feeding aids in the healing of lengthy bone fractures in a controlled animal model, according to Guarniero et al. [13]. According to Chen et al. [14], the food supply is sufficient for bone healing in small and medium-sized broken gaps. Still, in large fractured gaps, nonunion can be caused by either inadequate nutrition supply or an inadequate mechanical condition.

Fracture therapy and the traditional profession of bone setters both rely on antiinflammation as a fundamental premise. During inflammation, arachidonic acid metabolites and cytokines are released, increasing the synthesis of different mediators, such as swelling and pain relief. Nitric oxide (NO), a gas generated by the inducible nitric oxide synthase (iNOS), appears to have an essential role in inflammatory diseases like rheumatoid arthritis, as well, according to new research. Since macrophage NO generation is controlled by iNOS, an antiinflammatory agent might be used to minimize this reaction. Ultimately, the goal of bone repair is to return the broken bone to its preinjury strength level without fracturing or deforming it in any way. In preclinical investigations, it is critical to determine the impact of an intervention on bone regeneration by measuring bone strength following a fracture or lesion [15].

Plants and their extracts and poultices, together with a splint without a cast, are commonly used in traditional medicine to mend fractured bones. A resurgence of interest in traditional medicine has taken place recently. Biodynamic therapeutic substances derived from medicinal plants are plentiful. In Southeast Asia, the climbing tree *Cryptolepis buchanani* (Ganglong, Asclepiodaceae) has long been a source of traditional medicine. Climbing trees up to 200 m high, it is a medicinal plant native to marshy and wet places. Bone fractures in Arunachal Pradesh are historically treated using Ganglong, an indigenous herb. It can also be found growing as a creeper on the ground. Tribal people in Arunachal Pradesh traditionally utilize the plant's root, stem, and leaves to cure bone fractures. To determine the type of fracture, a local herbal practitioner places their palm, which they have developed through many years of experience, on the damaged area. Different sections of the plant are employed in different ways depending on the type of fracture. Banana leaves are smeared with a mixture of herb and mustard oil and left on for a week or longer, depending on the situation. Instead of using mustard oil, 100 g of paste is mixed with 200 mL of milk and administered orally three times daily for 5 days as a systemic treatment [16]. *C. buchanani* was also found to have antimicrobial properties [17]. *C. buchanani* extract has also been reported to have analgesic, antiinflammatory, and chondroprotective properties in the literature. The stem of *C. buchanani* has been shown to reduce muscular and joint discomfort. Researchers studied the antiinflammatory effects of 50% methanol extract B2 and leukotriene B4, generated by the COX and 5-lipoxygenase pathways. It also inhibits TNF-alpha generation by lipopolysaccharide-stimulated human monocyte cells [18]. The extract of *C. buchanani* was shown to be considered active against *Bacillus subtilis* and *Pseudomonas aeruginosa*; but, at lower concentrations, it had no appreciable inhibitory effect against *Escherichia coli* [19]. To protect the liver from acetaminophen-induced hepatotoxicity, *C. buchanani* was shown to have an ethanolic extract with hepatoprotective properties. The ethanol extract of *C. Buchnani* contains alkaloids and flavonoids that have been shown to have hepatoprotective properties. Liver damage and oxidative stress are both strongly protected by the ethanolic extract of *C. buchanani* leaf extract. Increased serum biochemical parameters such as serum glutamic oxaloacetic transaminase (GOT), glutamic pyruvic transaminase (GPT), and alkaline phosphatase (ALP) are shown in the serum of those who take the ethanolic extract of the *C. buchanani* leaf extract. Acetaminophen-treated rats had a dramatically decreased level of glutathione peroxidase, glutathione-S-transferase, and superoxide dismutase, which was enhanced by treatment with the extract [20].

It has long been recognized that *Cissus quadrangularis* (Harjor, family Vitaceae) possesses bone-healing capabilities, and it has been given both externally and internally as decoctions by bone setters. Vitamin C content has been shown to be high. In some regions of India and Sri Lanka, it is also consumed as a diet. A succulent of the Vitaceae family, it is known as Asthisamhari and may be found in the hottest parts of India. It may grow in plains, coastal locations, forests, and wasteland up to 500 m above sea level. There is a greenish tint to the surface, which is smooth, glabrous, and buff-colored. Taste and odor are absent from the sharp end, which has a reddish-brown color. The therapeutic benefits of the plant stem, leaves, and roots are reported. It is best to utilize the roots and stems for bone fracture repair. The stem is bitter, and it is used both orally and externally to treat back and spinal complaints. Osteoarthritis, osteoporosis, and rheumatoid arthritis are among the conditions for which the herb has been used in Ayurveda. Other medical qualities of the plant include its ability to treat asthma, burns, and insect bites. In addition to treating helminthiasis and anorexia, it is also effective in treating dyspepsia and colic, as well as treating hemorrhagic convulsions, piles, and anemia.

8.2.1 Icariin

Icariin is a kind of flavonoid categorized as a prenylated flavonol glycoside and is most commonly reported to cure bone diseases. Trauma, articular inflammation, and degeneration are the most common causes of osteochondral abnormalities. Joint disease and eventual complete joint destruction are caused by the biochemical breakdown and physical degeneration of articular cartilage. Osteoarthritis and other degenerative diseases of the joints can be challenging clinical conditions to treat since the cartilage itself is an avascular and aneural tissue with low regeneration and self-healing capabilities. Nonpharmacological, pharmacologic, and intra-articular therapy can be used to treat osteochondral abnormalities. With biocompatible, bioactive, and biodegradable materials that give structural support and molecular cues to drive healing, osteochondral defects can be improved. Tissue engineering utilizing cell-based treatment and a combination of materials is becoming increasingly extensively employed. Recent studies have shown that autologous conditioned serum (ACS) is a safe alternative therapy for osteoarthritis (OA). Believing that antiinflammatory cytokines may be concentrated in ACS, Meijer et al. (2003) reported a medical device known as OrthoKinew, which is used to generate and administer ACS with an antiinflammatory component [21]. Patients at risk of developing osteoarthritis could benefit from experimental therapies such as ACS intra-articular injections, according to some possible responders [22]. It is also claimed that an increase in tissue regeneration and reduction in degenerative processes can be achieved with the use of ACS. A Chinese patent drug known as "Xianlinggubao capsule" was used to make rabbit conditioned serum, and the proliferative effects of conditioned serum on primary rabbit chondrocytes were demonstrated. A key component of the Chinese patent capsule is the *Epimedium* plant, which is extensively used in traditional Chinese herbal therapy to treat arthritis. One of the key bioactive components of the *Epimedium* plant is the prenylated flavonol glycoside icariin (ICA). ICA outperforms other flavonoid drugs in stimulating osteoblast development and maturation. ICA has been shown to be a safe and powerful anabolic drug for chondrocytes, which can alter chondrocyte proliferation and inhibit extracellular matrix breakdown [23]. Accumulation of chondrocyte growth factors such as aggrecan, collagen II, and Sox9 might also be promoted by ICA [24]. ICA has been shown to have an osteoinductive impact on bone tissues when administered locally via biomaterials. In these studies, it has been claimed that the use of ICA-loaded biomaterials for cartilage tissue engineering is possible. Intra-articular injections of hyaluronic acid (HA) are commonly used to treat knee osteoarthritis. Synovial fluid contains a significant amount of it. HA is involved in wound healing, morphogenesis, inflammation, and cell proliferation as a key constituent of the cartilage's extracellular matrix. Injectable HA gels coupled with proteoglycan have been shown to reduce or prevent the onset of osteoarthritis following knee injury [25]. The gel can also be employed as a delivery vehicle for cartilage regeneration when combined with additional disease-modifying medicines such as chondroitin sulfate [26]. By injecting ICA into rabbits, the researchers in this work were able to create rabbit ICA conditioned serum (ICS). Protoglycan and collagen production was predicted to be enhanced in a cartilage healing model in vivo by combining the biomaterial ICS and HA.

8.2.2 Tetrandrine

Tetrandrine, a natural substance obtained from the plant *Stephania tetrandra*, is a bisbenzylisoquinoline alkaloid. An extensive range of pharmacologic activities are exerted by tetrandrine, the most notable of which include antiviral, anticancer, multidrug resistance reversal, and calcium channel blocking properties. Tetrandrine has recently been found to block endolysosomal two-pore channels, preventing Ebolavirus, SARS-CoV-2 viruses (severe acute respiratory syndrome coronavirus 2), MERS-CoV (Middle East respiratory syndrome—related coronavirus), or pseudoviruses from entering host cells. In China, a clinical trial (NCT04308317) is underway to investigate the use of tetrandrine as adjuvant therapy for COVID-19 patients [27]. Tetrandrine has also shown potent antiproliferative and cytotoxic activities against a variety of cancer cell lines, halting cell cycle progression, inducing proapoptotic signaling pathways, and reducing tumor cell motility. By inhibiting P-glycoprotein (P-gp), an efflux pump for xenobiotic drugs, tetrandrine has been demonstrated to resensitize chemoresistant tumors, which commonly causes therapeutic failure of tumor therapy. In addition to its several possible uses, tetrandrine is fascinating as a lead chemical because of its numerous pharmacologic properties. Unfortunately, the toxicity of this compound prevents it from finding widespread use in medicine. So far, tetrandrine and other bisbenzylisoquinolines have been associated with a number of hazardous side effects. The liver and lungs were the most commonly affected organs in animal studies. The toxic effects of tetrandrine have not yet been fully explained by scientists. Tetrandrine interaction with p38aMAPK (mitogen-activated protein kinase) was hypothesized by Li et al. (2019) to cause liver damage [28].

Tetrandrine-induced pulmonary and hepatic toxicity may be mediated by cytochrome P450 (CYP) enzymes, according to research [29]. Qi et al. (2013) believe that CYP2E1 is the major cause of rat hepatocyte mitochondrial dysfunction following tetrandrine exposure, which they attribute to reactive oxygen species produced during CYP2E1 metabolism. However, the molecular processes behind CYP2E1-mediated toxicity are unclear [29]. Jin et al. (2011) identify a CYP3A4- and CYP3A5-mediated metabolism that leads to a potentially unstable intermediate in a metabolic investigation. Tetrandrine's toxicity is thought to be caused by one structural feature in particular [30]. The methoxy group at C-12 in para-position to a benzylic methylene group is first demethylated to yield the matching phenol3 in the proposed metabolic route. A bio-nucleophilic intermediate known as para-quinone methide4 results from this phenol's enzymatic oxidation. There was evidence for the creation of the para-quinone methide4 after tetrandrine was incubated with human liver microsomes that also included glutathione. Bisbenzylisoquinolines and seco analogs like dauricine, berbamine, fangchinoline, cepha-ranthine, and muraricine have the discussed. A para-methoxybenzyl motif like tetrandrine or the equivalent para-hydroxybenzyl moiety may have an adverse hazardous profile. So it is critical to determine if and to what degree this structural motif causes cytotoxicity when oxidized by CYP3A4/5 enzymes [27].

Tetrandrine, a plant bisbenzylisoquinoline alkaloid, has antiviral, anticancer, and multidrug resistance reversal activity as well as calcium channel blocking activity, all of which make this alkaloid an intriguing therapeutic candidate [31,32]. Unfortunately, its toxicity, which mostly affects the liver and lungs, means that it cannot be used in therapeutic settings. Each of the five diastereomeric pairs that were synthesized and physiologically examined in terms of their toxicity as well as their antiproliferative as well as multidrug resistance reversal activities were analyzed. The methoxy group at C-12 in para-position to a benzylic methylene group, which is vulnerable to enzyme oxidation and, in turn, can react with bio-nucleophiles, was found to be the hazardous structural element, and new analogs were developed on the basis of this notion. This oxidative toxification process was meant to be prevented by the new chemicals' structure. The suspected problematic structural motif was absent from all analogs, although a loss in anticancer efficacy accompanied any considerable decrease in toxicity. The toxicity of RMS2, RMS4, and RMS8 to healthy cells was shown to be much higher than that of tetrandrine itself. The propagating mechanism of CYP3A4-mediated toxification involving the para-quinone methide4 is not the main source of cytotoxicity of tetrandrine and similar (bis)benzylisoquinoline alkaloids, as demonstrated by CYP3A4 overexpression in two cellular models for recombinant hepatitis investigations. The synthesized analogs were shown to have significant changes in biologic activity from tetrandrine. Even though most of the structural modifications preserved P-gp inhibitory power, seven compounds showed significantly higher antiproliferative capacity against drug-resistant leukemia cells and greater cytotoxicity to liver cancer cell lines as opposed to the standard tetrandrine. These drugs engaged on the intrinsic, mitochondria-initiated apoptosis route and/or on the Akt kinase activation mechanism. In terms of both their toxicity and their pharmacologic profile, chemicals RMS3 and RMS5 were determined to be the most promising because of their higher anticancer activities while exhibiting no additional damage to healthy liver cells. Nonmalignant blood and endothelial cells were used to confirm similar toxicity to primary cells. As a result, decreasing the therapeutic dose may be an effective way to prevent side effects, and our findings strongly propose that in vivo models be used to examine these consequences. Based on these promising results and recent progress in complete synthesis of bisbenzylisoquinoline alkaloids, future medicinal chemistry initiatives should focus on structure—activity relationships in this chemical family [27].

8.2.3 Ursolic acid

In secondary plant metabolites, triterpenoid acids are one of the most significant classes. The pentacyclic triterpenoids are represented by ursolic acid (UA) and its isomer oleanolic acid. Antidiabetic, antiinflammatory, antioxidant, antibacterial, and cancer-fighting activities are among the many essential pharmacologic characteristics of both biomolecules [33]. The Lamiaceae family has been shown to contain a significant concentration of UA in its chemistry [34]. In a recent investigation, we found a substantial concentration of UA in the *Clinopodium revolutum* (Lamiaceae), better known in Peru as "Flor de Arena," a popular therapeutic herb. It is used to treat gastritis, biliary calculi, stomach gas, and uric acid overproduction, among other ailments. There are 10 chiral centers in the UA molecule, making it a difficult chemical to produce in the lab. As a result, plants and fruit peels have been the only known UA sources. UA's purification is problematic since it shares a structure with its isomer and has comparable physicochemical characteristics.

High-performance liquid chromatography (HPLC), high-performance thin-layer chromatography (HPTLC), gas chromatography (GC), and a slew of additional analytical separation methods have all been created. Preparative scale separation of these two chemicals, on the other hand, has proven to be a significant hurdle [35]. Huaman et al. (2021) reported a technique that just requires the ethanolic extract of *C. revolutum* to be crystallized and recrystallized to get UA crystals [33]. Reproducibility is high, and costs are low, with no use of hazardous solvents or preparative chromatographic procedures required for this process. An experiment without activated carbon results in needle-shaped and very pure UA crystals. However, this experiment's yield is smaller than the one using activated carbon. Recrystallization can be avoided by doing the investigation using activated carbon. A larger yield but a somewhat poorer purity than in the experiment without activated carbon is the result. Also, the needle form of the UA crystals is not flawless. This process is faster than the earlier one in which the cuticular wax was removed with ethyl acetate, and recrystallization was necessary; however, the purity drops, and the crystals of UA are often amorphous. However, Fan et al. (2016) used apple peel as their raw material and performed ultrasound-assisted extraction using methanol, which they found to be successful, too [36]. Secondary metabolites cannot be purified in the same way since each plant has a unique matrix. As a result, the UA purification process must be optimized for each new source. The precise chemical structure of UA was determined by the use of spectroscopy. The functional groups associated with UA are clearly visible in infrared spectra. Nuclear magnetic resonance spectroscopy is the most helpful technique. The integration of the 1 H spectrum of UA's signals yielded a hydrogen atom count of 48 H. The DEPT experiment revealed that the molecule included seven CH_3 groups, nine CH_2 groups, seven CH groups, and seven C groups, which were confirmed by the 13CRMN analysis [33].

8.3 Influence of herbal plants as immunity boosters in the treatment of COVID-19 and other diseases

SARS-CoV-2 (COVID-19) infection is an acute respiratory illness that has emerged as a pandemic problem and will have significant implications on public health in 2019—20. When the first instance of COVID-19 was discovered in China's Hubei Province city of Wuhan, the virus quickly spread around the globe, infecting people in 215 nations. COVID-19 was classified as an international public health emergency on January 30 by the World Health Organization. India was the second most impacted country and the third most affected country on February 14, 2021, with more than 108,153,741 confirmed cases and 2,381,295 fatalities. Because of its high death rate and quick transmission by human-to-human contact, the number of COVID-19-affected patients has been gradually growing over the world to date. After the SARS-CoV epidemic of 2002 and the MERS-CoV epidemic of 2012, the COVID-19 outbreak in the 21st century was the third such outbreak [37]. COVID-19 are coronavirus-like, enveloped, positive ss-RNA viruses with genome sizes ranging from 26 to 32 kilobase pairs with genome sequence similarities to MERS-CoV and SARS-CoV [38,39].

The taxonomists' Coronavirus Study Group, under the auspices of the International Committee on Taxonomy of Viruses, named COVID-19 after its 82% similarity to the SARS-CoV genome sequence. Herbal medicinal plants were utilized to treat a variety of illnesses on the Indian subcontinent in the past. SARS-CoV cysteine proteases were found to be inhibited by a variety of medicinal plants, including *Angelica keiskei, Ecklonia cava, Salvia miltiorrhiza, Torreya nucifera (L.)*, an anti-SARS coronavirus 3C-like protease inhibitor, and *Lycoris radiata*, which all act as SARS-CoV 3CLpro inhibitors [40,41]. These herbs, along with others, have antiviral, antibacterial, antifungal, antiinflammatory, analgesic, antistress, antitumor, immunomodulatory, and neuroprotective benefits. Therefore, these herbs are used to treat a variety of ailments as a result of their beneficial properties. Traditional herbal remedies have been utilized to treat viral illness in China since the epidemic of COVID-19 began there. In a study of 214 COVID-19 patients, herbal remedies used in traditional Chinese medicine helped 90% of the patients recover from the COVID-19 viral illness [42]. In addition, several herbal medicinal plants were prescribed for COVID-19 patients based on their disease stage and symptom distinction to heal these viral disorders [43]. Islam et al. (2021) investigated the anti-COVID-19 disease effects of various plant metabolites, such as emodin (anthraquinone family), lopinavir (antiretroviral of the protease inhibitor class), lycorine (crystalline alkaloid), oseltamivir (neuraminidase inhibitors), hypericin (an anthraquinone derivative), etc. The research further highlights the possible use of herbal medicinal plant metabolites and other natural items to prevent or cure infections with COVID-19, as well as the mechanism by which they could act. Analysis of the COVID-19 structure led to the discovery of significant proteases including protease, major protease, and RNA-dependent RNA polymerase (RdRp). Viral genome assembly and replication are controlled by these proteases, which break down large polypeptides into smaller nonstructural proteins. COVID-19 infection's primary protease is the focus of a unified drug strategy, virtual screening, and high-throughput screening to identify novel drug drives. Scientists and researchers used docking-based drug design to identify an inhibitor like N3 and then designed the structure of COVID-19 viral protease, i.e., Mpro interacted with that chemical to stop this outbreak. On coronaviral transcription and replication machinery, RdRp is the most prominent section. The cryo-EM structure of COVID-19 infection full-length nsp12 complexes with cofactors nsp8 and nsp7, according to specialists, at 2.9 resolution. Remdesivir's relationship to this polymerase was discovered using a comparative research approach. There are novel antiviral medicines that target viral RdRp because of the structure. Currently, no particular treatment has been developed to treat patients infected with SARS-CoV-2, making this study focused only on the antiviral potential of medicinal plants against human SARS coronaviruses, which is the most catastrophic occurrence of the 21st century [37]. The potential of different herbal plants to cure COVID-19 has been explored in this section based on the available literature.

8.3.1 Azadirachta indica

Many phytochemicals in *Azadirachta indica* (commonly recognized as neem) have been demonstrated to have pharmacologic potential during the years of investigation. Triterpenes are the most therapeutically useful of these chemicals. Antipyretic, fungicidal, antihistamine, and antiseptic activities of nimbin (triterpene) have been demonstrated. The antiinflammatory and antioxidant properties of nimbin help to reduce damage by lowering the generation of reactive oxygen species [44]. Prostaglandin biosynthesis inhibitors flavonoids and endoperoxides are contained in neem, along with phosphodiesterases and other inflammation-related enzymes. Phytochemical examination of neem has verified the presence of triterpenes, flavonoids, and saponins in large concentrations, while other components like catechins and nimbin appear to be present in smaller amounts [45]. Toxins such as gallic acid and catechins are also discovered in neem extracts in the form of tannins and alkaloids [44,46]. According to a new study, neem leaf glycoprotein, a group of glycoproteins found in the leaf of the neem tree, has the ability to inhibit tumor development by influencing local and systemic immune responses [44,47]. An examination of leaf extracts (both aqueous and methane) by Dash et al. (2017) found substantial quantities of saponin, tannins, and glycosides in the aqueous extracts [48]. The alkaloids, tannins, and flavonoids in methanoic extracts were high. Previous investigations (nonmethanoic) revealed glycosides nimbanene, 6-desacetylnimbinene, nimbandiol, nimbolide, ascorbic acid, n-hexacosanol, and amino acid in leaf extracts, showing the wide range of compounds accessible, but they curiously place significant emphasis on the extraction procedure [6]. Proline is a contemporary medication for neurologic disorders including Alzheimer and Parkinson disease, type 2 diabetes mellitus, and polycythemia. With the varied polarity of each of the extracting solvents, the antioxidant capacity of each of the leaf extracts was tested in recent investigations by Hossai's group. Phytol, methyl isoheptadecanoate, and nonacosane were shown to be the most potent antioxidants in chloroform extracts. On the other hand, methanolic extracts have the least amount of antioxidant activity. mToluylaldehyde, methyl 14-methylpentadecanoate, lineoleoyl chloride, and methyl isoheptadecanoate were the primary ingredients in these extracts. Notably, the hexane extract had the most physiologically active compounds: methyl isoheptadecanoate, phytol, hexadecamethylcyclooctasiloxane, butyl palmitate nonadecane, isobutyl stearate, oxalic acid, heptacosane, eicosane, 7-hexyl-heptacosane, and octacosane. The same group quantified total phenolic compounds using gallic acid equivalents. So butanol has the greatest total phenolics (107.3 GA/g) and hexane the lowest (20.8 GA/g). Then they ultraviolet-measured total flavonoids in dry samples. The methanol extract had the greatest total flavonoid content (529.9 mg/100 g), whereas the butanol extract had the lowest (63.0 mg/100 g) [49–51].

Prenylated flavonoids were found in the methanolic extraction of the flowers. Compounds that were found to be absent from the leaves yet have an antimutagenic effect against TrpPI, TrpPII, and PhIP. Flowers include a wide range of chemicals, including flowerone, flowerine, diepoxyazadirol, and O-methylazadironolide, as one might anticipate. Triterpenoid (trichilenone acetate), flavanones, nimbaflavone, 3′prenylnaringenin, and

4(2hydroxyethyl) phenol are some of the other recognized compounds found in flowers [46]. Antimicrobial and insecticidal properties of neem-derived extracts have been discovered. In neem seeds, there is a compound tetranortriterpenoid limonoid known as azadirachtin, which is responsible for the poisonous effects on insects. Experiments with *Staphylococcus aureus* (a Gram-positive bacteria) and methicillin-resistant *Staphylococcus aureus* (a group of Gram-positive bacteria) showed that an ethanol extract of neem leaves has antibacterial action against both strains, and this was confirmed in subsequent studies.

Free radicals, also known as reactive oxygen species, are a key cause of inflammation because they damage numerous biologic components by removing electrons to reach a stable state, causing oxidative stress in the cell. As a result, sufficient chemicals (also known as antioxidants) are needed to stabilize or neutralize free radicals as a first step in preventing or stopping an escalation of oxidative stress, leading to a variety of disorders. Antioxidant molecules such as superoxide dismutase, catalase, glutathione peroxidase, glutathione, and nitric oxide dioxygenase will act in conjunction with the body's natural antioxidant defenses [52]. One easy method to include these substances in your diet is as dietary supplements. Neem extracts, in the form of teas and oils, are an economical and straightforward way to get antioxidants into your diet [53]. Although much debate and research surround the usefulness and safety of extracts, we may consider some preparations, such as those used in traditional medicine, to be safe. The possible advantages, on the other hand, differ from preparation to preparation. Keeping this in mind, it is important to remember that certain natural substances have the potential to exacerbate already existing pathologies. A wide range of research on neem has been published throughout the years to test its antioxidant properties and/or to evaluate its ability to enhance the body's natural defenses. Neem leaves and methanol are used in one such study to extract the plant's potential components. Using a rat model of induced intestinal ischemic-reperfusion damage, they evaluated the extract on rats for 7 days at a dose of 100−200 mg/kg as pretreatment. They compared the extract to untreated animals and animals treated with vitamin C (a recognized antioxidant) (IIRI). Myeloperoxidase in the serum was reduced in IIRI rats, but myeloperoxidase in the serum was reduced in the extract group. Non-IIRI nitric oxide levels remained stable (control: 0.036%, extract: 0.034%, and vitamin C: 0.042%), while IIRI levels dropped to 0.025% (mole/L); this was not true for non-IIRI samples at all. Extraction groups also improved glucose 6-phosphate dehydrogenase levels, so we came to the conclusion that the extract aids the body's natural defense mechanisms. The antiinflammatory properties of neem extracts are significant. Irritation is a pathophysiologic condition that affects several diseases, such as cancer and diabetes; it also affects other conditions, such as alcohol use and food digestion [54]. Neem contains the bioactive chemical limonoid, which is a primary component. One of the most well-known features of limonoid, a furanolactone, is its ability to reduce inflammation and its ability to activate the endogenous opioid pathways. When tested on damaged rat paws, Soares et al. found that limonoid derived from neem inhibited edema and fibrovascular tissue formation. They found that this was most effective at a dose of 120 mg/kg, with a specific inhibitory impact on key inflammatory molecules such as tumor necrosis factor-alpha (TNF-α) and interleukins (ILs) [55]. Epoxy-azadiradione is another chemical that has antiinflammatory properties. It has cytotoxic potential in various pathologies because it acts as a modulator of the macrophage migration inhibitory factor; it inhibits its tautomeric activity and the ability of NFk to translocate, preventing the release of cytokines such as IL-1α, IL-1β, IL-6, and TNF-α from proinflammatory macrophages [56,57].

8.3.2 Phyllanthus emblica

Phyllanthus emblica is endemic to central and southern India, Nepal, Sri Lanka, Burma, Pakistan, Bangladesh, Indonesia, Bhutan, China, and the Mascarene Islands. It was originally grown in Madagascar. There are a number of states in India where it may be found. These include the states of Tamil Nadu, Uttar Pradesh, Himachal Pradesh, Rajasthan, Madhya Pradesh, and Punjab. It may be planted everywhere along the coast and on hillsides up to 200 m in height, as well as in low-lying plains. The Phyllanthaceae family includes *P. emblica*, a medium-sized deciduous tree. An 8–18 m tall tree with light gray bark peeling in little irregular chunks may be found. Simple, subsessile leaves of a light green tint are seen on the branchlets. Pale yellow, globular-shaped fruits are 15–20 mm long and 18–25 mm broad, with six inconspicuous vertical furrows encasing six trigonous seeds in two-seeded three crustaceous cocci. Ripening results in a yellow mesocarp and a yellowish-brown endocarp [58]. When ripe, the fruits turn light brown. The fruit weighs 60–70 g on average. Lower leaflet axils are full of male flowers, whereas the female axils tend to be more sparsely populated with female flowers and some male flowers. February and May are the best months for flowers to bloom, while fruiting happens in December and January. Seeds or grafting can be used to propagate

P. emblica. Because the grafting procedure is dependent on the season, the highest success rate of 87.50% was observed in November, while the lowest success rate was reported in December at 66.69%. In contrast to seedlings, budded clones begin producing fruit after 5 years of planting. Soil with high salt levels, as well as arid and semidry locations, may all be used to grow it [59].

The nutritional value of *P. emblica* has been widely examined. Fruits of *P. emblica* (FPE) contain around 28% of the total tannins in the plant. Accumulating evidence suggests that tannins such as emblicanin A and B, which may be hydrolyzed, have powerful antioxidant effects [60]. Both emblicanin A and emblicanin B hydrolyze to produce gallic acid, ellagic acid, and glucose, respectively. FPE is fibrous and has a sour, bitter, and astringent flavor. Vitamin C concentrations in *P. emblica* fruit juice were greater than in oranges, tangerines, and lemons (478.56 mg/100 mL). Preservatives, pickles, chutneys, and vegetables may all be made with fruits of *P. emblica*. For murabba, fruits of *P. emblica* are also used to soak ripe fruits in concentrated sugar syrup for an extended length of time until the fruit's scent pours out of the syrup. Fresh juice may be made from ripe fruits, which is very handy in the summer. D-fructose, D-glucose, D-myoinositol, and free sugars were found in FPE ethanolic extract. D-arabinose, D-mannosyl, D-galacturonic acid, D-glucosyl, D-galactosyl, D-rhamnosyl, and D-xylosyl residues are found in the acidic water-soluble extract of fruits of *P. emblica*.

Additionally, it has been found to contain a number of essential amino acids and vitamins, including glutamic and proline, aspartic and alanine amino acids, as well as cysteine, cysteine, lysine, and nicotinic acid. Additionally, various other micro- and macronutrients nutrients, such as phosphorus and potassium, calcium and magnesium, as well as iron and manganese, are found [61]. The seed of this fruit also has a considerable quantity of minerals. The nutritional value of *P. emblica* fruits seeds was discovered to contain fixed oil (16%) as well as fatty acids such as linoleic acid (44%), oleic acid (28%), and linolenic acid (8.8%).

8.3.3 Picrorhiza kurroa

Bioactive components in the rhizome of *Picrorhiza kurroa,* such as picroside I and II, cucurbitacins, and apocynin, are responsible for its anticancer properties. Combined with other therapeutic plant extracts, *P. kurroa* effectively inhibited the development of human breast cancer cell lines. It has been claimed that methanolic and aqueous extracts of the plant can be used to treat hepatocellular carcinoma, prostate cancer, and breast cancer as well as to induce apoptosis in cancerous cells. *Bacillus subtilis* (a model organism for Gram-positive bacteria), *Staphylococcus aureus* (a member of the Firmicutes), and *Micrococcus luteus* (belongs to the family Micrococcaceae) were all killed by the ethanolic and methanolic extracts of *P. kurroa*, as were *E. coli* and *P. aeruginose*, which are Gram-negative bacteria. The antiviral activity of n-butanol extract of *P. kurroa* stems containing bis-iridoid and iridoid glycosides has been demonstrated utilizing TREx-HeLa-Vpr cells with no discernible cytotoxicity [62]. In inflammatory conditions, the extract of *P. kurroa* has been demonstrated to limit the proliferation of macrophages, neutrophils, and mast cells. Inflammatory cells can be inhibited by the bioactive components of *P. kurroa*, including apocynin, a catechol. Apocynin suppresses the neutrophil oxidative burst in vitro, but it has no effect on other bacterial elimination processes, including phagocytosis, chemotaxis, or intracellular removal. Antiallergy properties of the drosin component found in *P. kuroa's* rhizomes are used to treat a variety of conditions, including bronchial asthma, skin conditions like eczema, and others. When tested in vitro, *P. kurroa's* extract inhibits the production of histamine. As a result, the extract has also been found to reduce cholesterol levels in the livers of rats. Using indomethacin-induced ulcers in mice, *P. kurroa* has shown substantial antiulcerogenic activity [63]. Mucin production, prostaglandin synthesis, and cyclooxygenase enzyme and growth factor activation are all promoted by this supplement. The extract of *P. kurroa* has been shown to possess bioactive constituents iridoids and picroliv, which demonstrate antiviral action against the hepatitis B virus. Extracted *P. kurroa* demonstrates hepatoprotective efficacy against galactosamine, thioacetamide, rifampicin, and cadmium-induced liver damage in animal and cell cultures. *P. kurroa* has antidiabetic properties because it boosts gallbladder secretion, which aids the liver's fat digestion and metabolism [64]. It was reported that *Picrorhiza* rhizome hydro-alcoholic extract rejuvenated β cells, enhanced insulin production, and reduced hyperglycemic effects, as well as oxidative damage in rats. Accumulation of acetaminophen-caused hepatotoxicity in mice was studied using *P. kurroa* in conjunction with honey. The liver damage caused by acetaminophen was reduced by reducing the activities of serum glutamic pyruvic transaminase and serum glutamic-oxaloacetic transaminase [65]. The plant leaf extract was also examined for its antianemic capacity in a rat anemia model produced by phenylhydrazine and was shown to raise hemoglobin, red blood cell quantity, immature red blood cells without a nucleus, and the ratio of red blood cell volume to total blood volume. In addition to methoxsalen photochemotherapy, the plant has been found to aid in the repigmentation of vitiligo sufferers [66]. There were no toxicologic effects seen in Wistar rats when *P. kurroa* extract was given orally in a standardized formulation at a dosage of 2000 mg/kg body weight, as reported by Krishna et al. (2016) [67].

8.3.4 Ocimum tenuiflorum

In the treatment of gingival and periodontal disorders, chlorhexidine-based medicines have been employed as antibacterial adjuncts. As a result, long-term usage of chlorhexidine should be avoided because of its unattractive side effects, including tooth discoloration and bitter taste. Another drawback is the cytotoxicity of human gingival fibroblasts, periodontal ligament, and osteoblastic cells to this treatment. However, these electrostatic interactions account for the cytotoxic effects of chlorhexidine on mammalian cells, neutrophils, and wound-healing fibroblasts, as well as its antibacterial activity, which is owing to the positive charge of chlorhexidine attaching to the negative charge of bacteria. In addition, the outflow of chromium isotopes from gingival fibroblasts lowers the capacity of chromium to adhere to root surfaces. For this reason, there has been a quest for various natural products that may be safe and helpful for restoring normal health, as well as being cost-effective. Numerous herbal products are revered as "icons of herbs" because of their long tradition of medical use. It is known as "Holy basil," "Tulasi," or tulsi on the Indian subcontinent because of its spiritual significance. It is a fragrant Lamiaceae perennial with a wide distribution in Southeast Asia's tropical regions. It is referred to as "Shahesfaram" in Persian medicine and is used to treat mouth ulcers. Research on *Ocimum tenuiflorum's* scientific data shows that it has medicinal properties. Compositions of nutrients and other physiologically active substances in the plant's phytochemical makeup might vary greatly across the same species [68]. Other elements of *O. tenuiflorum*, including saponins, flavonoids, triterpenoids, and tannins, may also have biologic action in the stem and leaves. Involatile oil from the leaves contains 0.7% eugenol and 0.8% methyl eugenol, with eugenol accounting for 71% of the oil. Other polyphenolic substances with antioxidant and antiinflammatory properties, such as flavonoids and phenolic acids such as rosmarinic acid, apigenin, cirsilineol, apigenin, and isothymusin, have also been discovered [69]. The fixed oil of *O. tenuiflorum* leaf contains linoleic acid, which has been shown to inhibit both the lipoxygenase and cyclooxygenase pathways of the metabolism of arachidonate, which might be responsible for its antiinflammatory effect. *O. tenuiflorum* has also been reported to have a significant antibacterial activity because of eugenol (1-hydroxy 2-methoxy-4-allylbenzene) [9].

8.3.5 Withania somnifera

The most widely distributed species in the genus is *Withania somnifera*. From the Mediterranean to tropical Africa and the Canary and Cape Verde Islands to the Middle East and Arabia, including Afghanistan, Baluchistan, and Pakistan, it grows naturally in arid places like these: South Africa and the African continent as a whole as well as China, Nepal, and India. Throughout Europe, it is grown in gardens, and in South Australia and New South Wales, it has become a noxious plant [10]. When cultivated as a medicinal crop for its fleshy roots in India, it has a wide range of bioactive chemicals with several pharmacologic uses. The plant may be found in Punjab, Gujarat, Uttar Pradesh, Maharashtra, West Bengal, and Rajasthan in India's drier regions. A succulent and xerophytic shrub, *W. somnifera* grows to approximately 2 m tall and 1 m wide and is evergreen, woody, short, fragile, and perineal. Short, silver-gray hairs cover the tomentose branches, which are radially distributed from a central axis. The stems are brownish, ranging from upright to prostrate. This plant has opposite leaves that are green on the top and densely hairy on the underside, which are both virtually hairless. A faded, simple, glabrous green elliptic leaf and bell-shaped green flowers characterize this species. At the leaf nodes, a few inconspicuous bisexual blooms develop. As a calyx with five lobes, it is almost 5 mm in length, while the fruit is around 20 mm long, membranous with 5−10 ribs. 5−8 mm long, bright yellow to yellow-green, narrowly campanulate flower with five lobes. The five protruding stamens are a yellow-orange color. When ripe, the 5−8 mm in diameter, orange-red to crimson, hairless berry is wrapped in an inflated and membrane persistent calyx. The fruit has a large number of spherical seeds that are pale brown and kidney shaped. Fiber-like secondary branches arise from the main root and have a pungent odor and harsh, acidic flavor [10].

8.3.6 Piper nigrum

Piper nigrum, a well-known plant in traditional medicine, has several biologic qualities and is often employed in traditional medicines. However, the antioxidant and antimutagenic properties of fraction-based antioxidants have not yet been thoroughly studied. Sequential extraction in several solvents produced various extracts of the seeds from *P. nigrum*. A variety of assays were used to determine the antibacterial and antioxidant activity of each extract. The Ames Salmonella antimutagenic activity test was used to determine the most active percentage. EsβL-generating *Klebsiella pneumoniae* isolates have less antibacterial efficacy against methicillin-resistant *Staphylococcus aureus* (MRSA). *K. pneumoniae* had lower MIC values than MRSA did. For antimutagenic action against both direct and indirect mutagens, the most potent antioxidant extract (methanol extract) was further investigated. The highest tested concentration of methanol extract (200 g/plate) showed a varied amount of antimutagenic efficacy. The largest classes of chemicals found in the methanol extract were alkaloids, phenols, and flavonoids. The presence of different phytocompounds was discovered using gas chromatography-mass spectrometry. Two primary active phytocompounds (piperine and copaene) were identified to interact with the minor groove of DNA after molecular docking. Under physiologic settings, a molecular dynamics simulation demonstrated that both ligands were very stable with DNA. The capacity of phytocompounds to interact with DNA may reduce the interaction of mutagens, which might be one of the mechanisms of *P. nigrum* extract's antimutagenic effect. The antioxidant and antimutagenic properties of *P. nigrum* are highlighted in this study. For herbal medication research, the role of phytocompounds found in the bioactive extract has to be investigated further [70].

8.3.7 Zingiber officinale

Zingiber officinale (common name: ginger) is an herbaceous perennial plant native to Southern Asia and one of the Zingiberaceae family's spicy spices. For its characteristically spicy and pungent taste, the ginger rhizome is widely used as a spice in food and drink. It is utilized in a range of meals, as well as carbonated drinks, liquors, and sugar syrup preserves. There are several bioactive phenolics found in ginger, including gingerols, shogaol, paradols, and zingerones. Acute rheumatoid arthritis, muscular sprains, nausea, diarrhea, indigestion, fever, viral infections, and helminthiasis are treated with ginger in traditional medicine. It is used as a carminative and stimulant for the gastrointestinal tract in medicine. Ginger possesses antibacterial, antiviral, analgesic, and antipyretic effects, as well as increasing gastrointestinal motility [71].

One of the most prominent effects of ginger is its ability to stimulate the digestive system. Ginger acts as a sialagogue, increasing saliva production and making it easier to swallow. As a remedy for digestive issues, spices like ginger are commonly employed in traditional medicine or as a component in pharmaceutical formulations in animal research, the mechanism of ginger's digestive stimulating activity has been elucidated. Ginger has been shown to increase the formation of bile acid in the liver and its subsequent release into the bile stream. The significance of bile acids in fat digestion and absorption is well established [72]. Ginger has also been shown to have a protective impact on the gastrointestinal tract, with its favorable effects on mucosal glycoproteins reducing mucosal damage in experimental mice. Intestinal brush border membrane fluidity and permeability are altered by consuming dietary ginger, increasing the porous surface of the small intestine [73]. There have been a few studies on the effectiveness of ginger in lowering cholesterol and fat buildup in the body. Dietary ginger's lipid-lowering properties help in weight loss and, as a result, a decreased risk of cardiovascular disease. Compared to the control group, rats fed 0.5% ginger oleoresin combined with a 1% cholesterol diet for 20 days had lower blood and liver cholesterol levels and more excellent fecal cholesterol [74]. Several studies have shown ginger's antidiabetic properties. Ginger has been shown to reduce blood sugar levels in vitro, in vivo, and in humans. The antidiabetic action involves insulin release and sensitivity, as well as reversing altered glucose and lipid metabolism.

Gingerols and shogaols are the active compounds in ginger. Ginger has also been found to protect the liver, kidney, eye, and nervous system against diabetes-related problems [8]. Antioxidant properties and antiinflammatory properties of ginger are well-known. Ginger's pungent components [6]-gingerol and [6]-paradol, as well as other chemicals like zingerone, have been shown to inhibit cancer cell growth in vitro. Multiple pathways likely involved in ginger's chemopreventive potential have been demonstrated in a variety of experimental animals. In the last decade, several in vitro and in vivo investigations have shown dietary ginger's anticancer potential [75]. Given the various health and physiologic effects recognized to be exerted in a translational study, ginger deserves to be regarded a natural and required component of our daily diet, beyond its role in giving flavor to our meals.

8.3.8 Curcuma longa

Traditional medicine and daily cookery have employed *Curcuma longa*, or turmeric, for more than 6000 years as a spice and medicinal ingredient. It is a plant rhizome native to South and Southeast Asia, including Pakistan, China, Indonesia, and India. *C. longa* has also been found in Jamaica and Bangladesh. For centuries, the *Curcuma* genus has been widely utilized as a food preservative, coloring agent, and spice due to its strong therapeutic potential and about 70 identified species of medicinal plants. A member of the Zingiberaceae family, *C. longa* is widely cultivated throughout South East Asia, particularly in China and India. It is 91.44 cm tall, with lance-shaped leaves and yellow blooms that ripen in the thick rhizome or subterranean stem of this medicinal plant. *C. longa* rhizome is used to make the orange-colored medicinal powder that contains the phytochemical components commonly known as turmeric [76]. The phytochemical curcumin, also known as curcumin in Arab nations, saffron or Haridra (in Sanskrit and Ayurvedic) in India, and Jianghuang (yellow ginger) in China and Japan, is one of the primary causes of turmeric's yellow hue. Volatile oils, proteins, carbohydrates, and resins from *C. longa* are present in sufficient amounts. Curcuminoids make up around 2%–9% of this medicinal plant, with curcumin (76.9%), demethoxycurcumin (17.6%), bis-demethoxycurcumin (5.5%), and curcumin making up the rest [7,77].

8.4 Effect of herbal nanoformulation in the applications of tropical delivery

Since the dawn of time, natural materials and chemicals have been employed as herbal remedies. Phytochemicals and natural products are secondary metabolites formed from plants that can have a variety of biologic effects in humans, including anticancer qualities. Many of today's best-selling medications are natural ingredients or derivatives of natural sources. Microorganisms, plants that have been primary sources of natural products (e.g., paclitaxel from *Taxus brevifolia*), sea organisms, and mammals are the four groups of natural products as medical sources. Researchers have created various new delivery technologies, including liposomes and polymeric nanoparticles, to enhance the pharmacokinetics and pharmacodynamics of phytochemicals and natural substances using nanotechnology [78,79]. Natural chemicals and "nanomedicine and natural substances," as searched in PubMed in October 2017, turned up 54,236 and 77 results, respectively. *Nanomedicine* (London), *Nanomedicine NBM*, and the *International Journal of Nanomedicine* have all published large portions of these contributions, as have numerous other publications that have recently shifted their attention solely to nanotechnology and nanomedicine. Even while new research suggests that they can help prevent and treat cancer, the subject is still up for debate. Multitarget mechanisms of action, such as antimutagenic, antioxidant, and antiproliferative properties, are critical to phytochemical anticancer efficacy. The host's immunological response to cancer may also be modulated by them, lowering inflammation and increasing lymphocyte oncosurveillance. Multitargeted anticancer drugs such as phytochemicals may be useful since carcinogenesis is multifactorial and includes several signaling pathways. Natural goods and herbal medicines have been known to be utilized as natural medicinal cures throughout human history. The use of natural products to treat cancer, microbial infection, inflammation, and other disorders has just recently begun to be investigated by a variety of research organizations and physicians. Natural products' limited solubility and bioavailability have hampered scientific studies, making them unsuitable for treating cancer and other disorders. When it comes to improving medication delivery, biodistribution, biosolubility and bioavailability for phytochemicals and natural products in clinical practice, nanotechnology, or nanocarrier design may be a viable option. Research on the chemistry of natural products biosynthesis of nanocarriers, especially the synthesis of nanocompounds with precise sizes and shapes, might lead to the creation and enhancement of innovative nanoparticles that combine natural products for the treatment of sickness and cancer. When it comes to biology, medicine, and other medical professions, nanotechnology is a relatively young scientific field that has a wide range of applications. Nanomaterials in sizes ranging from 1 to 100 nm are used as coating materials or in the treatment and diagnosis of diseases and disorders. Due to the wide range of features and interactions that are specific to the nanoscale structure, nanotechnology has several advantages. Cancer, cardiovascular illness, and central nervous system disease are all disorders that might benefit from nanomedicine's rapid progress in diagnoses and treatment during the previous 15 years. The use of nanotechnology in medication delivery and tailored therapy has been particularly successful. Surface reactivity and insolubleness, a considerably increased surface area in ratio to mass, the capacity to agglomerate or alter size, and greater durability over conventional-scale substances are all properties of nanoparticles that are crucial to their utility. Nanomaterials may also offer considerable potential to increase the bioavailability and biodistribution of phytochemicals and natural products because of their quick manufacturing and inclusion into consumer items and medications. Polymer nanoparticles, solid lipid nanoparticles, crystal nanoparticles, liposomes, micelles, and dendrimers are among the best nanoparticles for medication delivery and biodistribution of phytochemicals and natural products. As a medication delivery vehicle, each one of these nanoparticles has its strengths and weaknesses [80]. It is possible to choose the type of nanoparticles employed in a certain delivery application depending on the phytochemical or natural product's physicochemical characteristics, hydrophilicity, or hydrophobicity. The liposomal aqueous compartment generated by the hydrophilic head groups of the phospholipids can be ideal for integrating one or more hydrophilic medicines [80]. In this context, as an alternative, the lipophilic tails of phospholipids constitute the drug-containing compartment in a micelle for lipophilic drugs; however, in circumstances when the lipophilic medication dissolves into the liposomal bilayer, liposomes have been employed. Liposome size, surface charge, and number of lamellae all have an impact on the biosolubility of phytochemicals, which may be further improved and optimized.

8.5 Summary

Herbs have a broad spectrum of phytochemical ingredients that contribute to their therapeutic effectiveness. Ayurveda is a system of ancient Indian medicine practiced for thousands of years. Evidence of the usage of medicinal plants in India dates back to the second millennium BC. Ayurveda is a scientific culture of healing that emerged from tribal and wandering healers in the lower Himalayas and Indo-Gangetic region. Traditional herbs such as *A. indica, P. emblica, O. tenuiflorum, P. nigrum, Z. officinale,* and *C. longa* were discussed. The use of these herbs for the treatment of a variety of critical conditions has been documented in the literature, which is highlighted in this chapter. Fracture therapy and the traditional profession of bone setters rely on antiinflammation as a fundamental premise. NO appears to have an essential role in inflammatory diseases like rheumatoid arthritis. An antiinflammatory agent might be used to minimize this reaction. *C. quadrangularis* possesses bone-healing capabilities. Ethanolic extract of *C. buchanani* leaf extract protects the liver from acetaminophen-induced hepatotoxicity. Increased serum biochemical parameters such as GOT, GPT, and GAP are shown in the serum of those who take the extract. The medicinal qualities of the plant stem, leaves, and roots are reported. Osteoarthritis, osteoporosis, and rheumatoid arthritis are among the conditions for which the herb has been used in Ayurveda. It is also effective in treating dyspepsia and colic.

The use of natural products to treat cancer, microbial infection, inflammation, and other disorders has just recently begun to be investigated. When it comes to improving medication delivery, biodistribution, biosolubility, and bioavailability for phytochemicals and natural products in clinical practice, nanotechnology may be a viable option. Nanomaterials offer considerable potential to increase the bioavailability and biodistribution of phytochemicals and natural products. Polymer nanoparticles, solid lipid nanoparticles, and crystal nanoparticles are among the best nanoparticles for medication delivery.

References

[1] V.L. Dhadge, M. Changmai, M.K. Purkait, Purification of catechins from Camellia sinensis using membrane cell, Food and Bioproducts Processing 117 (2019) 203–212.

[2] T.N. Baite, B. Mandal, M.K. Purkait, Ultrasound assisted extraction of gallic acid from Ficus auriculata leaves using green solvent, Food and Bioproducts Processing 128 (2021) 1–11.

[3] V. Singh, Medicinal plants and bone healing, National Journal of Maxillofacial Surgery 8 (1) (2017) 4–11.

[4] B. Debnath, D. Haldar, M.K. Purkait, Potential and sustainable utilization of tea waste: a review on present status and future trends, Journal of Environmental Chemical Engineering 9 (5) (2021) 106179.

[5] B. Debnath, D. Haldar, M.K. Purkait, A critical review on the techniques used for the synthesis and applications of crystalline cellulose derived from agricultural wastes and forest residues, Carbohydrate Polymers 273 (2021) 118537.

[6] M.A. Alzohairy, Therapeutics role of Azadirachta indica (neem) and their active constituents in diseases prevention and treatment, Evidence-Based Complementary and Alternative Medicine 2016 (2016).

[7] R.V. Lawand, S.V. Gandhi, Comparison of Curcuma caesia Roxb. with other commonly used Curcuma species by HPTLC, Journal of Pharmacognosy and Phytochemistry 2 (4) (2013) 126–131.

[8] Y. Li, et al., Preventive and protective properties of Zingiber officinale (ginger) in diabetes mellitus, diabetic complications, and associated lipid and other metabolic disorders: a brief review, Evidence-Based Complementary and Alternative Medicine 2012 (2012).

[9] S. Mallikarjun, et al., Antimicrobial efficacy of Tulsi leaf (Ocimum sanctum) extract on periodontal pathogens: an in vitro study, Journal of Indian Society of Periodontology 20 (2) (2016) 145.

[10] S. Paul, et al., Withania somnifera (L.) Dunal (Ashwagandha): a comprehensive review on ethnopharmacology, pharmacotherapeutics, biomedicinal and toxicological aspects, Biomedicine & Pharmacotherapy 143 (2021) 112175.

[11] M.A. Abd Jalil, A.N. Shuid, N. Muhammad, Role of medicinal plants and natural products on osteoporotic fracture healing, Evidence-based Complementary and Alternative Medicine : eCAM 2012 (2012), pp. 714512–714512.

[12] I.H. Kalfas, Principles of bone healing, Neurosurgical Focus 10 (4) (2001) 1–4.

[13] R. Guarniero, de Barros Filho, U. Tannuri, C.J. Rodrigues, J.D. Rossi, Study of fracture healing in protein malnutrition, Revista Paulista de Medicina 110 (2) (1992) 63–68.

[14] G. Chen, F. Niemeyer, T. Wehner, U. Simon, M.A. Schuetz, M.J. Pearcy, L.E. Claes, Simulation of the nutrient supply in fracture healing, Journal of Biomechanics 42 (15) (2009) 2575–2583.

[15] W.-S. Siu, et al., Evaluation of a topical herbal agent for the promotion of bone healing, Evidence-based Complementary and Alternative Medicine 2015 (2015).

[16] K. Tayung, N. Saikia, Cryptolepis buchanani—a less-known medicinal plant used in bone fracture, Indian Journal of Traditional Knowledge 2 (2003) 371–373.
[17] M. Khond, et al., Screening of some selected medicinal plants extracts for in-vitro antimicrobial activity, Middle-East Journal of Scientific Research 4 (4) (2009) 271–278.
[18] N. Hanprasertpong, et al., Analgesic, anti-inflammatory, and chondroprotective activities of Cryptolepis buchanani extract: in vitro and in vivo studies, BioMed Research International 2014 (2014).
[19] S. Jagtap, et al., Antimicrobial activity of some crude herbal drugs used for skin diseases by pawra tribes of Nandurbar district, Journal of Natural Products 1 (2010) 216–220.
[20] K. Padmalochana, M.D. Rajan, Evaluation of the antioxidant and hepatoprotective activity of Cryptolepis buchanani, Journal of Applied Pharmaceutical Science 3 (2) (2013) 99.
[21] H. Meijer, et al., The production of anti-inflammatory cytokines in whole blood by physico-chemical induction, Inflammation Research 52 (10) (2003) 404–407.
[22] A. Frizziero, et al., Autologous conditioned serum for the treatment of osteoarthritis and other possible applications in musculoskeletal disorders, British Medical Bulletin 105 (1) (2013) 169–184.
[23] M.-H. Liu, et al., Icariin protects murine chondrocytes from lipopolysaccharide-induced inflammatory responses and extracellular matrix degradation, Nutrition Research 30 (1) (2010) 57–65.
[24] L. Zhang, et al., Icariin promotes extracellular matrix synthesis and gene expression of chondrocytes in vitro, Phytotherapy Research 26 (9) (2012) 1385–1392.
[25] P.P. Srinivasan, et al., Injectable perlecan domain 1-hyaluronan microgels potentiate the cartilage repair effect of BMP2 in a murine model of early osteoarthritis, Biomedical Materials 7 (2) (2012) 024109.
[26] P. Chen, et al., The amelioration of cartilage degeneration by ADAMTS-5 inhibitor delivered in a hyaluronic acid hydrogel, Biomaterials 35 (9) (2014) 2827–2836.
[27] R. Schütz, et al., Synthesis, biological evaluation and toxicity of novel tetrandrine analogues, European Journal of Medicinal Chemistry 207 (2020) 112810.
[28] F. Li, et al., Molecular mechanisms involved in drug-induced liver injury caused by urate-lowering Chinese herbs: a network pharmacology study and biology experiments, PLoS One 14 (5) (2019) e0216948.
[29] X.-M. Qi, et al., ROS generated by CYP450, especially CYP2E1, mediate mitochondrial dysfunction induced by tetrandrine in rat hepatocytes, Acta Pharmacologica Sinica 34 (9) (2013) 1229–1236.
[30] H. Jin, et al., Pulmonary toxicity and metabolic activation of tetrandrine in CD-1 mice, Chemical Research in Toxicology 24 (12) (2011) 2142–2152.
[31] Y. Sakurai, et al., Two-pore channels control Ebola virus host cell entry and are drug targets for disease treatment, Science 347 (6225) (2015) 995–998.
[32] Q.-Y. Liu, E. Karpinski, P. Pang, Tetrandrine inhibits both T and L calcium channel currents in ventricular cells, Journal of Cardiovascular Pharmacology 20 (4) (1992) 513–519.
[33] M.A. Ludeña Huaman, et al., A simple method to obtain ursolic acid, Results in Chemistry 3 (2021) 100144.
[34] V. Saldaña-Bobadilla, et al., Tiquilia paronychioides (Phil.) AT Richardson (Boraginaceae): Una revisión etnobotánica, etnofarmacológica y, Ethnobotany Research and Applications 19 (25) (2020).
[35] R. Csuk, B. Siewert, A convenient separation of ursolic and oleanolic acid, Tetrahedron Letters 52 (49) (2011) 6616–6618.

[36] J.-P. Fan, D.-D. Liao, X.-H. Zhang, Ultrasonic assisted extraction of ursolic acid from apple pomace: a novel and facile technique, Separation Science and Technology 51 (8) (2016) 1344–1350.
[37] S.S. Islam, et al., Natural medicinal plant products as an immune-boosters: a possible role to lessen the impact of Covid-19, Case Studies in Chemical and Environmental Engineering 4 (2021) 100105.
[38] J.F.-W. Chan, et al., Genomic characterization of the 2019 novel human-pathogenic coronavirus isolated from a patient with atypical pneumonia after visiting Wuhan, Emerging Microbes & Infections 9 (1) (2020) 221–236.
[39] Y.-R. Guo, et al., The origin, transmission and clinical therapies on coronavirus disease 2019 (COVID-19) outbreak—an update on the status, Military Medical Research 7 (1) (2020) 1–10.
[40] Y.B. Ryu, et al., Biflavonoids from Torreya nucifera displaying SARS-CoV 3CLpro inhibition, Bioorganic & Medicinal Chemistry 18 (22) (2010) 7940–7947.
[41] J.-Y. Park, et al., Dieckol, a SARS-CoV 3CLpro inhibitor, isolated from the edible brown algae Ecklonia cava, Bioorganic & Medicinal Chemistry 21 (13) (2013) 3730.
[42] D. Hong-Zhi, et al., Traditional Chinese Medicine: an effective treatment for 2019 novel coronavirus pneumonia (NCP), Chinese Journal of Natural Medicines 18 (3) (2020) 206–210.
[43] Y.-H. Jin, et al., A rapid advice guideline for the diagnosis and treatment of 2019 novel coronavirus (2019-nCoV) infected pneumonia (standard version), Military Medical Research 7 (1) (2020) 1–23.
[44] M.R. Naik, et al., Study of anti-inflammatory effect of neem seed oil (Azadirachta indica) on infected albino rats, Journal of Health Research and Reviews 1 (3) (2014) 66.
[45] E. Hernández-Aquino, P. Muriel, Beneficial effects of naringenin in liver diseases: molecular mechanisms, World Journal of Gastroenterology 24 (16) (2018) 1679.
[46] S. Saleem, et al., A comprehensive review of phytochemical profile, bioactives for pharmaceuticals, and pharmacological attributes of Azadirachta indica, Phytotherapy Research 32 (7) (2018) 1241–1272.
[47] P. Kundu, et al., Chemical investigation of neem leaf glycoprotein used as immuno-prophylactic agents for tumor growth restriction, International Journal of Pharmacy and Pharmaceutical Sciences 7 (2015) 195–199.
[48] S.P. Dash, S. Dixit, S. Sahoo, Phytochemical and biochemical characterizations from leaf extracts from Azadirachta Indica: an important medicinal plant, Biochemistry & Analytical Biochemistry 6 (323) (2017), pp. 2161–1009.1000323.
[49] Z.S.S. Al-Hashemi, M.A. Hossain, Biological activities of different neem leaf crude extracts used locally in Ayurvedic medicine, Pacific Science Review A: Natural Science and Engineering 18 (2) (2016) 128–131.
[50] M.A. Hossain, et al., Identification and characterization of chemical compounds in different crude extracts from leaves of Omani neem, Journal of Taibah University for Science 7 (4) (2013) 181–188.
[51] H.S.K. Al-Jadidi, M.A. Hossain, Studies on total phenolics, total flavonoids and antimicrobial activity from the leaves crude extracts of neem traditionally used for the treatment of cough and nausea, Beni-Suef University Journal of Basic and Applied Sciences 4 (2) (2015) 93–98.
[52] M.K. Gautam, et al., Effects of Azardirachta indica on vascular endothelial growth factor and cytokines in diabetic deep wound, Planta Medica 81 (09) (2015) 713–721.
[53] C. Page, E.M. Hawes, Haemolytic anaemia after ingestion of neem (Azadirachta indica) tea, Case Reports 2013 (2013) bcr2013200890.
[54] X. Zeng, P. Zhang, Y. Wang, C. Qin, S. Chen, W. He, L. Tao, Y. Tan, D. Gao, B. Wang, Z. Chen, W. Chen, Y.Y. Jiang, Y.Z. Chen, CMAUP a database of collective

molecular activities of useful plants, Nucleic Acids Research 47 (D1) (2019) D1118–D1127, https://doi.org/10.1093/nar/gky965.
[55] D.G. Soares, et al., Anti-inflammatory and antinociceptive activities of azadirachtin in mice, Planta Medica 80 (08/09) (2014) 630–636.
[56] G. Shilpa, et al., Epoxyazadiradione purified from the Azadirachta indica seed induced mitochondrial apoptosis and inhibition of NFκB nuclear translocation in human cervical cancer cells, Phytotherapy Research 31 (12) (2017) 1892–1902.
[57] J.F. Islas, et al., An overview of neem (Azadirachta indica) and its potential impact on health, Journal of Functional Foods 74 (2020) 104171.
[58] K.H. Khan, Roles of Emblica officinalis in medicine-a review, Botany Research International 2 (4) (2009) 218–228.
[59] R. Saini, et al., Traditional uses, bioactive composition, pharmacology, and toxicology of Phyllanthus emblica fruits: a comprehensive review, Journal of Ethnopharmacology 282 (2022) 114570.
[60] S.K. Bhattacharya, et al., Effect of bioactive tannoid principles of Emblica officinalis on ischemia-reperfusion-induced oxidative stress in rat heart, Phytomedicine 9 (2) (2002) 171–174.
[61] N. Barthakur, N. Arnold, Chemical analysis of the emblic (Phyllanthus emblica L.) and its potential as a food source, Scientia Horticulturae 47 (1–2) (1991) 99–105.
[62] N.N. Win, et al., Bis-iridoid and iridoid glycosides: viral protein R inhibitors from Picrorhiza kurroa collected in Myanmar, Fitoterapia 134 (2019) 101–107.
[63] P. Debnath, et al., Picrorhiza kurroa: a promising traditional therapeutic herb from higher altitude of western Himalayas, Journal of Herbal Medicine 23 (2020) 100358.
[64] R.K. Verma, T. Paraidathathu, Herbal medicines used in the traditional Indian medicinal system as a therapeutic treatment option for overweight and obesity management: a review, International Journal of Pharmacy and Pharmaceutical Sciences 6 (2) (2014) 40–47.
[65] P. Gupta, et al., Synergistic protective effect of picrorhiza with honey in acetaminophen induced hepatic injury, Indian Journal of Experimental Biology 54 (2016) 530–536.
[66] S. Gianfaldoni, et al., Herbal compounds for the treatment of vitiligo: a review, Open access Macedonian journal of medical sciences 6 (1) (2018) 203.
[67] A.B. Krishna, et al., Single dose oral toxicity study of Picrorhiza kurroa rhizome extract in Wistar rats, Fundamental toxicological sciences 3 (1) (2016) 9–12.
[68] A. Jankish, et al., Comparative evaluation of antimicrobial and anti-gingivitis effect of Ocimum tenuiflorum Linn. gel with 0.2% chlorhexidine gel – randomized controlled clinical trial, Journal of Herbal Medicine 29 (2021) 100478.
[69] M. Kelm, et al., Antioxidant and cyclooxygenase inhibitory phenolic compounds from Ocimum sanctum Linn, Phytomedicine 7 (1) (2000) 7–13.
[70] M. Zahin, et al., Antioxidant, antibacterial, and antimutagenic activity of Piper nigrum seeds extracts, Saudi Journal of Biological Sciences 28 (9) (2021) 5094–5105.
[71] K. Srinivasan, Ginger rhizomes (Zingiber officinale): a spice with multiple health beneficial potentials, PharmaNutrition 5 (1) (2017) 18–28.
[72] K. Platel, K. Srinivasan, Digestive stimulant action of spices: a myth or reality? Indian Journal of Medical Research 119 (5) (2004) 167.
[73] U.N. Prakash, K. Srinivasan, Gastrointestinal protective effect of dietary spices during ethanol-induced oxidant stress in experimental rats, Applied Physiology Nutrition and Metabolism 35 (2) (2010) 134–141.
[74] U. Bhandari, J. Sharma, R. Zafar, The protective action of ethanolic ginger (Zingiber officinale) extract in cholesterol fed rabbits, Journal of Ethnopharmacology 61 (2) (1998) 167–171.

[75] C.-Z. Wang, L.-W. Qi, C.-S. Yuan, Cancer chemoprevention effects of ginger and its active constituents: potential for new drug discovery, The American Journal of Chinese Medicine 43 (07) (2015) 1351–1363.
[76] S. Sultana, et al., Molecular targets for the management of cancer using Curcuma longa Linn. phytoconstituents: a Review, Biomedicine & Pharmacotherapy 135 (2021) 111078.
[77] J.L. Funk, et al., Efficacy and mechanism of action of turmeric supplements in the treatment of experimental arthritis, Arthritis & Rheumatism 54 (11) (2006) 3452–3464.
[78] M. Gera, et al., Nanoformulations of curcumin: an emerging paradigm for improved remedial application, Oncotarget 8 (39) (2017) 66680–66698.
[79] P. Duarah, D. Haldar, M.K. Purkait, Technological advancement in the synthesis and applications of lignin-based nanoparticles derived from agro-industrial waste residues: a review, International Journal of Biological Macromolecules 163 (2020) 1828–1843.
[80] C. Enrico, Chapter 3 – nanotechnology-based drug delivery of natural compounds and phytochemicals for the treatment of cancer and other diseases, in: R. Atta ur (Ed.), Studies in Natural Products Chemistry, Elsevier, 2019, pp. 91–123.

CHAPTER 9

Pharmacologic and therapeutic aspects of various medicinal plants

9.1 Introduction

Two-thirds of the world's plant species are therapeutic. Chemical compounds with medicinal potential can be found in plants, and these plants can give new leads for pharmaceutical production. According to estimates from the World Health Organization, over 80% of the world's population practices traditional medicine, with herbal extracts and their active components accounting for a large portion of the therapy [1,2]. A lot of work is being put into discovering new properties in existing medicinal plants and their components. Herbal medicine has been practiced in India, China, Egypt, and Syria for over 5000 years, according to historical records. *Charaka Samhita*, *Rigveda*, *Atharva Veda*, and *Sushruta Samhita* are ancient Indian literature on human medicine. Humans learned to distinguish between edible and harmful plants through studying animals, according to the *Rigveda*. As a result, our ancient civilization's traditional and scientific traditions opened the path for creating herbal remedies. Ethnobotany, according to Morgenstern, is the study of indigenous plant use and its interaction with humans. Herbal cures exist in folk medicine from all cultures throughout the world. South Africa, for example, has incorporated the use of medicinal herbs into its fundamental healthcare system [3].

Herbs are a diverse range of plants having medicinal and culinary purposes. Researchers are particularly interested in herbs that have antiplatelet, anticancer, hypolipidemic, and immune-stimulating qualities, as these features may help lower the chances of cancer and cardiovascular disease [1]. Known for its medicinal and culinary properties, black cumin (*Nigella sativa* L.) is a common ingredient in many traditional medicines. Black cumin has a wide range of physiologically active compounds that

Advances in Extraction and Applications of Bioactive Phytochemicals
ISBN 978-0-443-18535-9
https://doi.org/10.1016/B978-0-443-18535-9.00002-8

include analgesic, anticancer, antiepileptogenic, antiinflammatory, antioxidant, antibacterial, antischistosomiasis, and immunomodulatory properties, as well as gastroprotective, hepatoprotective, and nephron protective properties [4]. In addition to *N. sativa*, *Abelmoschus manihot* (edible hibiscus), *Thespesia populnea* (Indian tulip tree, or milo), *Abutilon indicum* (Indian mallow), *Mucuna pruriens* (velvet bean), *Solanum surattense* (Surattense nightshade), and *Senna auriculata* (matura tea) have all been extensively studied for the treatment of various diseases.

A variety of medicinal plants are discussed in detail in this chapter, including their habitat, morphology, phytoconstituents content, and pharmacologic advantages. Characteristics of some of the primary bioactive chemicals present in the medicinal plants described are also emphasized.

9.2 Medicinal effect of *Nigella sativa* in different fields

N. Sativa is an annual plant that grows 20–90 cm tall and has finely split petals. The yellow, white, pink, blue, or purple blossoms are petite and delicate, with 5–10 petals. There are 3–7 linked follicles in the fruit, each containing many seeds. *N. Sativa* has been utilized for hundreds of years to cure respiratory, digestive, renal, and hepatic problems, as well as to improve the cardiovascular and immune systems. Avicenna's "*Canon of Medicine*" mentions black seeds helping the body recover from tiredness and disappointment. In Indian and Arabian traditions, black seeds and their oil have been utilized for many centuries as food and medicine. In Southeast Asian and Middle Eastern countries, the seeds are used to treat bronchitis, asthma, rheumatism, and other inflammatory illnesses. *N. Sativa* has been given the Arabic moniker "Habbatul barakah," which translates to "seed of blessing." Indigestion, loss of appetite, diarrhea, dropsy, amenorrhea, dysmenorrhea, worms, and skin eruptions are treated using a tincture made from the seeds. It works as an antiseptic as well as a local anesthetic. Internally, black seeds that have been roasted help to prevent vomiting [5].

Fig. 9.1 illustrates some primary compounds present in the *N. Sativa* seed and oil. Thymoquinone (TQ), thymol, proteins, oleic acid, phellandrene, and carbohydrates are all major chemical elements of *N. Sativa*. The primary components of black seeds have previously been extracted and identified as oleic acid, linoleic acid, palmitic acid, and trans-anethole. According to Kumar et al. (2010), the plant is rich in quinones and phenolics [7]. Harzallah et al. (2011) extracted 48 distinct compounds from

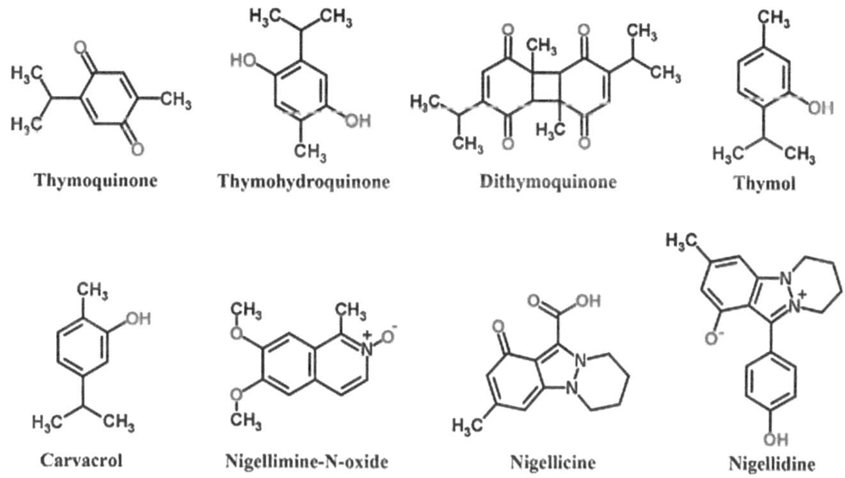

Figure 9.1 TQ and other chemical components of *N. Sativa* seed extracts and oils. *(Reproduced with permission from Majdalawieh et al. [6].)*

black seed oils, the majority of which were TQ [8]. According to Benkaci-Ali et al. (2013), the seeds of *N. Sativa* produce a variety of chemicals, the majority of which are monoterpene hydrocarbons [9]. Recent research has reported that the plant contains an array of biochemicals, primarily phenols, terpenes, and flavonoids [10].

N. Sativa seeds have a variety of therapeutic qualities. The plant has been used to treat asthma, hypertension, stomach problems, liver diseases, immunologic disorders, cancer, neurologic disorders, and a variety of other ailments in herbal therapy. In a modified paper disc diffusion technique, the antibacterial impact of pulverized black seeds was investigated. With pure water as a control, a dose of 300 mg/mL repressed the growth of *Staphylococcus aureus* clearly, and this repression was validated using the positive control azithromycin. The inhibition achieved with Hadramout *N. Sativa* ground seeds was more significant than with Ethiopian *N. Sativa* ground seeds. TQ and melanin, two major active components of *N. Sativa*, are thought to be responsible for the positive inhibition [11]. Various raw extracts of *N. Sativa*, consisting of 16 Gram-negative and 6 Gram-positive samples, were tested for antibacterial activity against a range of bacterial strains. Antibiotic resistance was found in these isolates, particularly in the Gram-negative strains. *N. Sativa* crude extracts had a significant effect against certain test species. A combination of water and alkaloid extracts proved to be the most potent. When it came to Gram-positive and

Gram-negative isolates, the latter were more seriously damaged [12]. Hannah et al. (2008) investigated *N. Saliva's* antibacterial efficacy against methicillin-resistant *Staphylococcus aureus*. The ethanolic extract of *N. Sativa* at a dosage of 4 mg/disc was sensitive to all methicillin-resistant *Staphylococcus aureus* strains tested, with a MIC range of 0.2–0.5 mg/mL [13]. Its antibacterial properties and the efficacy of triple therapy in eliminating *Helicobacter pylori* in patients with nonulcer dyspepsia were studied. It was discovered that *N. Sativa* seeds had anti-*H. Pylori* activity equivalent to triple treatment. On 11 human pathogenic bacteria, TQ's antibacterial activity and biofilm inhibition potencies were studied. TQ has a bactericidal action against a variety of human pathogenic microorganisms, including Gram-positive cocci [14].

N. Sativa extracts in methanolic form show the highest antifungal action, followed by extracts in chloroform, against several strains of *Candida albicans*. The antifungal activity of aqueous extracts was nonexistent. *C. albicans* colonies were found in the liver, spleen, and kidneys after intravenous inoculation of the bacterium. Immediately after inoculation, the plant extract had a significant impact on the development of the organism in all organs examined. According to the study, *N. Sativa* seed aqueous extract inhibited candidiasis growth in mice. The plant extract reduced *Candida* in kidneys by five times, liver by eight times, and spleen by 11 times in groups of mice. Histopathologic investigation of the relevant organs corroborated these findings. *Trichophyton interdigitale*, *Epidermophyton floccosum*, *Trichophyton mentagrophytes*, and *Microsporum canis* were tested using the Agar diffusion technique. Between 10–40 and 0.125–0.250 mg/mL, respectively, the *N. Sativa* ether extract and TQ had MICs, while those of griseofulvin varied from 0.00095 to 0.01550 mg/mL. For the treatment of fungal skin diseases, folk medicine relies on the use of *N. Sativa* as a source of antifungal medicines [15]. The antifungal efficacy of the black cumin seed quinines, dithymoquinone, thymohydroquinone, and TQ against six dairy spoilage yeast species was investigated in vitro using a broth microdilution technique. There were considerable antifungal effects of thymohydroquinone and TQ compared with preservatives frequently used in milk products at two pH levels (4.0 and 5.5) [16]. Ns-D1 and Ns-D2, two new antifungal defensins, were identified and sequenced from *N. Sativa* seeds. A variety of phytopathogenic fungi were shown to be resistant to the antifungal action of the Ns-D1 and Ns-D2 defensins [17].

9.2.1 Treatment for asthma

More than 0.3 billion people worldwide suffer from asthma, a respiratory illness with hereditary or environmental causes. In many regions of the world, the seeds, oil, and herbal tea of *N. Sativa* have all been utilized to treat acute and chronic asthma symptoms. Boskabady et al. (2010) reported that daily use of boiling *N. Sativa* seed extracts alleviated asthma symptoms in asthmatic patients [18]. In another trial, 15 asthmatic patients were given boiling extracts, which increased bronchodilatory responses. Patients' asthmatic problems improved to some extent after they received 1–2 g of *N. Sativa* per day for a period of 2 weeks [19]. Using a 500-mg capsule twice per day, Koshak et al. (2017) concluded that the seed oil helped patients with controlled asthma treated with the oil [20]. Ethanolic extracts and oil dramatically decreased histamine release and alleviated asthmatic symptoms in rats in animal studies. When guinea pigs were given *N. Sativa* oil instead of a control group, airway inflammation was decreased, and asthma was managed [21]. *N. Sativa* appears to contain these qualities that contribute to significant asthma control since typical anti-asthmatic drugs serve as dilating agents of the airways in addition to their antiinflammatory actions.

9.2.2 Role in diabetes control

Various research has been undertaken throughout the years better to understand the role of *N. Sativa* in diabetes control. For example, one of the studies explored the therapeutic potentials of alpha-lipoic acid (α-LA), L-carnitine, and *N. Sativa*, or a combination of them, in the glucose and lipid metabolism of diabetic rats treated with 65 mg/kg streptozotocin (STZ). Because of its capacity to specifically target and kill insulin-producing pancreatic islet β cells, STZ is the most often employed agent in experimental diabetes. C-peptide, homeostatic model assessment, and pyruvate dehydrogenase activity were all tested to investigate glucose metabolism. α-LA and *N. Sativa* both lowered high blood glucose levels. The combination of three substances resulted in a considerable rise in insulin and C-peptide concentrations. The combination of α-LA, L-carnitine, and *N. Sativa* would significantly increase carbohydrate metabolism in diabetic rats, increasing the rate of diabetes mellitus (DM) treatment success [22]. In streptozotocin-diabetic rats, the effects of *N. Sativa* aqueous extract and oil, as well as TQ, were examined. Tests were conducted to evaluate insulin and glucose concentrations in the blood, superoxide dismutase (SOD) levels, and malondialdehyde (MDA) concentrations in pancreatic tissue. Any subcellular alterations were observed by using electron microscopy. Diabetic patients have higher amounts of MDA in tissues and serum glucose, but insulin and SOD levels are lower. STZ's toxicity was mitigated by TQ's ultrastructural effects, which included mitochondrial vacuolization and disintegration, as well as segregated nucleoli and heterochromatin aggregates (showing DNA damage). *N. Sativa*'s aqueous extract reversed STZ's effects in a similar way, but with a less amount. There was an improvement in insulin levels, but after 10 days of treatment, glucose concentrations in diabetics were much lower than those in the untreated diabetic group, although insulin levels were not significantly elevated. It is hypothesized that TQ and *N. Sativa* extract have therapeutic and protective effects against STZ-diabetes by lowering oxidative stress, which preserves pancreas cells. Due to improved cell ultrastructure, the hypoglycemic effect may have been caused by higher insulin levels. TQ and *N. Sativa* may be effective in the treatment of diabetes and the prevention of oxidative stress in cells [23].

Diabetes is one of the most common causes of mortality in individuals all over the world; however, prevention and a healthy lifestyle can lower the risk of subsequent illnesses. Globally, it affects around 400 million individuals and will reach 600 million by 2050. The benefits of *N. Sativa* for diabetics are widely documented. Using *N. Sativa* capsules reduced blood glucose levels and other indicators in type 2 diabetic patients. In a comparative trial, oral *N. Sativa* supplementation reduced glucose concentration and dyslipidemia in patients. Also, *N. Sativa* oil improved lipid profiles and glycemic control in type 2 diabetes studies. Oral *N. Sativa* supplementation helped diabetic patients regulate cholesterol and other indicators. Reflections on the effects of seed extracts and oils on diabetic rats and other model organisms are common [24].

9.2.3 Efficacy against different types of cancer

There have been several reports on the usefulness of *N. Sativa* seeds in the treatment of various malignancies. Still, more research is needed to thoroughly understand the underlying processes of the plant's anticancer properties. Studies on rats, rabbits, and in rare cases, humans using *N. Sativa* as a cancer prevention medication have yielded promising results. According to Fathy et al. (2018), ethanolic extracts inhibited the development of tumors and carcinomas in rat models. Proliferating cell lines in the breast cancer cell line (human) investigation were killed by *N. Sativa*, demonstrating anticancer properties [25]. Shanmugam et al. (2018) stated that the anticancer activities of *N. Sativa* were linked to TQ, a significant component of the plant. Using human ovarian cancer cell lines as a model, researchers found that *N. Sativa* seed extracts had antiproliferative effects. Different extracts of *N. Sativa* were found to have antiproliferative effects on HeLa cell lines in recent research. *N. Sativa* extracts, oils, and pulp have been shown in various research to have antioxidative and anticancer effects in model organisms. Its chemical ingredient TQ, which is antiproliferative, antioxidant, protective, and gene regulatory, is the key to *N. Saliva*'s ability to fight cancer [4].

9.2.4 Common effects

TQ, thymol, and nigellone are all pharmaceutically significant compounds in *N. Sativa*, making it a potential source of therapeutics for a variety of ailments. Its antianalgesic, antiinflammatory, antiasthmatic, wound-healing, rheumatoid arthritis—corrective, antioxidative, and immune-stimulant activities have been demonstrated in its extracts, oil, and supplements. In animal studies, the extract of *N. Sativa* and oil have been shown to have positive effects on obesity, lipid profile, and insulin regulation. Al Mofleh et al. (2008) revealed that *N. Sativa* has antiulcerative effects in rats [26]. *N. Sativa* seeds have been found to have beneficial effects on animals with heart disease and cardiotoxicity. In rats, Parhizkar et al. (2016) found that *N. Sativa* improved the menstrual and postmenopausal cycles of rats, as well as their reproductive health [27]. Male rats' sperm counts increased in direct connection to *N. Sativa* oil consumption, according to research. *N. Sativa* dramatically enhanced renal function and avoided cytotoxicity in rats during five-week research. When mice were given *N. Sativa* oil, it was shown to protect them against reactive oxygen species and cause convulsions. The antitoxin and antiherpetic properties of black seed have also been demonstrated in other research investigations [4].

9.3 Selective plants in the treatment of different diseases

9.3.1 Abelmoschus manihot

The most significant medicinal plant in the Malvaceae family is *A. Manihot*, found in New Caledonia, India, China, and Papua New Guinea. For hundreds of years, nearly all portions of the *A. Manihot* medicinal plants have been widely used as traditional medicine. *A. Manihot* leaf extract has been discovered to have analgesic and antioxidant properties, while stem extract has an antiinflammation effect. *A. Manihot's* medicinal properties have been linked to the prevention of heart attack and ischemic brain damage, as well as the improvement of kidney function and the treatment of diabetic mellitus. *A. Manihot* is currently a key ingredient in Huang Kui capsule, China's most popular medicine for treating diabetic nephropathy and chronic glomerulonephritis. Pan et al. (2018) used the UPLC−MS/MS technique to identify five main flavonoid components in various *A. Manihot*, including hyperoside, quercetin, myricetin, isoquercitrin, and rutin [28]. Mass spectrometric analysis revealed that the concentration of five flavonoid constituents is organized as follows: flower > leaf > stem > root.

The UPLC-TQ-MS/MS approach was used by Du et al. (2015) to identify 12 bioactive chemicals from the parts of *A. Manihot* plant, including 2′-deoxyinosine, 2′-deoxyuridine, uracil, inosine, 2′-deoxyadenosine, adenine, guanine, cytidine, and 2′-deoxyadenosine-5′-monophosphate [29]. Even though the varying patterns of these bioactive chemicals have been studied, the processes underlying their change remain unknown and require further investigation. There were 297.43 ± 0.48 mg gallic acid equivalent/g of total phenolic content in *A. Manihot* leaf extract and 117.31 ± 0.38 mg quercetin equivalent/g of total flavonoid content in the extract, according to the study by Taroreh et al. (2016) [30]. In another study, *A. Manihot* stem methanol extract was studied in ICR mice at several doses, comprising 500, 1000, 1500, 2000, and 2500 mg/kg of extract. After 14 days of extract administration, mice were observed. During the 14 days of observation, no mice died or showed any behavioral abnormalities such as ataxia or hyperactivity. The plant extract exhibits no negative effects at any level, proving that it is safe for human consumption [31].

9.3.2 Abutilon indicum

Fragrant *A. indicum*, also known as Atibaia or Indian mallow, is a Malvaceae family aromatic plant that grows mostly in India, Sri Lanka, Pakistan, and Bangladesh. Anthelminthic, antiinflammatory, antimicrobial, antifertility, antiemetic, antiasthmatic, and antipyretic activities are found in *A. Indicum*. Wounds, ulcers, infections (urinary and vaginal), piles, diabetes, and hemorrhoids can be treated with the extracts. In the local area, it is used to treat a number of ailments, including fevers and colds as well as mumps, tuberculosis, eye irritation, toothache, sore gums, and gonorrhea [3]. Flavorings such as luteolin and chrysoeriol 7-O-β−glucopyransoside have been discovered by Matlawska and Sikorska. Extracts of *A. indicum* flowers included quercetin 3-O-α–glucopyransoside, apigenin 7-O-β–glucopyransoside, luteolin 7-O-β–glucopyransoside, chrysoeriol, and quercetin 3-O–rhamnopyranosyl(1–6)–glucopyransoside [32].

The development of nanotechnology as a strong tool for medical treatment has made it feasible to develop new and innovative medical therapies. Because of their biocompatibility and efficacy in treating an extensive range of diseases, nanoparticles derived from plants are becoming increasingly popular. By boosting intracellular reactive oxygen species formation, *A. Indicum* silver nanoparticles (AI Ag-NPs) killed COLO 205 cells, resulting in apoptosis, even at low concentrations (IC_{50} values between 4 and 3 g/mL) [33]. After 24 and 48 h, the AI Au-NPs (gold nanoparticles) showed cytotoxicity in HT-29 colon cancer cell lines (IC_{50} values of 210 and 180 g/mL, respectively). Catalytic and antioxidant activities are also exhibited by AI Ag-NPs and AI Au-NPs, in addition to their antibacterial properties [34]. Orally given AI Ag-NPs and AI Au-NPs were biocompatible and nontoxic in Wistar rats as studied by Mata et al. (2018), paving the way for their potential use in biomedicine [35]. It was shown that aqueous extracts of *A. Indicum* leaf might protect against the liver damage caused by carbon tetrachloride and paracetamol in studies by Porchezhian et al. (2005) [36]. In severely diabetic rats, aqueous extracts of *A. Indicum* plants at 1.0 g/kg dramatically reduced blood glucose levels, dropping from 567.81 ± 24.06 (control) to 506.89 ± 11.42 (treated) in 30 min [37].

9.3.3 Thespesia populnea

T. populnea (L.) is a Malvaceae tree that is mostly found in tropical and coastal parts of India, as well as in the United States. The "Indian tulip tree" is the moniker given to it by locals. The pharmacologic effects of *T. Populnea* have been documented in ancient Ayurvedic writings dating back thousands of years. A variety of plant components have traditionally been used to treat skin infections, liver illnesses, dysentery, and cholera, among other things [38]. Gonorrhea and urethritis are treated with bark oil and vegetable oil. As a traditional medicine, it is utilized to treat wounds, ulcers, and boils, as well as to treat fracture wounds. Hepatoprotective, antiinflammatory, antinociceptive, and antidiarrheal effects were reported by Shah et al. (2011) in their study [39]. Gossypol, a key component of *T. Populnea,* has antiviral and anticancer properties. Gossypol rats and humans both demonstrated antiinflammatory and antifertility effects from it. Gossypol is being tested as an anticancer treatment in advanced cancer patients because of its strong affinity for the apoptotic proteins Bcl-2 and Bcl-xL [40]. *T. Populnea*'s duramen has yielded quinones such thespone, mansonone-d, mansonone-H, and thespesone [41].

T. Populnea extracts were shown to protect cardiac cells from oxidative damage. According to Pandanaboina et al. (2014), administering rats ethanolic leaf extracts of *T. Populnea* decreased oxidative damage to the kidneys and liver [42]. The study reported that during alcohol-induced oxidative stress, treatment with *T. Populnea* extract protects the heart tissue, reducing the amount of oxidative damage that occurs to the cardiac tissue. The sinusoids, central vein, hepatocytes, and renal glomeruli that had been damaged owing to alcohol intake were all restored in histologic tests of the liver. When applied to the wound site, *T. Populnea* fruit aqueous extracts exhibited enhanced wound healing and a decrease in re-epithelization time from 24.33 to 19.17 days, with 79.17% of tissue rea-eration by the 8th day [43]. For 7 days, Vasudevan and parle administered *T. Populnea* bark ethanolic extracts orally to mice, resulting in a reduction in transfer latency and an increase in step-down latency. It was also shown that a 7-day course of therapy with *T. Populnea* prevented the rats from suffering from memory loss caused by common medications like diazepam and scopolamine. The results indicated that *T. Populnea* bark might improve memory and hence be useful in treating Alzheimer disease [44].

9.3.4 Solanum surattense

S. surattense is a perennial Solanaceae family herbal plant. It may be found across India's tropical areas. *S. surattense*, also well-known as Surattense or yellow nightshade, has traditionally been used to cure a variety of diseases, including diabetes, asthma, fever, and cough, particularly in South India. Constipation, leprosy, and asthma are all treated with *S. surattense*. Antimalarial and free radical scavenging properties are also present. Fruits of *S. surattense* were shown to have a significant antidiabetic effect in rats that had been given diabetes medication [45,46]. A combination of antibacterial and wound-healing properties was demonstrated by the ethanolic and methanolic extracts of *S. surattense*. Antioxidant properties of *S. surattense* leaf extract were demonstrated by Muruhan et al.'s phytochemical research, which indicated the presence of alkaloids, triterpenoids, glycosides, flavonoids, and sterols in the alcoholic leaf extract. Plant extracts were tested for antioxidant properties using DPPH and ABTS assays. To sum it all up, 46.7 mg gallic acid equivalents were found in the plant extract. Antioxidant properties may be attributed to a high concentration of phenolic chemicals [47].

Sheeba et al. (2010) found that ethanolic extracts of *S. surattense* have antibacterial efficacy against various bacteria, including *Bacillus subtilis*, *Escherichia coli*, *Salmonella typhi*, and *Vibrio cholerae*. It was tested for antibacterial activity at 25, 50, 100, 25, and 500 μg leaf extract concentrations. The extract was antibacterial against *Pseudomonas aeruginosa* except at 25 g and had no effect on *Shigella dysenteriae* at any concentration [48]. Antidiabetic effects of *S. surattense* alcoholic leaf extract were studied in STZ induced diabetic rats at a concentration of 100 mg/kg body weight for 45 days by Sridevi et al. (2011). Rats with diabetes had higher blood glucose levels and lower insulin levels. The liver, kidneys, and plasma all had possibly increased levels of cholesterol, phospholipids, triglycerides, and free fatty acids. Diabetic rats have altered lipoprotein and fatty acid compositions in their blood. Low and extremely low-density lipoproteins had higher cholesterol levels, while high-density lipoproteins had lower cholesterol levels. There has been an overall drop in linoleic, arachidonic, protein, and albumin levels and an increase in palmitic and stearic acid levels. Diabetes-induced rats were given *S. surattense* at a dose of 100 mg/kg body weight daily for 45 days, and all of the following parameters returned to normal. In this study, *S. surattense* extracts were found to have antihyperlipidemic effects, perhaps because they include numerous phytoconstituents, including sterols and triterpenes as well as alkaloids and flavonoids [49].

9.3.5 Mucuna pruriens

Cowitch or velvet bean is the common name for the tropical legume *M. Pruriens*, a member of the Fabaceae family. Food, cattle feed, and cover crops are all being grown out of just one species of plant. It is common for traditional remedies to be made from leaves, seeds, and roots [50]. *M. pruriens* has a wide range of therapeutic qualities, including antidiabetics, antiinflammation, analgesia, neuroprotection, arousal, and antioxidant. This plant's high alkaloid content makes it an attractive first-line therapy for Parkinson disease in Ayurvedic medicine. It is a precursor to many neurotransmitters such as noradrenaline, dopamine (DOP), and adrenaline. Neurotransmission is impeded as DOP concentration decreases in the brain. To correct neuronal transmissions, DOP is converted into levodopa (LD) after it crosses the blood–brain barrier [51]. In dried *M. pruriens* seeds, the median LD concentration was around 5.29% [52]. *M. pruriens* leaf methanolic extract has antisickling (membrane-stabilizing) properties, according to Anosike et al. (2019), who used it to treat sickle cell anemia [2]. Chalé et al. (2014) revealed that the peptide fraction derived from *M. pruriens* beans had antihypertensive and antioxidant properties [53]. *M. pruriens* seed extract was shown to be effective in the treatment of erectile dysfunction in male Wister rats, as revealed by Duangnin et al. (2017) [54].

It was shown that the seed extract of *M. pruriens* (three injections at a dosage of 21 mg/kg in rats) had a protective effect against the snake venom of *Naja sputatrix* (84%) and *Calloselasma rhodostoma* (33%) in rats [50]. In both normal and diabetic rat models produced with STZ, Bhaskar et al. (2008) found that an aqueous extract of *M. pruriens* seed extract was hypoglycemic. Glucose levels dropped from $240.5 \pm 7.2\%$ to $90.6 \pm 5.6\%$ following 21 days of oral administration of 100 and 200 mg/kg body weight of the extract. Within 2 h, the glucose level in control rats dropped from around $127.5 \pm 3.2\%$ mg to $75.6 \pm 4.8\%$ mg [55]. The effects of *M. pruriens* seeds on male infertility were investigated by a group of researchers. The participants in the study were 75 healthy fertile men (controls) and 75 persons who were undergoing infertility evaluation. After eating the seeds, the researchers measured the levels of reproductive hormones and catecholamine parameters in the patients' bodies before and after they ate the seeds. The consumption of 5 g of *M. pruriens* seed powder with milk for 3 months increased sperm concentration in oligozoospermic males, according to the research [56].

9.3.6 Senna auriculata

An herb belonging to the Fabaceous family, *Senna auriculata* (L.) Roxb. can develop up to 1.2–3.0 m in height. The medicinal properties of numerous components of this plant have been documented. Sugar-related illnesses and rheumatoid arthritis can be treated using the bark's antidiuretic properties. The bark is also used as an antifungal and antiparasitic. This plant's leaves can help with anything from leprosy to ulcers to throat irritation to chyluria to ocular difficulties to dysentery to inflammations to chronic purulent conjunctivitis and even skin diseases like eczema to acne. Asthma sufferers use the leaves and roots of *S. auriculata*. Patients with diabetes, congestion, and bladder infections use the tea Kalpa, which contains plant components from *S. auriculata*, to relieve their symptoms. Hepatoprotective and antihyperlipidemic properties are also claimed to be present in it [57]. Therapeutical studies have shown that *S. auriculata* contains flavonoids, polysaccharides, alkaloids, as well as tannins that may be useful in the treatment of conditions such as asthma, conjunctivitis, ulcerative colitis, diabetes, cancer, kidney, and liver disease [58]. In addition to luteolin, quercetin, kaempferol, and kaempferol-3-O-rutinoside, Juan-Badaturuge et al. discovered other bioactive antioxidant compounds from *S. auriculata*. Several previously recognized antidiabetic substances were found in the investigation. For the first time, kaempferol-3-O-rutinoside, a significant antioxidant molecule, has been discovered in this plant [59].

S. auriculata flower methanolic extracts showed antiviral efficacy against a variety of viral strains, including feline herpes (infects domestic and wild cats), feline corona (common viral illness of cats), herpes simplex-2 (genital herpes), herpes simplex-1 (oral herpes), vaccinia (causes fever, rash, and head and body aches), and vesicular stomatitis (primarily affects cattle, horses, and swine), according to Arthanari et al. (2013) [60]. Using the human colon cancer HCT 15 cell line, Esakkirajan et al. (2014) discovered that *S. auriculata* leaves had an anticancer component. 4,5,6,7-hexahydro7,4-dichlorobenzylidene[h] [1,4,8]. Triazecin8(1H)-one at a concentration of 20 g/mL suppressed human colon cancer cell HCT 15 by half after 24 h incubation. An anticancer chemical produced from the leaves of *S. auriculata* has been shown to be effective against human colon cancer cells. Based on the results of the in vitro investigation, it appears that the bioactive components may possess anticancer effects and might thus be employed therapeutically [61].

9.4 Medicinal efficacy of phytochemicals

As previously said, researchers have looked at a broad variety of plants for the treatment of different essential ailments such as cancer, Alzheimer, and Parkinson diseases. Quercetin, ferulic acid, curcumin, and myricetin, among other phytochemicals, have been intensively studied for the treatment of the disorders indicated earlier [62–65]. This section of the chapter gives a brief overview of these chemicals.

9.4.1 Quercetin

In foods such as onions, apples, citrus fruits, cherries, and green leafy vegetables, there is a bioactive flavonoid component called quercetin (2-(3,4-dihydroxy phenyl)-3,5,7-trihydroxychromen-4-one). The chemical structure of quercetin is illustrated in Fig. 9.2A. When mixed with fatty acids (oils and fats), it dissolves easily. It is common to find quercetin linked to sugar, alcohol, or other phenolic acids in leaves. When the glycosyl group is attached to quercetin, the resulting quercetin glycosides have a greater water solubility than the quercetin aglycone. Antioxidant and

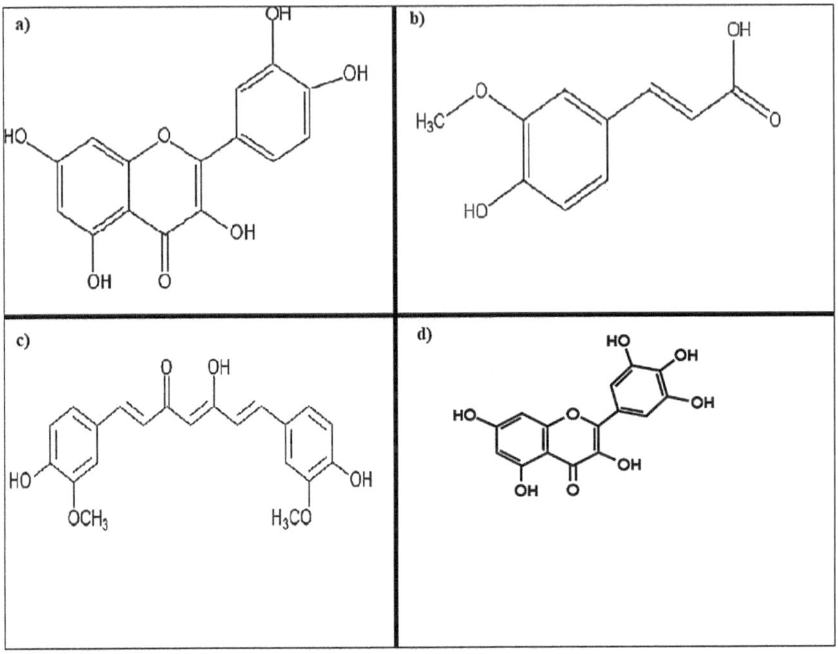

Figure 9.2 Chemical structure of (A) quercetin, (B) ferulic acid, (C) curcumin, and (D) myricetin.

anticancer effects, as well as apoptosis-inducing capabilities, are well known for quercetin. Quercetin's antioxidant and chelating properties may be enhanced by the presence of several hydroxyl groups in its molecular arrangement, as evidenced by numerous studies. Quercetin's biologic and pharmacologic properties have previously shown that it may inhibit the development of degenerative disorders such atopic dermatitis, myocarditis, renal fibrosis, and neurodegenerative diseases, as well as in the treatment of cardiovascular and cancer-related illnesses [66]. Cell growth and inhibition rates in U2OS and Saos2 human metastatic osteosarcoma cells were reduced by quercetin, which inhibited PTHR1 activity [67].

9.4.2 Ferulic acid

Corn, tomatoes, and rice bran all have high levels of the phytochemical ferulic acid (FA). The Shikimate pathway in plants is responsible for the synthesis of phenylalanine and tyrosine. Cancer, diabetes, cardiac disease, and neurologic illnesses are just a few of the conditions that it has been shown to be effective in treating. Even more remarkable, FA has both prooxidant (acid) and antioxidant capabilities, as well as a broad spectrum of antibacterial activity against all microorganisms. The chemical structure of the FA is illustrated in Fig. 9.2B. FA has been shown to protect the male genital system from arsenic-induced toxicity and reduce testicular damage and oxidative stress, according to Guvvala and colleagues. *Nfe2l2*, *Ppargc1a*, and *StAR* genes were also regulated to increase sperm quality [68].

Protease secretion and oxidation intermediate synthesis all contribute to the development of oxidative stress, which finally causes tissue degradation, accelerated aging, necrosis, and cell apoptosis, including cancer development. Nonenzyme antioxidant systems and enzyme antioxidant systems are the two types of antioxidant systems found in the human body. Researchers have recently discovered that FA, in addition to its antioxidant properties, also inhibits the formation of reactive oxygen species and participates in a variety of signaling pathways. The molecular pathways involved in the antioxidant effect of FA are described in Fig. 9.3.

Nuclear factor-erythroid-related factor 2 (Nrf2) is a redox-sensitive transcription regulator that regulates stress induction and activation of a range of cell protection genes. HO-1 is a rate-limiting enzyme in heme catabolism and a key medium via which Nrf2 can exert its antioxidant

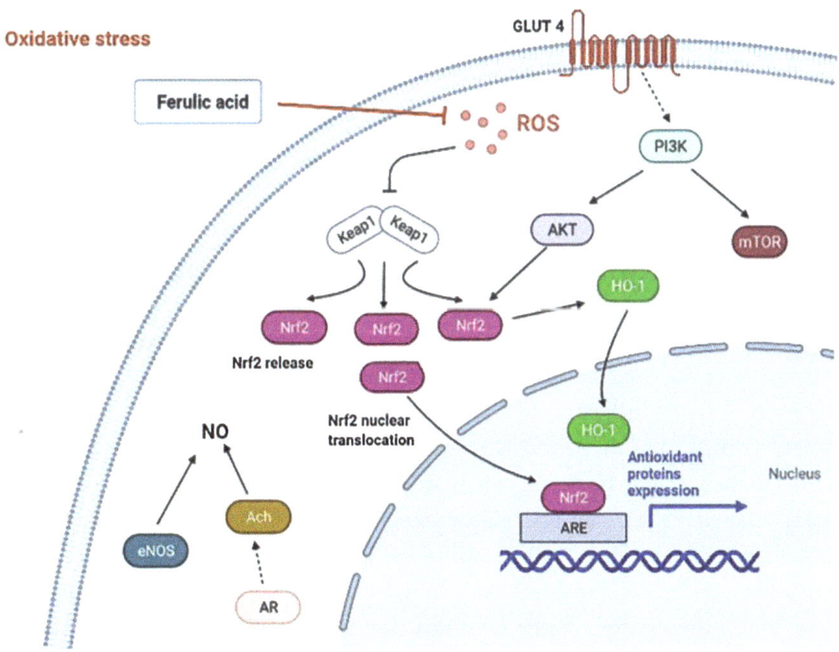

Figure 9.3 Molecular mechanisms involved in ferulic acid's antioxidant action. *(Reproduced with permission from Dan et al. [62].)*

activity. Studies on animals suggest that the Nrf2/HO-1 cascade response has a major impact on pathophysiologic processes such as oxidative stress in diseases such as diabetes and ischemia. With nicotinamide adenine dinucleotide phosphate (NADPH) as a cofactor, aldose reductase catalyzes the conversion of aldehydes or ketones to matching alcohols. NADPH is linked to oxidative stress and is involved in the onset and progression of diabetes problems as well as a number of oxidative stress illnesses [62].

9.4.3 Curcumin

Curcumin, a yellow, polyphenolic natural chemical utilized in traditional medicine for millennia, is turmeric's pharmacologically active component. The chemical structure of curcumin is illustrated in Fig. 9.2C. Even at large dosages, curcumin appears to have little toxicity, but the therapeutic effects of curcumin are frequently seen at lower daily dosing levels. Curcumin interacts directly with proteins including inflammatory molecules, cell survival proteins, and the proteasome to have many therapeutic actions and regulate different cell signaling pathways. Curcumin also interacts with DNA and RNA, as well as metal ions. It can also interact with other factors, including as NF-B, AP-1, beta-catenin, and the signal transducer and activator of transcription protein, through indirect means. Due to its unique chemical structure, curcumin demonstrates a wide spectrum of pharmacologic and biologic properties.

In animal models, curcumin has been proven to protect against fatal diseases like Alzheimer disease, Parkinson disease, depression, and ischemic stroke. Curcumin has been shown to play a function in preventing stomach cancer in several trials. In 1987, the anticancer properties of curcumin were first discovered. Cancer cell proliferation, cell cycle arrest and apoptosis, inhibition of protein-kinase and production of death receptors all contribute to curcumin's anticancer properties [69]. Curcumin has been shown to reduce tumorigenesis and tumor growth in animal models of gastric cancer. As indicated by the drastically reduced triglyceride level in rat liver, Mahmoud et al. found that curcumin protects liver cells in rats fed a high-fat diet. It has been shown that curcumin possesses anticancer properties against HeLa cervical cancer cells, as revealed by Ghasemi et al. (2019). Curcumin had an IC_{50} value of 34.23 M/mL, which substantially inhibited cancer cell proliferation. Rats on a high-fat diet were found to have much lower triglyceride levels in their livers, which was corroborated in this study. The invasion, proliferation, and increased mortality of cervical cancer cells can all be decreased by curcumin therapy [65].

9.4.4 Myricetin

Flavonoid chemical myricetin is found in a wide variety of food plants, including grapes and oranges, as well as berries and teas. Polyhydroxyflavonol is a polyhydroxyflavonol molecule made of light yellow crystals that is readily soluble in alcohol, acetonitrile, ethanol, and other polar solvents. It has the chemical formula $C_{15}H_{10}O_8$ (Fig. 9.2D) and a relative molecular mass of 318.24, which makes it a polymer. As an antiinflammatory and antioxidant, myricetin also possesses anticancer potential. Cancer cell lines such as gastric cancer, esophageal carcinoma, ovarian cancer, colon cancer, and cervical cancer have shown that myricetin has a function in inhibiting cancer development and promoting apoptosis. To combat type 2 diabetes, it inhibited both α-amylase and α-glucosidase (T2DM) [70]. Zhang et al. (2019) evaluated myricetin's protective effectiveness in blood–brain barrier in vitro models of brain microvessel endothelial ischemia/reperfusion damage. Oxygen glucose deprivation and reperfusion (OGD/R) may produce inflammation-related cytokines such as IL-1β, TNF-α, and IL-6 in human brain microvessel endothelial cells (HBMECs). Myricetin might suppress IL-1β, TNF-α, and IL-6 levels in OGD/R-injured HBMECs [64].

9.5 Summary

The widespread use of herbal medicines to supplement conventional medical care is garnering worldwide acclaim. A large number of medications are derived directly from plants, while the rest are chemically modified natural substances. In vitro and in vivo studies on *N. Sativa* oil and extracts have indicated that TQ and alpha-hederin, two of the plant's most active constituents, have significant antidisease effects and have been determined to be generally safe as have other original research publications. In addition to *N. sativa*, *A. manihot*, *T. populnea*, *A. indicum*, *M. pruriens*, *S. surattense*, and *S. auriculata* have all been extensively studied for the treatment of various diseases. *S. auriculata* has a wide range of medicinal characteristics (antidiabetic, antileprosy, antiasthma, anticancer, antioxidant, wound healing, and hepatoprotective, among others) and is well accepted by the Indian populace. In addition, the most current studies on each of the medicinal plants examined are included in the chapter. People nowadays are becoming more conscious of the negative side effects of allopathic drugs, which is a step toward better understanding and using natural plant products for human benefit.

References

[1] V.L. Dhadge, M. Changmai, M.K. Purkait, Purification of catechins from Camellia sinensis using membrane cell, Food and Bioproducts Processing 117 (2019) 203–212.
[2] C.A. Anosike, O.N. Igboegwu, O.F.C. Nwodo, Antioxidant properties and membrane stabilization effects of methanol extract of Mucuna pruriens leaves on normal and sickle erythrocytes, Journal of Traditional and Complementary Medicine 9 (4) (2019) 278–284.
[3] M. Prasathkumar, et al., Therapeutic and pharmacological efficacy of selective Indian medicinal plants – a review, Phytomedicine 1 (2) (2021) 100029.
[4] A. Majeed, et al., Nigella sativa L.: uses in traditional and contemporary medicines – an overview, Acta Ecologica Sinica 41 (4) (2021) 253–258.
[5] A. Ahmad, et al., A review on therapeutic potential of Nigella sativa: a miracle herb, Asian Pacific Journal of Tropical Biomedicine 3 (5) (2013) 337–352.
[6] A.F. Majdalawieh, M.W. Fayyad, Immunomodulatory and anti-inflammatory action of Nigella sativa and thymoquinone: a comprehensive review, International Immunopharmacology 28 (1) (2015) 295–304.
[7] S.K. Tiruppur Venkatachallam, et al., Chemical composition of Nigella sativa L. seed extracts obtained by supercritical carbon dioxide, Journal of Food Science & Technology 47 (6) (2010) 598–605.
[8] H.J. Harzallah, et al., Chemical composition, antimicrobial potential against cariogenic bacteria and cytotoxic activity of Tunisian Nigella sativa essential oil and thymoquinone, Food Chemistry 129 (4) (2011) 1469–1474.
[9] F. Benkaci-Ali, et al., Chemical composition of the essential oil of Nigella sativa seeds extracted by microwave steam distillation, Journal of Essential Oil Bearing Plants 16 (6) (2013) 781–794.
[10] Y. Mazaheri, et al., A comprehensive review of the physicochemical, quality and nutritional properties of Nigella sativa oil, Food Reviews International 35 (4) (2019) 342–362.
[11] H.A. Bakathir, N.A. Abbas, Detection of the antibacterial effect of Nigella sativa ground seeds with water, African Journal of Traditional, Complementary and Alternative Medicines: AJTCAM 8 (2) (2011) 159–164.
[12] N.M. Morsi, Antimicrobial effect of crude extracts of Nigella sativa on multiple antibiotics-resistant bacteria, Acta Microbiologica Polonica 49 (1) (2000) 63–74.
[13] A. Hannan, et al., Anti bacterial activity of Nigella sativa against clinical isolates of methicillin resistant *Staphylococcus aureus*, Journal of Ayub Medical College, Abbottabad 20 (3) (2008) 72–74.
[14] K. Chaieb, et al., Antibacterial activity of Thymoquinone, an active principle of Nigella sativa and its potency to prevent bacterial biofilm formation, BMC Complementary and Alternative Medicine 11 (1) (2011) 1–6.
[15] S.H.M. Aljabre, et al., Antidermatophyte activity of ether extract of Nigella sativa and its active principle, thymoquinone, Journal of Ethnopharmacology 101 (1–3) (2005) 116–119.
[16] K. Halamova, et al., In vitro antifungal effect of black cumin seed quinones against dairy spoilage yeasts at different acidity levels, Journal of Food Protection 73 (12) (2010) 2291–2295.
[17] E.A. Rogozhin, et al., Novel antifungal defensins from Nigella sativa L. seeds, Plant Physiology and Biochemistry 49 (2) (2011) 131–137.
[18] M. Boskabady, N. Mohsenpoor, L. Takaloo, Antiasthmatic effect of Nigella sativa in airways of asthmatic patients, Phytomedicine 17 (10) (2010) 707–713.
[19] A.M. Salem, et al., Effect of Nigella sativa supplementation on lung function and inflammatory mediators in partly controlled asthma: a randomized controlled trial, Annals of Saudi Medicine 37 (1) (2017) 64–71.

[20] A. Koshak, et al., Nigella sativa supplementation improves asthma control and biomarkers: a randomized, double-blind, placebo-controlled trial, Phytotherapy Research 31 (3) (2017) 403–409.
[21] M.A. Rafique, et al., Nigella Sativa essential oil prevents airway inflammation in ovalbumin sensitized Guinea-pigs, Annals of King Edward Medical University 24 (4) (2018).
[22] R.H.M. Salama, Hypoglycemic effect of lipoic acid, carnitine and Nigella sativa in diabetic rat model, International Journal of Health Sciences 5 (2) (2011) 126.
[23] N.E. Abdelmeguid, et al., Effects of Nigella sativa and thymoquinone on biochemical and subcellular changes in pancreatic β-cells of streptozotocin-induced diabetic rats, Journal of Diabetes 2 (4) (2010) 256–266.
[24] E. Nourbar, et al., Effect of hydroethanolic extract of Nigella sativa L. on skin wound healing process in diabetic male rats, International Journal of Preventive Medicine 10 (2019).
[25] M. Fathy, T. Nikaido, In vivo attenuation of angiogenesis in hepatocellular carcinoma by Nigella sativa, Turkish Journal of Medical Sciences 48 (1) (2018) 178–186.
[26] I.A. Al Mofleh, et al., Gastroprotective effect of an aqueous suspension of black cumin Nigella sativa on necrotizing agents-induced gastric injury in experimental animals, Saudi Journal of Gastroenterology 14 (3) (2008) 128.
[27] S. Parhizkar, L.A. Latiff, A. Parsa, Effect of Nigella sativa on reproductive system in experimental menopause rat model, Avicenna Journal of Phytomedicine 6 (1) (2016) 95.
[28] X.-X. Pan, et al., Characterization and immunomodulatory activity of polysaccharides from the stems and leaves of Abelmoschus manihot and a sulfated derivative, International Journal of Biological Macromolecules 107 (2018) 9–16.
[29] L.-y. Du, et al., Comparative characterization of nucleotides, nucleosides and nucleobases in Abelmoschus manihot roots, stems, leaves and flowers during different growth periods by UPLC-TQ-MS/MS, Journal of Chromatography B 1006 (2015) 130–137.
[30] M. Taroreh, et al., Antioxidative activities of various fractions of gedi's leaf extracts (Abelmoschus manihot L. medik), Agriculture and Agricultural Science Procedia 9 (2016) 271–278.
[31] P. Jain, S. Bari, S. Surana, Acute oral toxicity of Abelmoschus manihot and Wrightia tinctoria in mice, Pharmacognosy Journal 3 (25) (2011) 78–81.
[32] I. Matławska, M. Sikorska, Flavonoid compounds in the flowers of Abutilon indicum (L.) sweet (Malvaceae), Acta Poloniae Pharmaceutica 59 (3) (2002) 227–229.
[33] R. Mata, J.R. Nakkala, S.R. Sadras, Biogenic silver nanoparticles from Abutilon indicum: their antioxidant, antibacterial and cytotoxic effects in vitro, Colloids and Surfaces B: Biointerfaces 128 (2015) 276–286.
[34] R. Mata, J.R. Nakkala, S.R. Sadras, Polyphenol stabilized colloidal gold nanoparticles from Abutilon indicum leaf extract induce apoptosis in HT-29 colon cancer cells, Colloids and Surfaces B: Biointerfaces 143 (2016) 499–510.
[35] R. Mata, et al., In vivo bio-distribution, clearance and toxicity assessment of biogenic silver and gold nanoparticles synthesized from Abutilon indicum in Wistar rats, Journal of Trace Elements in Medicine & Biology 48 (2018) 157–165.
[36] E. Porchezhian, S. Ansari, Hepatoprotective activity of Abutilon indicum on experimental liver damage in rats, Phytomedicine 12 (1–2) (2005) 62–64.
[37] C. Krisanapun, et al., Aqueous extract of Abutilon indicum Sweet inhibits glucose absorption and stimulates insulin secretion in rodents, Nutrition Research 29 (8) (2009) 579–587.
[38] R. Ilavarasan, et al., Antioxidant activity of *Thespesia populnea* bark extracts against carbon tetrachloride-induced liver injury in rats, Journal of Ethnopharmacology 87 (2–3) (2003) 227–230.

[39] A.S. Shah, K.R. Alagawadi, Anti-inflammatory, analgesic and antipyretic properties of *Thespesia populnea* Soland ex. Correa seed extracts and its fractions in animal models, Journal of Ethnopharmacology 137 (3) (2011) 1504–1509.
[40] G.L.S. Viswanatha, et al., Antidiarrheal effect of fractions from stem bark of *Thespesia populnea* in rodents: possible antimotility and antisecretory mechanisms, Asian Pacific Journal of Tropical Medicine 4 (6) (2011) 451–456.
[41] S.C. Pandanaboina, et al., Alterations in antioxidant enzyme activities and oxidative damage in alcoholic rat tissues: protective role of *Thespesia populnea*, Food Chemistry 132 (1) (2012) 150–159.
[42] S.L. Rajbanshi, C.S. Pandanaboina, Alcohol stress on cardiac tissue—Ameliorative effects of *Thespesia populnea* leaf extract, Journal of Cardiology 63 (6) (2014) 449–459.
[43] A. Nagappa, B. Cheriyan, Wound healing activity of the aqueous extract of *Thespesia populnea* fruit, Fitoterapia 72 (5) (2001) 503–506.
[44] M. Vasudevan, M. Parle, Pharmacological actions of *Thespesia populnea* relevant to Alzheimer's disease, Phytomedicine 13 (9–10) (2006) 677–687.
[45] S. Mickymaray, et al., Screening and antibacterial efficacy of selected Indian medicinal plants, Asian Pacific Journal of Tropical Biomedicine 6 (3) (2016) 185–191.
[46] T. Thirumalai, et al., Effect of Solanum surattense seed on the oxidative potential of cauda epididymal spermatozoa, Asian Pacific Journal of Tropical Biomedicine 2 (1) (2012) 21–23.
[47] S. Muruhan, S. Selvaraj, P.K. Viswanathan, In vitro antioxidant activities of Solanum surattense leaf extract, Asian Pacific Journal of Tropical Biomedicine 3 (1) (2013) 28–34.
[48] E. Sheeba, Antibacterial activity of Solanum surattense burm. F, Kathmandu University Journal of Science, Engineering and Technology 6 (1) (2010) 1–4.
[49] M. Sridevi, P. Kalaiarasi, K. Pugalendi, Antihyperlipidemic activity of alcoholic leaf extract of Solanum surattense in streptozotocin-diabetic rats, Asian Pacific Journal of Tropical Biomedicine 1 (2) (2011) S276–S280.
[50] N.H. Tan, et al., The protective effect of Mucuna pruriens seeds against snake venom poisoning, Journal of Ethnopharmacology 123 (2) (2009) 356–358.
[51] L. Misra, H. Wagner, Alkaloidal constituents of Mucuna pruriens seeds, Phytochemistry 65 (18) (2004) 2565–2567.
[52] E. Cassani, et al., Mucuna pruriens for Parkinson's disease: low-cost preparation method, laboratory measures and pharmacokinetics profile, Journal of the Neurological Sciences 365 (2016) 175–180.
[53] F.G.H. Chalé, et al., ACE inhibitory, hypotensive and antioxidant peptide fractions from Mucuna pruriens proteins, Process Biochemistry 49 (10) (2014) 1691–1698.
[54] N. Duangnin, et al., In vitro and in vivo investigation of natural compounds from seed extract of Mucuna pruriens lacking L-DOPA for the treatment of erectile dysfunction, Asian Pacific Journal of Tropical Medicine 10 (3) (2017) 238–252.
[55] A. Bhaskar, V. Vidhya, M. Ramya, Hypoglycemic effect of Mucuna pruriens seed extract on normal and streptozotocin-diabetic rats, Fitoterapia 79 (7–8) (2008) 539–543.
[56] K.K. Shukla, et al., Mucuna pruriens improves male fertility by its action on the hypothalamus–pituitary–gonadal axis, Fertility and Sterility 92 (6) (2009) 1934–1940.
[57] S.Z.A. Khader, et al., Modulatory effect of dianthrone rich alcoholic flower extract of Cassia auriculata L. on experimental diabetes, Integrative Medicine Research 6 (2) (2017) 131–140.
[58] G. Sharmila, et al., Ultrasound assisted extraction of total phenolics from Cassia auriculata leaves and evaluation of its antioxidant activities, Industrial Crops and Products 84 (2016) 13–21.
[59] M. Juan-Badaturuge, S. Habtemariam, M.J. Thomas, Antioxidant compounds from a South Asian beverage and medicinal plant, Cassia auriculata, Food Chemistry 125 (1) (2011) 221–225.

[60] S. Arthanari, et al., In vitro antiviral and cytotoxic screening of methanolic extract of Cassia auriculata flowers in HeLa, Vero, CRFK and HEL cell lines, Drug Invention Today 5 (1) (2013) 28–31.
[61] M. Esakkirajan, et al., Apoptosis mediated anti-proliferative effect of compound isolated from Cassia auriculata leaves against human colon cancer cell line, Spectrochimica Acta Part A: Molecular and Biomolecular Spectroscopy 127 (2014) 484–489.
[62] D. Li, et al., Ferulic acid: a review of its pharmacology, pharmacokinetics and derivatives, Life Sciences 284 (2021) 119921.
[63] K. Wadhwa, et al., New insights into quercetin nanoformulations for topical delivery, Phytomedicine (2022) 100257.
[64] S. Zhang, et al., Myricetin ameliorated ischemia/reperfusion-induced brain endothelial permeability by improvement of eNOS uncoupling and activation eNOS/NO, Journal of Pharmacological Sciences 140 (1) (2019) 62–72.
[65] F. Ghasemi, et al., Curcumin inhibits NF-kB and Wnt/β-catenin pathways in cervical cancer cells, Pathology, Research & Practice 215 (10) (2019) 152556.
[66] C.-Y. Lan, et al., Quercetin facilitates cell death and chemosensitivity through RAGE/PI3K/AKT/mTOR axis in human pancreatic cancer cells, Journal of Food and Drug Analysis 27 (4) (2019) 887–896.
[67] S. Li, et al., Quercetin suppresses the proliferation and metastasis of metastatic osteosarcoma cells by inhibiting parathyroid hormone receptor 1, Biomedicine & Pharmacotherapy 114 (2019) 108839.
[68] P.R. Guvvala, et al., Ellagic and ferulic acids protect arsenic-induced male reproductive toxicity via regulating Nfe2l2, Ppargc1a and StAR expressions in testis, Toxicology 413 (2019) 1–12.
[69] M. Moballegh Nasery, et al., Curcumin: a potential therapeutic natural product for adenocarcinomas, Phytochemistry Letters 49 (2022) 45–55.
[70] Z. Yao, et al., Dietary myricetin intake is inversely associated with the prevalence of type 2 diabetes mellitus in a Chinese population, Nutrition Research 68 (2019) 82–91.

CHAPTER 10

Applications of plant-derived metal nanoparticles in pharmaceuticals

10.1 Introduction

The design and building of functioning systems at the molecular level is the focus of nanoscience. Nanotechnology is an applied science that focuses on the synthesis and implementation of the smallest feasible materials and technologies. Basic nanoscience is the study of how to make new materials at the atomic scale by modifying existing ones. Materials with at least one dimensional structure less than 100 nm are commonly referred to as "nanoscaled" [1,2]. Biologic imaging, filtration, nanocomposites, drug delivery, and tumor hyperthermia are just few of the various uses for nanoparticles (NPs) in the biomedical field. Metal NPs are among the many different types of NPs that have a range of therapeutic and pharmacologic applications. Most commonly, in the rapidly developing multidisciplinary subject of nano biotechnology, gold (Au) and silver (Ag) NPs are majorly explored for biomedical applications [3,4]. AuNPs, for example, have been studied for a variety of pharmacologic and therapeutic uses, including immunoassay, protein assay, cancer nanotechnology (particularly cancer cell detection), and capillary electrophoresis. Even in a biologic screening test, AuNPs are useful indicators. Moreover, AuNPs are employed in a variety of ways in the medical industry. AgNPs, meanwhile, demonstrate potential antibacterial properties against pathogenic organisms including *Escherichia coli, Vibrio cholerae, Bacillus subtilis*, syphilis, typhus, *Pseudomonas aeruginosa,* and *Staphylococcus aureus*. Other metal NPs, including as copper (Cu), palladium (Pd), platinum (Pt), and iron (Fe), are also being investigated for diverse applications [5—8].

The synthesis of NPs may be classified as either a top-down or bottom-up process depending on the technique used. Researchers' primary

Advances in Extraction and Applications of Bioactive Phytochemicals
ISBN 978-0-443-18535-9
https://doi.org/10.1016/B978-0-443-18535-9.00001-6

attention in recent years has shifted to developing effective green chemistry methods for the manufacture of metal NPs to establish a sustainable synthesis process for the production of well-characterized NPs. Owing to their increasing success and convenience in producing NPs, green synthesis methods are becoming increasingly popular in this field [9,10]. In addition, the biosynthesis of metal NPs is a process that uses no harsh, hazardous, or costly ingredients. AgNPs made through chemical reduction, for example, might absorb harsh substances from their surroundings, raising concerns about their toxicity.

In view of that, researchers have come up with a variety of innovative methods for producing metal NPs using biosynthesis processes. Phytosynthesis of metallic NPs, for example, involves the utilization of plants with the potential for phytomining and phytoremediation of heavy metals. Plant extracts have created a new age of rapid and harmless approaches for producing NPs through biosynthesis. There have been various publications on the production of metal NPs by plant leaf extracts and their potential use in medicine, all of which have received widespread attention. The applications of biosynthesized metal NPs are widely explored in the field of pharmaceuticals, which is illustrated in Fig. 10.1. The advancement in the production of metal NPs for pharmaceutical applications is discussed in this section. In addition, the utilization of the mentioned metal particles in different pharmaceutical applications is briefly reviewed.

10.2 Biosynthesis of metallic nanoparticles for pharmaceutical application

NPs can be synthesized in three ways: physically, chemically, or biologically. Laser irradiation, thermal breakdown, and electrolysis are some of the physical processes utilized to synthesize NPs. High temperatures are used to synthesize materials using the thermal decomposition technique. It is common for physical approaches to require expensive vacuum systems or equipment to prepare NPs, which is a drawback in and of itself. The chemical reduction approach, which employs reducing agents like sodium citrate or sodium borohydride, is the most often used method for synthesizing NPs chemically. Chemical synthesis provides a number of benefits; however, the use of hazardous compounds on NP surfaces and nonpolar solvents in the production procedure restricts their use in therapeutic domains. As a result, a number of scientists have worked to devise new ways to synthesize NPs that are safe for humans, animals, and the environment.

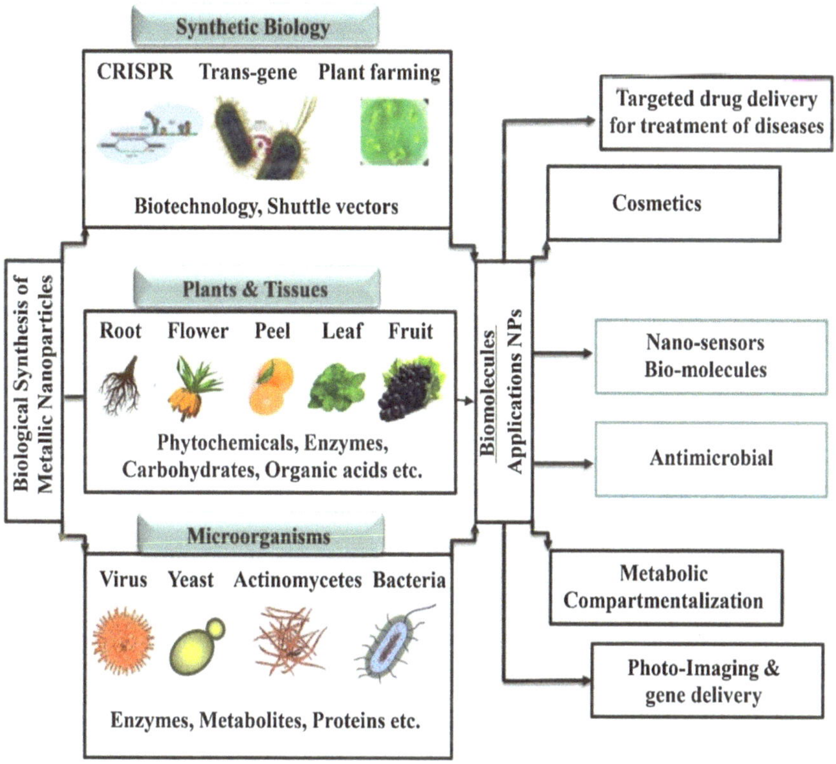

Figure 10.1 The green synthesis of metal NPs utilizing various biologic sources and their biologic applications. *(Reproduced with permission from Behzad et al. [11]).*

Researchers have discovered that NPs may be produced by using biologic methods. Biomaterials such as bacteria, yeast, fungus, macroalgae, microalgae, viruses, and plant biomass/extracts are used in the biologic production of NPs. Because of the growing success and simplicity of NP synthesis, the utilization of numerous biologic entities is quickly expanding in this field. In the last several years, researchers have claimed progress in the biosynthesis of metallic nanosized rod-like structures, as well as wire-like structures and flower-like structures. They might be used in various ways, including therapy, diagnostics, the creation of surgical nanodevices, and the production of commercial products. Plant biomass/extracts have certain inert benefits over other microscopic creatures in the creation of NPs among other biologic components. Biomolecules (including proteins, enzymes, and organic acids) found in plant biomass play a role in the production of metallic NPs [12,13].

10.2.1 Silver nanoparticles

Ag biosynthesis using plant extracts has been widely researched, and it has proven to be a simpler and faster technique than laborious and time-consuming microbial synthesis procedures. Furthermore, the scientific community is interested in the synthesis of AgNPs because of their many uses, which include spectrally selective coating for absorption of solar energy, surface increased Raman scattering for imaging, and a variety of other medicinal applications. For the synthesis of AgNPs, several plants and their various parts were used. Silver nitrate salt ($AgNO_3$) and plant extract/biomass are the main building blocks of plant biosynthesis. According to the following reaction, the emergence of a brownish-yellow hue after a brief contact time verifies the creation of AgNPs:

$$\text{Ag} + \text{NO}_3^- + \text{Plant molecule(OH, COOH, etc.)} \rightarrow \text{Ag}^0\text{nanoparticles} \tag{10.1}$$

When it comes to plant-assisted extracellular production of AgNPs, Shankar et al. performed a study employing geranium (*Pelargonium graveolens*) leaf assistance. The researchers observed that when $AgNO_3$ solution was applied to leaf extract, the Ag ions were rapidly reduced, resulting in solution-soluble, incredibly stable, crystalline AgNPs (16–40 nm) [14]. A fungus species, *Fusarium oxysporum*, was also shown to reduce Ag ions more slowly than the geranium leaf extract, according to the study's findings. Later, Huang et al. demonstrated that dried *Cinnamomum camphora* leaf extract could be used to make triangular or spherical AgNPs (55–80 nm in size). According to the findings, the leaf extract's water-soluble heterocyclic and polyol components were mostly responsible for decreasing Ag ions in the experiment [15]. To synthesize AgNPs, Leela et al. analyzed leaf extracts from a variety of plants in 2008. They found that *Helianthus annuus* (*H. annus*) had the greatest ability to reduce Ag ions and the fastest rate of reduction [16]. To synthesize AgNPs, Ahmad et al. used an extract made from the common medicinal herb basil (*Ocimum sanctum*). AgNPs between 10 and 5 nm in size were found to be extremely stable by the researchers [17]. The extract of *Podophyllum hexandrum* leaf was utilized to synthesize AgNPs by Jeyaraj et al. Spherical-shaped particles ranging from 12 to 40 nm in diameter were formed after 2.5 h of interaction at 60°C and pH 4 [18]. *Acacia nilotica* pod extract was utilized to produce AgNPs at pH 5, 6, 7, 8, and 9. Surface plasmon resonance measurements demonstrated that pH had no effect on the structure of AgNPs (409–430 nm). Particle size distribution may be expanded by reacting with a pH range of 5−9, as seen by a hypsochromic shift [19]. The reaction temperature is also vital. Using *Couroupita guianensisl*, AgNPs were synthesized at seven distinct reaction temperatures. From the experiment it is revealed that no AgNPs could be produced below 37°C [20].

10.2.2 Gold nanoparticles

Due to their unique features and applications in nanoelectronics, nanodevices, nonlinear optics, biomedicine, and catalysis, AuNPs have also piqued the interest of researchers in the field of biosynthesis using plant extracts. Furthermore, AuNPs have the potential to serve as excellent scaffolding for delivering drugs and genetic material. Unique properties such as monodispersity, variable core size, the huge surface-to-volume ratio, and facile functionalization with nearly any chemical or biomolecule enable targeting, transporting, and tailoring the delivery process [21]. For the majority of the aforementioned applications, AuNPs synthesized in an environmentally acceptable and chemical-free manner are recommended. The bioreduction of chloroauric acid ($HAuCl_4$) to AuNPs follows the procedure shown here in general:

$$H^{+}Au3^{+}4Cl^{-}\ 4H_2O$$
$$+ \text{Plant molecule}(OH,\ COOH,\ \text{etc.}) \rightarrow Au^{0}\ \text{nanoparticles}$$

The aforementioned reaction causes the suspension to become ruby red, indicating that AuNPs have formed in the solution. Shankar et al. were the first to reveal that geranium leaves (*Pelargonium graveolens*) may be used to make AuNPs [22]. They discovered that terpenoids in the leaves served as capping agents and reduced, allowing chloroaurate ions to be rapidly reduced to stable AuNPs of varying sizes. Using various types of plants including neem (*Azadirachta indica*) leaf extract and lemongrass (*Cymbopogon citratus*) plant extract, the same research group showed the production of AuNPs in subsequent years [23]. Black tea leaf extract was used by Begum et al. to create spheres, trapezoids, prisms, and rod-shaped AuNPs. Tea polyphenols, particularly flavonoids, were responsible for the leaf extract's exceptionally effective reduction potential [24]. Song et al. found that leaf broths from *Magnolia kobus* and *Diospyros kaki* could produce environmentally friendly metallic AuNPs (5−300 nm) with various hexagonal, triangular, pentagonal, and spherical forms in just a few minutes (at 95°C, up to 90% conversion) [25]. Babu et al. observed that an ethanolic extract of

Mentha arvensis leaves generated hexagonal and spherical AuNPs with an average size of 39 ± 15 nm [26]. At ambient temperature, pear fruit extract biosynthesized triangular and hexagonal AuNPs (200−500 nm). Plate-like AuNPs morphologies were formed when pear fruit extract was subjected to chloroaurate ions because of phytochemicals including saccharides, organic acids, proteins, and amino acids. *Garcinia combogia* fruit extract was utilized in 2014 to produce spherical and anisotropic AuNPs [27]. The form of the AuNPs was determined by the amount of extract and the temperature of the reaction. *Pistacia integerrima* leaf gall extract was shown by Islam et al. to reduce ions to AuNPs. Polyphenols' hydroxyl and carboxylic acid groups were to blame for the drop in toxicity. They also demonstrated great potential for enzyme inhibition, antifungal, antibacterial, antinociceptive, muscle relaxant, and sedative actions, as well as stability in a variety of pH solutions and high temperatures [28].

To synthesize AuNPs, microorganisms might be used. For instance, the yeast *Magnusiomyces ingens* LH-F1 was grown until it reached the logarithmic growth phase under aerobic conditions and an ambient temperature of 30°C. The cell suspension was treated with HAuCl4, and the resulting AuNPs were seen. Green synthesis of AuNPs was also carried out using microorganisms such as HS-11 and filamentous mesophiles [13].

10.2.3 Copper nanoparticles

Cu is the most used coinage metal because of its low cost, simplicity of usage, and excellent conductivity. As a result, it has found a lot of use in electrical devices, heterogeneous catalysis, mechanical alloys, thermal processes, and optical materials. It is reported that CuNPs are important as micronutrients and biopesticides, such as bactericides, fungicides, and lampricides, against plant infections in a number of studies [29]. In addition, CuNPs are also being studied for their antibacterial and catalytic properties in the biomedical and organic chemistry disciplines, respectively. CuNPs may be synthesized via green techniques, which are commonly used for diverse applications. Cu^{2+} may be reduced to Cu° by biomolecules in plant extracts, resulting in green CuNPs [30]. For starters, metal ion concentration influences synthesis rate, shape, and CuNP size. *Eucalyptus globulus* (*E. globulus*) leaf extract was used in a 1:10 dilution ratio to produce CuNPs by Iliger et al. [5]. At a concentration of 10 mM, the as-fabricated CuNPs had diameters of 60−75 nm and were triangular in structure. Chinnathambi et al. used the same ratio but a lower concentration of Cu^{2+} (1 mM) to produce smaller CuNPs (10−12 nm) [31]. Sarwar et al. noticed a significant rise in CuNP size at a concentration of Cu^{2+} as low as 0.1 mM [32]. It is apparent that a lower Cu^{2+} concentration has the benefit of inhibiting the clustering of CuNPs, and that this has the potential to be beneficial. The minute concentration of Cu^{2+} ions, on the other hand, is insufficient to cause nucleation, which results in a sluggish reaction rate.

10.2.4 Other metallic nanoparticles

Platinum nanoparticles (PtNPs) are utilized as catalysts and in a wide range of biologic applications. In comparison to Ag and Au, there are far fewer publications on PtNPs. When platinum solution and plant biomass combine, the following reaction normally occurs:

$$H_2Pt + 6Cl^- \; 6H_2O + \text{Plant molecule(OH, COOH, etc.)} \rightarrow Pt^0\text{nanoparticles}$$

Song et al. used *Diopyros kaki* leaf extract as a reducing agent for extracellular production of PtNPs (2–12 nm) from an aqueous chloroplatinic acid hexahydrate ($H_2PtCl_6H_2O$) solution [33]. They converted 90% of Pt ions into NPs at 95°C and a leaf broth content >10%. Biochemical synthesis of PtNPs with a diameter of 2.4 nm was attained by Zheng et al. using an extract from *Cacumen platycladi*. The reaction conditions involve the use of 90%, 70% plant extract, 0.5 mM starting Pt^{2+} concentration, and a reaction period of 25 h [34]. Reducing sugars and flavonoids was also shown to have an important function in the reduction of Pt ions. To synthesize PtNPs from an aqueous H_2PtCl_66H2O solution, Soundarrajan et al. employed the extract of *Ocimum sanctum*. Compounds in plants, including ascorbic acid, terpenoids, gallic acid, specific proteins, and amino acids, were shown to reduce Pt in certain experimental procedures [35]. PtNPs (4 nm) were synthesized in a single step utilizing plant polyphenols extracted from *Terminalia chebula* aqueous extract, according to Kumar et al. [7]. The decrease of Pt^{4+} to Pt^0 and subsequent stabilization was found to be due to oxidized polyphenols in the plant extract.

Palladium nanoparticles (PdNPs) are another type of widely explored metal NPs that are commonly utilized in chemiresistor-type sensing devices and as catalysts in different processes and plasmonic wave directing. Using plant biomass, palladium chloride ($PdCl_2$) may be reduced to PdNPs.

$$Pd + Cl_2^- + \text{Plant molecule}(-C=C,\ -C=O,\ \text{etc.}) \rightarrow Pd^0\text{nanoparticles}$$

At room temperature, Nadagouda et al. performed the production of Pd nanocrystals utilizing coffee and tea extract [36]. According to the researchers, the produced NPs were 20–60 nm in size and crystallized in face-centered cubic symmetry. Following that, Sathishkumar et al. reported the manufacture of PdNPs (15–20 nm) using *Cinnamom zeylanicum* bark extract [37]. Despite the fact that the specific process was unknown to the scientists, they assumed that terpenoids played a key role in the production of PdNPs. To create PdNPs, Yang et al. utilized *Cinnamomum camphora* leaf extract as a bioreductant. The average particle size measured by the researchers was 3.2–6.0 nm, and they concluded that polyols, as well as heterocyclic components, were responsible for the decrease of Pd ions and the stability of PdNPs [38]. Kora et al. used a plant polymer, gum ghatti, to synthesize PdNPs from $PdCl_2$ (*Anogeissus latifolia*). The emergence of a strong brown hue in the solution showed the synthesis of PdNPs, and the prepared PdNPs were spherical in shape, polydisperse, and had an average particle size of 4.8 ± 1.6 nm [6].

10.3 Factors influencing the production of metallic nanoparticles from plant extract

Plant-mediated biosynthesis is affected by a variety of factors, including the kind of plant involved, which influences the synthesis, characterization, and use of NPs. Some of the most critical considerations are illustrated in Fig. 10.2.

10.3.1 pH

Plant-mediated synthesis of NPs relies heavily on the pH of the medium. It has been shown that the solution medium's pH has an effect on the size and form of the NPs prepared. The formation of nucleation centers, which rise in pH, is responsible for this occurrence. Metal ion reduction to metal NPs increases with nucleation center size. At the same time, the pH of the solution affects the activity of the functional groups in the plant extract/biomass, as well as the rate of metal salt reduction. For instance, according to Armendariz et al., the size of AuNPs generated by *Avena sativa* depends on the solution pH. They found that sizable AuNPs (25–85 nm) developed at pH 2. At pH 3 and 4, however, considerable amounts of smaller NPs developed [39]. AuNPs are thought to favor aggregation over nucleation at low pH (pH 2), leading to the formation of bigger NPs. As a result, a more significant number of Au^{2+} complexes bound to the plant biomass at pH 3

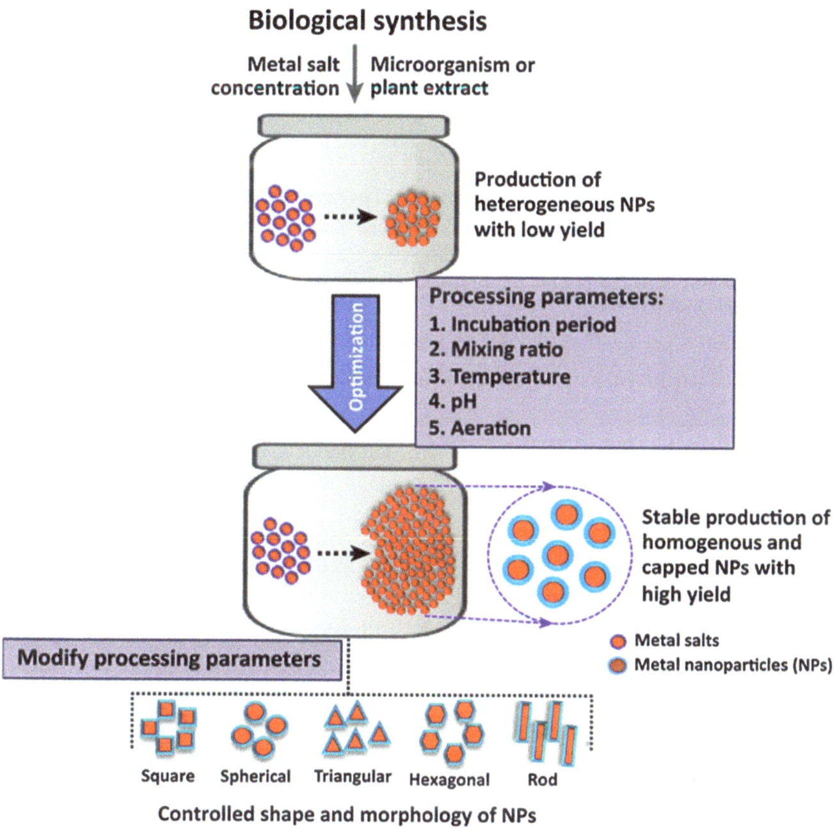

Figure 10.2 Factors affecting the production of metallic nanoparticles from plant extract. *(Reproduced with permission from Behzad et al. [11]).*

and 4, where more functional groups (carbonyl and hydroxyl) were accessible. Using *Cacumen platycladi* leaf extract, Zhan et al. investigated the influence of pH on the production of AuNPs using leaf extracts [40]. AuNPs became smaller as pH rose, but the strength of their absorption peaks became stronger. They also discovered that high pH speeds up the chloroaurate ion reduction rate, increases homogeneous nucleation, and reduces anisotropy development. Slow reduction rates under acidic conditions, on the other hand, led to heterogeneous nucleation and secondary nucleation of seeds for the formation of smaller AuNPs. The reduction rates of Au and Ag ions at pH 3.3 and 10.8 were also studied by Jacob et al. In their experiments, researchers found that Ag ions significantly reduced more slowly than Au ions decreased at pH 3.3, leading to a 2-day precipitation of NPs as a result [41].

Nonetheless, at pH 10.8, both metal ions experienced simultaneous decreases, and a single surface plasmon resonance (SPR) band was identified. The transmission electron microscope imaging revealed a uniform electron density, indicating the formation of alloyed NPs. They went on to say that a high pH value aided in the creation of AgO^- and AgO, which interact strongly with hydroxyl groups in plant extracts and therefore efficiently coat the surface of NPs.

10.3.2 Temperature

Another critical component determining the shape, size, and pace of NP formation is temperature. The development of nucleation centers increases with increasing temperature, in a manner similar to that of pH, which in turn increases the pace of biosynthesis. Sneha et al. investigated the influence of temperature on the production of AuNPs using a leaf extract of the Piper betel plant [42]. TEM scans revealed mostly nano-triangles at temperatures as high as 200°C, but smaller nanoplatelets and NPs with diameters ranging from 5 to 500 nm were visible at temperatures as low as 30–40°C. At 50 and 60°C, the researchers observed that, despite the presence of nano-triangles and octahedral platelets, the shape and size of the produced NPs were relatively constant. According to Sheny et al., the optimal temperature for bimetallic Au–Ag synthesis was determined by testing leaf extracts of *Anacardium occidentale* at various reduction temperatures [43]. To produce stable NPs at low reaction temperatures, more leaf extract was needed, according to the authors, than at high reaction temperatures. Biosynthesis at 100°C needed just 0.06 mL of leaf extract, whereas synthesis at 27°C required 2.5 mL of leaf extract. They also found that NPs generated at high temperatures were more stable and more significant in size than those created at lower temperatures. Iravani et al. prepared the reaction mixture (*Pinus eldarica* bark extract and $AgNO_3$) at various temperatures (25, 50, 100, and 150°C) in an attempt to examine the influence of temperature [44]. The absorbance of AgNPs increased, but their size shrank when the reaction temperature was raised, according to the researchers.

10.3.3 Reaction time

The amount of time the suspension media is incubated affects the size, shape, and extent of NPs formation utilizing plant-based biomaterials. Unlike microorganisms, seed extract of *Coriandrum sativum* produced

AgNPs in 1–2 h, compared to 2–4 days, according to Nazeruddin et al. [45]. Another study found that the production of AuNPs using a hybrid petal catalyst took only 5 min. Plant-mediated NP biosynthesis is typically faster than microorganism-mediated NP biosynthesis; however, several researchers have observed improved yield rates at high reaction times. *Chenopodium album* leaf extract-based synthesis of AgNPs and AuNPs began after 15 min of the reaction, according to Dwivedi et al. [46]. Researchers showed that both AgNPs and AuNPs had sharper peaks when the contact duration was increased. The form and size of the NPs might change depending on the length of the reaction period, according to a few studies. Li et al. found that a 5-h reaction period produced AgNPs with a spherical and polycrystalline form (10 nm) when utilizing *Capsicum annuum* L. extract to synthesize AgNPs. The size of NPs increased with the increase in response time from 9 to 13 h to 25 and 40 nm accordingly [47].

10.3.4 Concentration of plant extract

NPs synthesis is typically influenced by the amount of plant biomass/extract used. Several researchers have shown that increasing the biomass dose increases NPs formation while altering their shape. Due to this reason, optimizing biomass dose for a process is so important. Leaf extract of aloe vera was utilized by Chandran et al. to alter the size and form of produced AuNPs. Depending on the extract concentration, the majority of the AuNPs were triangular and ranged in size from 50 to 350 nm. Nanogold triangles of bigger sizes were formed when the extract was added to the $HAuCl_4$ solution in small doses. There was also a drop in nano-triangle to spherical ratio as the extracted content increased [48].

10.4 Application of metallic nanoparticles in pharmaceuticals

10.4.1 Antibacterial

The toxicity of AgNP to bacteria is caused by Ag ions liberated into an aqueous medium during partial oxidation. Ag ions and NPs react with the plasma membrane, disrupting cellular activities such as permeability and respiration, eventually leading to lysis. Exposure to AgNP can disrupt DNA replication and ribosome denaturation [4]. Against *E. coli*, Cui et al. discuss the methods by which AuNP functions as an antibacterial agent [49]. A drop in cellular ATP levels was seen due to AuNP collapsing membrane potential, which substantially inhibited ATPase action. One of the side effects of AuNP exposure was that tRNA binding to the ribosomal subunit was hindered. The cell wall structure of bacteria can influence their sensitivity to antimicrobial drugs. Microorganisms with a multilayer cell wall are known as Gram-negative bacteria (G^-), whereas microorganisms with a single-layer cell wall are known as Gram-positive bacteria (G^+). This classification is based on their cell wall structure. The antibacterial activity of NPs prepared via biologic route has been studied in both types of bacteria. For the biogenesis of NPs with demonstrated antibacterial properties, a range of biologic materials has been employed. Fungal, bacterial, and algal biomass, as well as botanical extracts from roots, leaves, bark, and tubers, are among the materials used. Vigneshwaran et al. presented one of the earliest publications on the antibacterial properties of biosynthesized NPs. The researchers synthesized AgNPs utilizing the edible fungus *Pleurotus sajor-caju* and tested them against *Staphylococcus aureus* (G+) and *Klebsiella pneumoniae* (G^-) with great success [50]. *Pestalotia* sp., an endophytic fungus isolated from *Syzygium cumini* leaves, was utilized to synthesize AgNPs extracellularly and the antibacterial activities of AgNPs against *S. aureus* (ATCC-25,923) and *Salmonella typhi* were reported by Raheman et al. [51]. The combination of biosynthesized AgNPs and commercially available antibiotics gentamycin and sulphamethizole resulted in synergistic effects. In two researches by Sadhasivam et al., the antimicrobial capabilities of bacteria-biosynthesized NPs were demonstrated. *Staphylococcus epidermidis* and *Staphylococcus aureus* were shown to be resistant to the antibacterial capabilities of *Streptomyces hygroscopicus* cells utilized for the production of AgNPs and AuNPs [52]. The microalgal strains *Chaetocerus calcitrans, Isochrysis galbana, Chlorella salina,* and *Tetraselmis gracilis* generated antibacterial AgNPs in a study by Merin et al. using algae-based NP biosynthesis [53]. Clearing zone assays demonstrated that these NPs have antibacterial activity against *Proteus vulgaris, K. pneumoniae, P. aeruginosa*, and *E. coli*. Sulfated polysaccharides obtained from the marine red alga *Porphyra vietnamensis* were used by Venkatpurwar et al. to synthesize AgNPs. *S. aureus* (G+) was less resistant to AgNPs generated in this investigation, *E. coli* (G−) was significantly more effective [54]. A marine alga, *Galaxaura elongata*, was used by Abdel-Raouf et al. to synthesize antimicrobial AuNPs using powder or ethanolic extract [3]. Algal compounds that may be used as reducing agents or NP capping agents were identified through spectroscopic investigations carried out by these researchers. It has been shown that plant tissues and extracts may be employed as reducing agents in numerous studies of biosynthesized antibacterial NPs. To eliminate pathogenic or dangerous molecules from biosynthesized NPs, purification may be necessary, especially for materials intended for usage in vivo. Botanical extracts that have been thoroughly analyzed and are known to be safe can be used for biosynthesis [55]. When it comes to the production of NPs, green tea extract (made from the leaves of *Camellia sinensis*) is a popular choice. AgNPs with a shown antibacterial action against *Vibrio harveyi* were prepared by Vaseeharan et al. using tea extract. Antimicrobial AgNPs have been synthesized using other plant extracts. *E. coli* biofilm-forming *E. coli*, *Proteus vulgaris*, *Vibrio paraheamolyticus*, and *Listeria monocytogenes* were all inhibited by AgNPs synthesized from the stem callus extract of bitter apple (*Citrullus colocynthis*) [56]. *Salmonella enteritidis*, *Proteus mirabilis*, and *Staphylococcus aureus* were all found to be completely dormant. AgNPs were biosynthesized by Kaviya et al. utilizing extract from the navel orange peel (*Citrus sinensis*), which proved antibacterial against *E. coli*, *Pseudomonas*, and *Staphylococcus aureus* [57]. It has been shown that the Chinese yam (*Dioscorea batatas*) rhizome extract may be utilized to synthesize antibacterial AgNPs. Antibiotics and phytosynthesized NPs have been shown to have synergistic antibacterial properties [58]. Ghosh et al. created AgNPs from tuber extract of *Dioscorea bulbifera* before testing the antibacterial synergy of the compounds with an array of commercially available antibiotics and seven different bacterial strain types and subtypes [59]. For example, when streptomycin and AgNPS are utilized in conjunction against *E. coli*, they discovered an 11.8-fold improvement in inhibitory efficacy. Antibacterial AuNPs have also been synthesized using plant extracts. To make AuNPs that were effective against *S. aureus*, Kumar et al. employed the *Terminalia chebula* tree extract [60]. For the production of AuNPs and AgNPs, Ali et al. employed *Mentha piperita* leaf extract, which they found to have antibacterial properties against *S. aureus* and *E. coli* bacteria. Biosynthesized metallic NPs that are immobilized on cotton fabric offer a wide range of vital uses as a wound dressing material [61]. Duran et al., for example, described the extracellular synthesis of AgNPs mediated by the fungus *Fusarium oxysporum* in a cell culture system [62]. In this study, AgNPs were integrated into cotton textiles to limit *S. aureus* growth. Although immobilized AgNPs in the fabric have many advantages, one restriction is that they lose their Ag ions and, in some cases, their AgNPs, when the fabric is washed. A study conducted by El-Rafie et al. revealed the use of immobilized biogenic AgNPs on cotton fabric [63]. Specifically, AgNPs were produced using *Fusarium solani* and then applied to cotton textiles using an acrylate-based binder in this research. After 20 washing cycles, the cotton fabric demonstrated significant antimicrobial efficacy against *S. aureus* and *E. coli*, with an approximate 90% antimicrobial efficiency. As part of their research, Tripathi et al. investigated the synthesis of AgNPs in aqueous extracts from the leaves of *Azadirachta indica*, as well as their subsequent immobilization on cotton fabric [64]. With washing in distilled water, these researchers observed a bactericidal effect against *E. coli* and *Staphylococcus aureus* bacteria. It has also been reported that the production of AgNPs from extract of *Eucalyptus citriodora* and *Ficus bengalensis* leaf, as well as their loading into cotton fibers, was carried out by Ravindra et al. Cotton fibers were soaked in AgNP-containing leaf extract for 24 h, shaken, and then, using a modified disc diffusion method, they were evaluated for resistance to *E. coli* [65].

AgNPs made from *Curcuma longa* tuber extract and powder were also evaluated for antibacterial activity against *E. coli* before being immobilized on cotton fabric. AgNPs were resuspended in water or polyvinylidene fluoride (PVDF) and sprayed over presterilized cotton fabric. The antibacterial activity of cloth treated with NPs in PVDF was decreased, but the reusability was substantially longer. Biosynthesized AgNPs embedded into nonwoven textiles have recently been shown to offer antibacterial properties. Yang et al. used mango peel extract to make AgNPs and tested their antibacterial efficiency against *E. coli*, *S. aureus*, and *B. subtilis* when they were immobilized on nonwoven textiles [66]. Sundaramoorthi et al. presented an extracellular preparation of biosynthesized AgNPs utilizing the fungus *Aspergillus niger* for wound healing [67]. Following excision in a rat model, the AgNPs' efficacy was confirmed. The findings validated Ag's antibacterial properties as well as AgNPs' potential to influence wound-healing cytokines. Following excision in animal models, the medicinal plant *Indigofera aspalathoides* was utilized to synthesize AgNPs that were investigated in wound-healing applications. In addition, biogenic AgNPs produced from *Chrysanthemum morifolium* have been introduced to clinical ultrasound gel. On an ultrasonic probe, the gel was tested for bactericidal and instrument sterility properties [12].

10.4.2 Antiviral

Biosynthesized NPs' antiviral activity has been reported sparingly, despite the pervasiveness of viruses in medicine and agriculture. The antiviral activity of AgNPs generated intracellularly in *Aspergillus ochraceus* was described by Vijayakumar et al. The plaque count technique was used in the study to test the efficiency of AgNPs embedded in a carbonaceous matrix against M13 phage [68].

Other researchers have detailed the use of zero-valent cerium, which is created by adding aqueous Ce(III) to cultures of *Leptothrix discophora* or *Pseudomonas putida*, to prevent the spread of viruses [69]. Antivirus activity against bacteriophage UZ1 was effective using the cerium in its as-prepared state. *Lactobacillus fermentum* bacteria were utilized as both a reducing agent and a scaffold for AgNPs in another investigation by the same team. Their antiviral efficacy against murine norovirus 1 and bacteriophage UZ1 was tested. A NanoCeram electropositive filter was used to investigate the continuous antiviral capability of AgNPs implanted in *Lactobacillus* bacteria in an aquatic setting. The cell-embedded NP filter had a significantly higher antiviral activity than the original filter, according to the study. UZ1 bacteriophage inactivation was also demonstrated by De Gusseme et al. utilizing cell-embedded NPs on PVDF membrane [70].

10.4.3 Anticancer

Biosynthesized NPs have been shown to be cytotoxic to a variety of cancer cell types. AuNPs produced from phytochemicals found in grapes were used in investigations published by Amarnath et al. [71]. Using these AuNPs, we were able to induce apoptosis in human breast cancer cells (HBL-100) after exposure. Mishra et al. documented the production of AuNP by the fungus *Penicillium brevicompactum* using the supernatant, live-cell filtrate, and biomass as starting materials [72]. The cytotoxic effects of biosynthesized NPs were investigated in this study utilizing C2C12 mouse myoblast cancer cells. In another investigation, guava and clove extracts were utilized to lower the amount of Au and Ag salts [73]. HEK-293, HeLa, and HT-29 cancer cell lines treated with biosynthesized AuNPs showed anticancer action; however, AgNPs did not. AgNPs, on the other hand, have been linked to anticancer activity in other studies. When *Piper longum* leaf was used to reduce and limit antitumoral AgNP biosynthesis, Jacob et al. published their findings. It was shown that these particles had a great cytotoxic impact on cancer cell lines such as HEp-2. *Citrullus colocynthis* callus extract was also used to make AgNPs that were efficient against HEp-2 cells in the lab.

AgNPs biosynthesized from *Melia azedarach*, a deciduous tree from the mahogany family, showed comparable efficacy against HeLa cells in a lymphoma animal model. Jeyaraj et al. provided a detailed assessment of AgNPs' influence on malignant cell lines [74]. The cytotoxicity of biogenic AgNPs against human breast cancer cells was investigated in vitro using the 3-(4,5-dimethylthiazol-2-yl)-2,5-diphenyltetrazolium bromide (MTT), acridine orange/ethidium bromide, and Hoechst techniques, as well as the COMET assay. CuNPs were synthesized extracellularly using *Euphorbia nivulia* stem latex [75]. CuNPs are hazardous to A549 (human lung cancer) cells in a dose-dependent manner, according to this study. The anti-metastatic effect of biologically produced AuNPs in the human fibrosarcoma cell line HT-1080 was recently revealed [76]. Biosynthetic AuNPs exhibited no harmful effects on HT-1080 cells; however, the study found that AuNPs hinder cell migration by interfering with the actin polymerization process.

10.4.4 Antioxidant

The production of metal NPs with increased antioxidant and antibacterial properties is gaining relevance in biochemical applications. Antioxidants are reported to defend cells against detrimental effects induced by the reactive oxygen species, thereby lowering the occurrences of several degenerative illnesses such as cancer, neurodegeneration, and heart disease. A study published in 2015 by Nakkla et al. described the production of AgNP and AuNP utilizing *Costus pictus* leaf extract and their in vitro antioxidant and catalytic properties. The NPs showed outstanding catalytic and free radical scavenging abilities [77]. Alcoholic 2,2-diphenyl-1-picrylhydrazyl (DPPH) solutions exhibit a deep violet hue and a prominent absorption band at 517 nm, both hallmarks of the DPPH test. To reduce the amount of DPPH produced, antioxidants must absorb either one hydrogen atom or one electron. Its color changes from violet to light yellow as a result of the DPPH reduction, and this drop in absorbance may be seen using spectrophotometry. The seeds of *Pimpinella anisum* were used to synthesize AgNPs and AuNPs, which were tested for DPPH scavenging by Zayed et al. As expected, the results demonstrated that the scavenging ability of all samples against the DPPH free radical increased with increasing concentrations. *P. anisum* extract and AuNPs have lower DPPH antioxidant activity than AgNPs [78].

10.4.5 Other applications

Many other applications of metal NPs have been revealed in recent years. An extensive range of disease-causing insects and parasites can benefit from the use of biosynthesized NPs. Varying lotus leaf extracts (*Nelumbo nucifera*) were used to produce AgNPs with different larvicidal properties. *Anopheles subpictus* and *Culex quinquefasciatus*, two well-known malaria and lymphatic filariasis vectors, were tested for antilarval activity in the study [79].

Gnanadesigan et al. conducted a similar investigation on AgNPs biosynthesized using extract of mangrove leaf against *Aedes aegypti* and *C. quinquefasciatus larva* [80]. AgNPs derived from henna (*Lawsonia inermis*) leaf extract were found to be effective against the human head louse Pediculus humanus capitis and the sheep body louse Bovicola ovis. The study used both a direct contact approach (P. *humanus*) and an impregnated filter paper method to test lousicidal activity (*B. ovis*). Furthermore, the acaricidal activity of an aqueous extract of an evergreen tree (*Manilkara zapota*) and AgNPs made using this extract against the cattle tick were evaluated [12].

Drug delivery is another prominent use of metal NPs in the pharmaceutical industry. NPs synthesized via a biologic route can interact with mammalian tissues and change their function. Metallic NPs, for example, can disrupt the antioxidant defense system, resulting in the buildup of reactive oxygen species, mitochondrial damage, and cell death. The capping agent significantly influences the in vivo consequences of metal NP exposure, so this effect may be targeted. The identical AgNPs with various capping agents have been found to be both cytotoxic and noncytotoxic [12]. For instance, the targeted delivery of anticancer drugs to cancer cells can be minimized by the use of stable noble metal NPs as carriers. Due to its affinity for thiols (−SH) and amines ($-NH_2$), gold may be easily changed. As a result, chemotherapeutic and targeted biomolecules may easily be applied to the NP surface [81]. Using a variety of capping agents, the cytotoxic capability of metallic NPs may be used for both drug delivery and cancer cell targeting. Although biosynthesized NPs may be used for therapeutic purposes or as carriers for other agents, their importance in nanomedicine is growing.

10.5 Limitations and future perspectives

Many recent studies have shown that plants may be used as efficient precursors for the production of metal NPs while being environmentally benign. The use of plant extracts to synthesize NPs, on the other hand, has yet to be fully explored. To fully comprehend the mechanism of NP production and stability by plant extracts, further research is required. Despite the substantial advances achieved in this subject, a number of concerns remain unresolved. The limitations and challenges associated with the synthesis of plant NPs are illustrated in Fig. 10.3. Despite the immense potential of metal NPs generated using plant extracts, the precise synthetic process parameters must yet be refined.

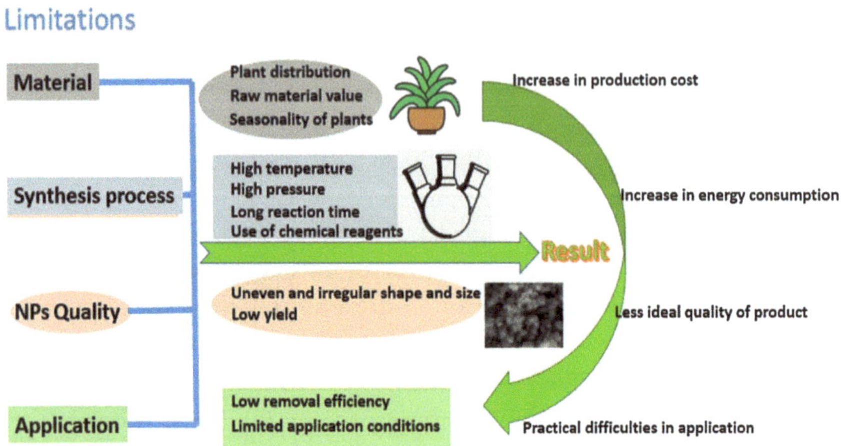

Figure 10.3 Limitations and challenges associated with the synthesis of metal NPs. *(Reproduced with permission from Ying et al. [13]).*

Meanwhile, the key synthetic pathways must be clarified, and researchers have significant difficulty in comprehending the chemical components involved in the synthesis and stability of metal NPs. Numerous researchers have examined plants that can be grown locally and in abundance for the green synthesis of NPs. Despite the fact that these studies reveal that local plants may be completely used, industrial-level global production of green-synthesized nanoscale metals remains a challenge. It is exclusively found in the Cyrenaica, southern Aegean Sea, Cyprus, and southern Turkey regions, where *Lithodora hispidula* (Sm.) Griseb leaf is present. PdNPs may be synthesized using other materials, such as *Sapium sebiferum* and *Euphorbia* plants [82]. Another significant issue related to the synthesis of metal NPs is the energy-intensive synthesis procedure that is required. Another limiting aspect is the inconsistency in the quality of the metal NPs synthesized from plant extracts. NPs generated by various extracts vary greatly in size and shape, and the attributes identified are inadequate. According to recent studies, there are large variances in particle size, making green technology unsuitable for large-scale manufacturing and making particle size controlling throughout production a huge difficulty.

The process by which active molecules in extracts cling to the surfaces of metal NPs, as well as the identification of real molecular active groups in the molecules, must be investigated in more depth. Moreover, as metal NP applications grow at an exponential pace, the accumulation of these particles in the environment becomes a source of concern, mandating a focus on in vivo toxicology as well as long-term repercussions for people, animals, and the environment. Future studies on the challenges encountered should assist researchers to make greater use of green synthesis in our society's growth and progress.

10.6 Summary

Metal NPs, including nanogold, silver, copper, platinum, and palladium, have been synthesized in recent years utilizing plant extracts. A wide range of uses for metal NPs, including catalysis, water purification, medicine, antibacterial and anticancer agents (in addition to bioengineering and sensors), and medical imaging are just a few examples. Importantly, the synthesis method does not use any harmful chemical reagents. The resultant metal NPs are free of toxic chemicals, making them particularly useful in medicinal applications where nontoxicity is necessary. Plant extracts also include several unique bioactive compounds that aid in the creation of metal NPs and improve their stability. This study has focused on the synthesis of these frequently used metal NPs. The rapid growth of green chemistry and nanotechnology has encouraged the use of green synthetic approaches to produce nanomaterials from plants. In contrast to fungus and bacteria, plants (and especially plant extracts) can decrease metal ions far more quickly.

Furthermore, plant extracts are preferable to plant biomass or living plants for industrial scale-up and manufacturing of well-dispersed metal NPs using a safe and straightforward green process. Metal NPs may be produced using a plant extract—mediated approach, which has the benefits of cheap cost and nontoxicity, as well as easy scale-up and environmental friendliness. It was established that pH, temperature, reaction duration, and plant dosage all had a significant impact on metal NP formation. Despite the immense potential of metal NPs generated using plant extracts, the specific preparation process parameters must yet be refined. Some research has suggested that plant biomass functional groups may be involved in the formation of NPs. There has been a dramatic increase in NP biosynthesis research over the past few years, and it looks to be on the verge of a major expansion into pharmaceutical applications. It is expected that the fundamental biosynthesis mechanisms will be further developed, as will the ability to create new biosynthetic NP forms.

References

[1] P. Duarah, D. Haldar, M.K. Purkait, Technological advancement in the synthesis and applications of lignin-based nanoparticles derived from agro-industrial waste residues: a review, International Journal of Biological Macromolecules 163 (2020) 1828–1843.

[2] D. Haldar, M.K. Purkait, Micro and nanocrystalline cellulose derivatives of lignocellulosic biomass: a review on synthesis, applications and advancements, Carbohydrate Polymers 250 (2020) 116937.

[3] N. Abdel-Raouf, N.M. Al-Enazi, I.B. Ibraheem, Green biosynthesis of gold nanoparticles using Galaxaura elongata and characterization of their antibacterial activity, Arabian Journal of Chemistry 10 (2017) S3029–S3039.

[4] K. Chaloupka, Y. Malam, A.M. Seifalian, Nanosilver as a new generation of nanoproduct in biomedical applications, Trends in Biotechnology 28 (11) (2010) 580–588.

[5] K.S. Iliger, et al., Copper nanoparticles: green synthesis and managing fruit rot disease of chilli caused by Colletotrichum capsici, Saudi Journal of Biological Sciences 28 (2) (2021) 1477–1486.

[6] A.J. Kora, L. Rastogi, Green synthesis of palladium nanoparticles using gum ghatti (Anogeissus latifolia) and its application as an antioxidant and catalyst, Arabian Journal of Chemistry 11 (7) (2018) 1097–1106.

[7] K.M. Kumar, B.K. Mandal, S.K. Tammina, Green synthesis of nano platinum using naturally occurring polyphenols, RSC Advances 3 (12) (2013) 4033–4039.

[8] P. Mondal, A. Anweshan, M.K. Purkait, Green synthesis and environmental application of iron-based nanomaterials and nanocomposite: a review, Chemosphere 259 (2020) 127509.

[9] P. Mondal, M.K. Purkait, Preparation and characterization of novel green synthesized iron—aluminum nanocomposite and studying its efficiency in fluoride removal, Chemosphere 235 (2019) 391–402.

[10] P. Mondal, M.K. Purkait, Green synthesized iron nanoparticles supported on pH responsive polymeric membrane for nitrobenzene reduction and fluoride rejection study: optimization approach, Journal of Cleaner Production 170 (2018) 1111–1123.

[11] F. Behzad, et al., An overview of the plant-mediated green synthesis of noble metal nanoparticles for antibacterial applications, Journal of Industrial and Engineering Chemistry 94 (2021) 92–104.

[12] A. Schröfel, et al., Applications of biosynthesized metallic nanoparticles — a review, Acta Biomaterialia 10 (10) (2014) 4023–4042.

[13] S. Ying, et al., Green synthesis of nanoparticles: current developments and limitations, Environmental Technology and Innovation 26 (2022) 102336.

[14] S.S. Shankar, A. Ahmad, M. Sastry, Geranium leaf assisted biosynthesis of silver nanoparticles, Biotechnology Progress 19 (6) (2003) 1627–1631.

[15] J. Huang, et al., Biosynthesis of silver and gold nanoparticles by novel sundried Cinnamomum camphora leaf, Nanotechnology 18 (10) (2007) 105104.

[16] A. Leela, M. Vivekanandan, Tapping the unexploited plant resources for the synthesis of silver nanoparticles, African Journal of Biotechnology 7 (17) (2008).

[17] N. Ahmad, et al., Rapid synthesis of nanoparticles using medicinal particles of basil, Colloids and Surfaces B: Bionterf 81 (2010) 81–86.

[18] M. Jeyaraj, et al., An investigation on the cytotoxicity and caspase-mediated apoptotic effect of biologically synthesized silver nanoparticles using *Podophyllum hexandrum* on human cervical carcinoma cells, Colloids and Surfaces B: Biointerfaces 102 (2013) 708–717.

[19] T.N. Jebakumar Immanuel Edison, M.G. Sethuraman, Electrocatalytic reduction of benzyl chloride by green synthesized silver nanoparticles using pod extract of Acacia nilotica, ACS Sustainable Chemistry and Engineering 1 (10) (2013) 1326–1332.

[20] Y. Ping, et al., Green synthesis of silver nanoparticles using grape seed extract and their application for reductive catalysis of Direct Orange 26, Journal of Industrial and Engineering Chemistry 58 (2018) 74–79.

[21] G. Han, et al., Drug and gene delivery using gold nanoparticles, NanoBiotechnology 3 (1) (2007) 40–45.

[22] S.S. Shankar, et al., Bioreduction of chloroaurate ions by geranium leaves and its endophytic fungus yields gold nanoparticles of different shapes, Journal of Materials Chemistry 13 (7) (2003) 1822–1826.

[23] S.S. Shankar, et al., Controlling the optical properties of lemongrass extract synthesized gold nanotriangles and potential application in infrared-absorbing optical coatings, Chemistry of Materials 17 (3) (2005) 566–572.

[24] N.A. Begum, et al., Biogenic synthesis of Au and Ag nanoparticles using aqueous solutions of Black Tea leaf extracts, Colloids and Surfaces, B: Biointerfaces 71 (1) (2009) 113–118.

[25] J.Y. Song, H.-K. Jang, B.S. Kim, Biological synthesis of gold nanoparticles using Magnolia kobus and Diopyros kaki leaf extracts, Process Biochemistry 44 (10) (2009) 1133–1138.

[26] P.J. Babu, et al., Synthesis of gold nanoparticles using Mentha arvensis leaf extract, International Journal of Green Nanotechnology: Physics & Chemistry 2 (2) (2010) P62–P68.

[27] A. Rajan, M. MeenaKumari, D. Philip, Shape tailored green synthesis and catalytic properties of gold nanocrystals, Spectrochimica Acta Part A: Molecular and Biomolecular Spectroscopy 118 (2014) 793–799.

[28] N.U. Islam, et al., Pistacia integerrima gall extract mediated green synthesis of gold nanoparticles and their biological activities, Arabian Journal of Chemistry 12 (8) (2019) 2310–2319.

[29] T. Mehdizadeh, A. Zamani, S.M.A. Froushani, Preparation of Cu nanoparticles fixed on cellulosic walnut shell material and investigation of its antibacterial, antioxidant and anticancer effects, Heliyon 6 (3) (2020) e03528.

[30] M. Nasrollahzadeh, et al., In situ green synthesis of Cu nanoparticles supported on natural Natrolite zeolite for the reduction of 4-nitrophenol, Congo red and methylene blue, IET Nanobiotechnology 11 (5) (2017) 538–545.

[31] A. Chinnathambi, T. Awad Alahmadi, S. Ali Alharbi, Biogenesis of copper nanoparticles (Cu-NPs) using leaf extract of Allium noeanum, antioxidant and in-vitro cytotoxicity, Artificial Cells, Nanomedicine, and Biotechnology 49 (1) (2021) 500–510.

[32] N. Sarwar, et al., Citric acid mediated green synthesis of copper nanoparticles using cinnamon bark extract and its multifaceted applications, Journal of Cleaner Production 292 (2021) 125974.

[33] J.Y. Song, E.-Y. Kwon, B.S. Kim, Biological synthesis of platinum nanoparticles using Diopyros kaki leaf extract, Bioprocess and Biosystems Engineering 33 (1) (2010) 159–164.

[34] B. Zheng, et al., Plant-mediated synthesis of platinum nanoparticles and its bioreductive mechanism, Journal of Colloid and Interface Science 396 (2013) 138–145.

[35] C. Soundarrajan, et al., Rapid biological synthesis of platinum nanoparticles using Ocimum sanctum for water electrolysis applications, Bioprocess and Biosystems Engineering 35 (5) (2012) 827–833.

[36] M.N. Nadagouda, R.S. Varma, Green synthesis of silver and palladium nanoparticles at room temperature using coffee and tea extract, Green Chemistry 10 (8) (2008) 859–862.

[37] M. Sathishkumar, et al., Phyto-crystallization of palladium through reduction process using Cinnamom zeylanicum bark extract, Journal of Hazardous Materials 171 (1–3) (2009) 400–404.
[38] X. Yang, et al., Green synthesis of palladium nanoparticles using broth of Cinnamomum camphora leaf, Journal of Nanoparticle Research 12 (5) (2010) 1589–1598.
[39] V. Armendariz, et al., Size controlled gold nanoparticle formation by Avena sativa biomass: use of plants in nanobiotechnology, Journal of Nanoparticle Research 6 (4) (2004) 377–382.
[40] G. Zhan, et al., Synthesis of gold nanoparticles by Cacumen Platycladi leaf extract and its simulated solution: toward the plant-mediated biosynthetic mechanism, Journal of Nanoparticle Research 13 (10) (2011) 4957–4968.
[41] J. Jacob, T. Mukherjee, S. Kapoor, A simple approach for facile synthesis of Ag, anisotropic Au and bimetallic (Ag/Au) nanoparticles using cruciferous vegetable extracts, Materials Science and Engineering: C 32 (7) (2012) 1827–1834.
[42] K. Sneha, et al., Counter ions and temperature incorporated tailoring of biogenic gold nanoparticles, Process Biochemistry 45 (9) (2010) 1450–1458.
[43] D. Sheny, J. Mathew, D. Philip, Phytosynthesis of Au, Ag and Au–Ag bimetallic nanoparticles using aqueous extract and dried leaf of Anacardium occidentale, Spectrochimica Acta Part A: Molecular and Biomolecular Spectroscopy 79 (1) (2011) 254–262.
[44] S. Iravani, B. Zolfaghari, Green synthesis of silver nanoparticles using Pinus eldarica bark extract, BioMed Research International 2013 (2013).
[45] G. Nazeruddin, et al., Coriandrum sativum seed extract assisted in situ green synthesis of silver nanoparticle and its anti-microbial activity, Industrial Crops and Products 60 (2014) 212–216.
[46] A.D. Dwivedi, K. Gopal, Biosynthesis of silver and gold nanoparticles using *Chenopodium album* leaf extract, Colloids and Surfaces A: Physicochemical and Engineering Aspects 369 (1–3) (2010) 27–33.
[47] S. Li, et al., Green synthesis of silver nanoparticles using *Capsicum annuum* L. extract, Green Chemistry 9 (8) (2007) 852–858.
[48] S.P. Chandran, et al., Synthesis of gold nanotriangles and silver nanoparticles using Aloevera plant extract, Biotechnology Progress 22 (2) (2006) 577–583.
[49] Y. Cui, et al., The molecular mechanism of action of bactericidal gold nanoparticles on *Escherichia coli*, Biomaterials 33 (7) (2012) 2327–2333.
[50] N. Vigneshwaran, et al., Silver– protein (core– shell) nanoparticle production using spent mushroom substrate, Langmuir 23 (13) (2007) 7113–7117.
[51] F. Raheman, et al., Silver nanoparticles: novel antimicrobial agent synthesized from an endophytic fungus Pestalotia sp. isolated from leaves of *Syzygium cumini* (L), Nano Biomed Eng 3 (3) (2011) 174–178.
[52] S. Sadhasivam, P. Shanmugam, K. Yun, Biosynthesis of silver nanoparticles by Streptomyces hygroscopicus and antimicrobial activity against medically important pathogenic microorganisms, Colloids and Surfaces B: Biointerfaces 81 (1) (2010) 358–362.
[53] D.D. Merin, S. Prakash, B.V. Bhimba, Antibacterial screening of silver nanoparticles synthesized by marine micro algae, Asian Pacific journal of tropical Medicine 3 (10) (2010) 797–799.
[54] V. Venkatpurwar, V. Pokharkar, Green synthesis of silver nanoparticles using marine polysaccharide: study of in-vitro antibacterial activity, Materials Letters 65 (6) (2011) 999–1002.
[55] K.P. Kumar, W. Paul, C.P. Sharma, Green synthesis of gold nanoparticles with Zingiber officinale extract: characterization and blood compatibility, Process Biochemistry 46 (10) (2011) 2007–2013.

[56] B. Vaseeharan, P. Ramasamy, J. Chen, Antibacterial activity of silver nanoparticles (AgNps) synthesized by tea leaf extracts against pathogenic Vibrio harveyi and its protective efficacy on juvenile Feneropenaeus indicus, Letters in Applied Microbiology 50 (4) (2010) 352–356.

[57] S. Kaviya, et al., Biosynthesis of silver nanoparticles using Citrus sinensis peel extract and its antibacterial activity, Spectrochimica Acta Part A: Molecular and Biomolecular Spectroscopy 79 (3) (2011) 594–598.

[58] P. Nagajyothi, K. Lee, Synthesis of plant-mediated silver nanoparticles using Dioscorea batatas rhizome extract and evaluation of their antimicrobial activities, Journal of Nanomaterials 2011 (2011).

[59] S. Ghosh, et al., Synthesis of silver nanoparticles using Dioscorea bulbifera tuber extract and evaluation of its synergistic potential in combination with antimicrobial agents, International Journal of Nanomedicine 7 (2012) 483.

[60] K.M. Kumar, et al., Terminalia chebula mediated green and rapid synthesis of gold nanoparticles, Spectrochimica Acta Part A: Molecular and Biomolecular Spectroscopy 86 (2012) 490–494.

[61] D. MubarakAli, et al., Plant extract mediated synthesis of silver and gold nanoparticles and its antibacterial activity against clinically isolated pathogens, Colloids and Surfaces B: Biointerfaces 85 (2) (2011) 360–365.

[62] N. Durán, et al., Antibacterial effect of silver nanoparticles produced by fungal process on textile fabrics and their effluent treatment, Journal of Biomedical Nanotechnology 3 (2) (2007) 203–208.

[63] M. El-Rafie, et al., Antimicrobial effect of silver nanoparticles produced by fungal process on cotton fabrics, Carbohydrate Polymers 80 (3) (2010) 779–782.

[64] A. Tripathi, et al., Antibacterial applications of silver nanoparticles synthesized by aqueous extract of Azadirachta indica (Neem) leaves, Journal of Biomedical Nanotechnology 5 (1) (2009) 93–98.

[65] S. Ravindra, et al., Fabrication of antibacterial cotton fibres loaded with silver nanoparticles via "Green Approach", Colloids and Surfaces A: Physicochemical and Engineering Aspects 367 (1–3) (2010) 31–40.

[66] N. Yang, W.-H. Li, Mango peel extract mediated novel route for synthesis of silver nanoparticles and antibacterial application of silver nanoparticles loaded onto nonwoven fabrics, Industrial Crops and Products 48 (2013) 81–88.

[67] V. Kalaiselvan, A. Rajasekaran, Biosynthesis of silver nanoparticles from Aspergillus Niger and evaluation of its wound healing activity in experimental rat model, International Journal of PharmTech Research 4 (2009) 1523–1529.

[68] P. Vijayakumar, B. Prasad, Intracellular biogenic silver nanoparticles for the generation of carbon supported antiviral and sustained bactericidal agents, Langmuir 25 (19) (2009) 11741–11747.

[69] B.D. Gusseme, et al., Virus removal by biogenic cerium, Environmental Science and Technology 44 (16) (2010) 6350–6356.

[70] B. De Gusseme, et al., Virus disinfection in water by biogenic silver immobilized in polyvinylidene fluoride membranes, Water Research 45 (4) (2011) 1856–1864.

[71] K. Amarnath, et al., Facile synthesis of biocompatible gold nanoparticles from Vites vinefera and its cellular internalization against HBL-100 cells, Cancer nanotechnology 2 (1) (2011) 121–132.

[72] A. Mishra, et al., Microbial synthesis of gold nanoparticles using the fungus Penicillium brevicompactum and their cytotoxic effects against mouse mayo blast cancer C2C12 cells, Applied Microbiology and Biotechnology 92 (3) (2011) 617–630.

[73] D. Raghunandan, et al., Anti-cancer studies of noble metal nanoparticles synthesized using different plant extracts, Cancer nanotechnology 2 (1) (2011) 57–65.

[74] S.J.P. Jacob, J. Finub, A. Narayanan, Synthesis of silver nanoparticles using Piper longum leaf extracts and its cytotoxic activity against Hep-2 cell line, Colloids and Surfaces B: Biointerfaces 91 (2012) 212–214.
[75] M. Valodkar, et al., Biocompatible synthesis of peptide capped copper nanoparticles and their biological effect on tumor cells, Materials Chemistry and Physics 128 (1–2) (2011) 83–89.
[76] P. Karuppaiya, et al., Anti-metastatic activity of biologically synthesized gold nanoparticles on human fibrosarcoma cell line HT-1080, Colloids and Surfaces B: Biointerfaces 110 (2013) 163–170.
[77] J.R. Nakkala, et al., Comparative study of antioxidant and catalytic activity of silver and gold nanoparticles synthesized from Costus pictus leaf extract, Journal of Materials Science and Technology 31 (10) (2015) 986–994.
[78] M.F. Zayed, et al., In-vitro antioxidant and antimicrobial activities of metal nanoparticles biosynthesized using optimized *Pimpinella anisum* extract, Colloids and Surfaces A: Physicochemical and Engineering Aspects 585 (2020) 124167.
[79] T. Santhoshkumar, et al., Synthesis of silver nanoparticles using *Nelumbo nucifera* leaf extract and its larvicidal activity against malaria and filariasis vectors, Parasitology Research 108 (3) (2011) 693–702.
[80] M. Gnanadesigan, et al., Biosynthesis of silver nanoparticles by using mangrove plant extract and their potential mosquito larvicidal property, Asian Pacific Journal of Tropical Medicine 4 (10) (2011) 799–803.
[81] C.R. Patra, et al., Fabrication of gold nanoparticles for targeted therapy in pancreatic cancer, Advanced Drug Delivery Reviews 62 (3) (2010) 346–361.
[82] E. Turunc, et al., Green synthesis of silver and palladium nanoparticles using Lithodora hispidula (Sm.) Griseb. (Boraginaceae) and application to the electrocatalytic reduction of hydrogen peroxide, Materials Chemistry and Physics 202 (2017) 310–319.

CHAPTER 11

Patents on naturally derived pharmaceuticals

11.1 Introduction

The study, development, and marketing of functional bioactive components and nutraceuticals are gaining popularity across the world. Consumer knowledge of the link between nutrition, health, and illness has led to an increase in the intake of plant-derived bioactive components in the last 2 decades [1,2]. Humans have always been on the lookout for natural goods that can boost biologic functioning and help people live longer, better, and fitter lives. Plants are one of nature's greatest assets, with a long history of usage as traditional food and medicine dating back to antiquity. The global growth in human health issues, on the other hand, has always posed a serious challenge to medical science. As a result, the desire to deal with natural foods has risen at the same time. In addition, numerous researches have been undertaken to extract other useful components from the plants for diverse applications, ranging from water treatment to generating live-saving medications [3–5].

Nonnutritive plant-based bioactive components with disease-preventive characteristics are known as phytochemicals. Phytochemical consumption in the diet promotes health benefits and protects the body from sickness. Because of their many uses, these plant-derived bioactive components have lately gained a lot of attention. Components of ancient systems of medicine, contemporary medications, nutraceuticals, dietary supplements, folk remedies, pharmaceutical intermediates, and chemical entities for synthesized pharmaceuticals can all be found in medicinal plants. Phytochemicals can be found in a variety of foods, including whole grains, fruits and vegetables, and nuts. These phytochemicals, alone or in combination, offer enormous therapeutic promise in the treatment of a variety of illnesses. Because of their positive impacts on human health, phytochemicals with nutraceutical qualities found in food are extremely important. Cancers, coronary heart disease, diabetes, high blood pressure, inflammation, microbial, viral, and

Advances in Extraction and Applications of Bioactive Phytochemicals
ISBN 978-0-443-18535-9
https://doi.org/10.1016/B978-0-443-18535-9.00008-9

parasite infections, psychotic illnesses, spasmodic conditions, ulcers, osteoporosis, and related disorders and other diseases are all protected by them.

Phytochemicals have a high antioxidant capacity and are of great interest because of their positive effects on human health. They also provide other significant health advantages to consumers, including antiinflammatory, antimetabolic, anticancer, antineuralgic, and wound-healing advantages. The antioxidant property of the phytochemical has been widely explored in recent years. In vitro antioxidants and in vivo antioxidants are the two types of natural antioxidants. Polyphenols, anthocyanidins, flavonoids, glucosinolates, isoflavonoids, phytoestrogens, limonoids, terpenoids, carotenoids, phytosterolsand, and fibers are among the phytochemicals described as having possible health advantages [6–8].

High-tech enterprises and economic prosperity are built on innovation. Modern macroeconomic growth models emphasize the importance of innovation and the competition that fosters it, as well as the interaction between small entrants and large incumbents. Simultaneously, a vast body of microeconomic data suggests that research and development is underinvested, with social rates of return being more than twice as high as private rates. This is one of the most compelling arguments for government support of innovation, and patent rights are one of the most important governmental tools available. It is critical to know if patents are a viable innovation incentive and, more crucially, whether they function equally effectively for small and large businesses, as well as in diverse competitive settings.

The topic of patents has gained a lot of traction recently and has received a lot of coverage in the media. If you get much of your knowledge on patents from the media, you may have a mistaken picture of what patents are, what they do, and the benefits and drawbacks.Therefore, it is essential to acquire knowledge on patents by consulting the appropriate sources. It is becoming increasingly necessary for scientists who make discoveries to comprehend the significance of patents in today's world and to thoroughly understand the patent system to ensure that the goals they set for their discoveries can be met [9].

The objective of this chapter is to present a complete overview of patents produced in the previous 2 decades that relate to the extraction of phytochemicals and their application in the food and pharmaceutical industries, as well as in other fields. This chapter contains patents relating to the development of novel extraction methods and the applications of these technologies in various fields. The purpose of this chapter of the book is to encourage researchers to identify new research gaps and attempt to bridge such gaps using their knowledge and expertise.

11.2 Patents on naturally derived pharmaceuticals

11.2.1 Extraction of pharmaceutically active components from plant materials

Extracting pharmaceutically active constituents from plant materials and synthesizing a botanical drug substance (BDS) for inclusion in medication is the focus of this patent (US7344736B2). BDS purity is also an issue, as it might be used in pharmaceuticals. BDSs containing cannabinoids extracted from cannabis are particularly relevant here.

In 2008, Whittle et al. were awarded this patent. Methods for extracting herbal medicine substances from medicinal cannabis have been revealed by the research team. Three stages are involved in the procedure. The first step is to decarboxylate chopped cannabis (2–3 mm in diameter) by heating it to 100–150°C for an extended period of time. At a packing density of 0.3, CO_2 extraction was carried out at supercritical conditions of 600 bar at 35°C for 4 h; however, different combinations of temperature and pressure ranging from 10 to 35°C were also possible in step two. In the final step, filtration removes the waxy particles after 24 h of ethanolic precipitation at 20°C.

In 1822, Baron Cagniard de le Tour discovered that when certain materials were heated in a closed glass container, the gas–liquid barrier vanished, paving the way for the development of supercritical fluid extraction (SFE). The first time a substance's critical point was determined was through this early research. It is possible for a material to exist in gas, liquid, and solid phases if it is heated above the critical point. Later, it was discovered that substances might be utilized as sophisticated solvents for the extraction and fractionation of complicated combinations by heating and pressing them to or above their critical temperatures and pressures. Plant and fish oils have both been processed using this method, which is commonly utilized in the fuel oil processing industry.

It is more enticing to use SFE than traditional solvents because of the ability to regulate the solvent power (E°) by changing pressure and temperature above the critical point, as opposed to traditional solvents. There are three lines in a typical pressure-temperature diagram for a material that defines the equilibrium between two phases. The triple point is where these lines intersect. The lines describe the transition between gas, liquid, and solid states, and the spots along the line establish the phase equilibrium. The boiling point (vapor pressure) curve, for instance, begins at the triple point and finishes at the critical point. At this point, the critical area begins, and a supercritical fluid is defined as any material that is over its critical pressure and temperature. Thus, the temperature at which pressure may convert a gas to liquid is known as the critical temperature. Whereas, the greatest pressure at which an increase in temperature may transform a liquid into a normal gas is known as the critical pressure. There is just one phase in the so-called critical area, and it exhibits some of the characteristics of both a gas and a liquid.

CO_2, with a critical temperature of 31.1°C and a critical pressure of 73.8 bar, has been chosen as the applicant's preferred solvent. The great degree of selectivity that may be accomplished was a crucial criterion in the initial selection of liquid CO_2 as the solvent for the creation of a high potency standardized extract of the cannabis plant. Solvating power in the CO_2 system has been demonstrated to be essentially a function of density and temperature, with solvent density being the more critical component. Subcritical rather than supercritical cannabis extraction is preferred by the applicant, contrary to what was expected. By regulating temperature and pressure below the supercritical temperature and pressure, the applicant has been able to separate certain lipophilic or hydrophilic fractions rich in cannabinoids with other components readily separated to provide a pharmaceutically acceptable BDS. As a result, chemicals in botanical raw materials that are recognized to be active agents can be isolated from their complicated combinations. As a result of adopting subcritical conditions, selective extraction is possible. The application, on the other hand, discovered that using SFE as the solvent, in addition to solubilizing the desired cannabinoids, also solubilized additional nontarget compounds that were difficult to separate out in a subsequent clean-up process.

Decarboxylation, extraction with liquid CO_2, and reducing the proportion of nontarget materials in the extract are all included in one aspect of the invention. The extraction with liquid CO_2 is carried out under subcritical conditions at a temperature between 5 and 15°C and a pressure between 50 and 70 bar during the liquid CO_2 extraction step. Further, the inventor claimed that the technique of the invention could be utilized to extract cannabinoids from cannabis plant material. The ideal use of the procedure is to generate a BDS, such as a marijuana extract [10].

11.2.2 Pharmaceutical and therapeutic compositions derived from *Garcinia mangostana* L plant

This invention pertains to pharmacologic, therapeutic, nutritional, cosmetic, and dermatological formulations obtained from the *Garcinia mangostana* L plant's pericarp (rind), as well as the innovative extraction procedures utilized to make such compositions. The invention is concerned with a 0.01%–80% mixture of a xanthone-rich mangosteen pericarp (rind) extract in innovative combinations for pharmacologic, cosmetic, medicinal, or dermatological formulations that provide significant health advantages. In addition, the invention pertains to unique extraction procedures that result in the creation of the invention's innovative compositions.

In 2006, Alex Moffett and Parag Shah were awarded this patent. *G. mangostana*, an abundant source of natural xanthones, is used in the present invention to create an antioxidative composition having highly concentrated xanthone components used topically for the treatment of various human illnesses and disorders. In addition to its popular name, the mangosteen plant is also known by a variety of other names in other languages. Its spherical, dark-purple to red-purple, and smooth exterior is topped by the large calyx at the stem end, which is adorned with four to eight triangular, flat remains of the stigma in a rosette at the apex. Red in cross-section and purplish-white on the interior, the rind contains bitter yellow latex and a purple staining fluid that is 6–10 mm thick and red in cross-section. Snow-white, luscious, delicate flesh is divided into four to eight triangular parts (actually the arils of the seeds). As many as five completely grown ovoid-oblong seedlings, which are about 2.5 cm long and 1.64 cm broad, are attached to the fruit.

Pharmaceutical, therapeutic, cosmetic, and dermatologic formulations generated from the *G. mangostana* L (mangosteen) plant pericarp are the subject of this invention. Among the first goals of the invention is to create naturally xanthone-rich pharmaceuticals and cosmetic products that are easy to make and formulate while also providing health benefits such as reducing the effects of photo-oxidation, which can lead to cancer and aging when exposed to ultraviolet (UV) radiation. UVA (320–400 nM), UVB (280–320 nM), and UVC (less than 280 nM) wavelengths are used to classify the three types of UV radiation. A unique extraction procedure yielding remarkable antioxidative health effects from mangosteen's pericarp/rind has resulted in novel compositions ranging from around 0.1% to nearly 80% xanthone-rich concentrate combination. Antioxidant-rich, antiseptic, antibacterial, and antiviral properties abound in the compositions of the present invention, which are also simple to make, have a positive impact on the body's immune system, and promote wound healing.

Also, in accordance with one of the invention's second objectives is the provision of a method to produce pharmaceuticals and therapeutic and nutritional products derived from the *G. mangostana* L plant that are rich in natural xanthones and that provide the therapeutic effects of the mangosteen pericarp (rind), either alone or with other complementary and enriching components. Preparation of highly concentrated extracts and less concentrated extracts, as well as their blending or admixture, are the imaginative methods used to create the various compositions. Tannings are also lowered by these methods relative to their naturally occurring amounts in the xanthone-rich extracts. The concentration of tannins can be controlled independently of the concentration of xanthones by dissociating the relative degree of concentration of xanthones and tannins. Tannin's antioxidant effectiveness can be maximized while avoiding its harmful, perhaps lethal effects at high doses by modifying or controlling its concentration on its own.

Techniques for treating or preventing skin problems caused by solar exposure and the generation of reactive oxygen species were the goal of this research. Additionally, the *G. mangostana* xanthone-rich extract is coupled with other agents that offer therapeutic or cosmetic advantages for the skin, as a goal of this invention, increasing the efficiency and benefit that each agent would provide alone [11].

11.2.3 Hot-melt extruded compositions containing plant-derived phenolic materials and processes for the preparation thereof

The invention is concerned with composition delivery systems and techniques in pharmaceutical applications, and more specifically with compositions for enhancing the stability, solubility, and in vivo administration of plant-derived phenolic compounds.

Plant-derived phenolic compounds need to be stabilized, solubilized, and delivered into the body in a more efficient manner. For example, bioflavonoids and anthocyanidins are powerful antioxidants found in plants that have the potential to improve the health of humans and other living organisms. It is difficult to transfer these molecules into living organisms, and target tissues in a regulated manner suffer from low solubility in aqueous systems and are susceptible to oxidation, both thermal and light-induced. There are a few chemicals that, based on their melting points and their potential integration into low-melting-point medicinal carriers, do not appear to be ideal candidates for this type of application.

Many diverse materials, devices, dosage forms, and systems have been produced using hot-melt extrusion (HME). Compounds with low aqueous solubility would otherwise have poor bioavailability when fed to people and animals; however, by adding suitable excipients and HME, compounds with increased solubility and bioavailability have been produced. When it comes to making solid dispersions, newer HME technologies such as solvent evaporation may be a better alternative. To name a few advantages, the removal of solvents, a more comprehensive range of product shapes, and improved medication delivery efficiency are all essential factors.

HME processing temperatures are limited by the stability of the excipients utilized because many of them are thermally unstable. As a result, the majority of HME processing takes place at or around the melting point or glass transition temperature of the principal excipient or excipients employed in HME formulations. Many of the other excipients in the formulation, including the physiologically active ingredient of interest, such as some medicines and plant-derived phenolic compounds, are unstable when handled at high temperatures. Plant phenolic materials, such as trans-resveratrol and quercetin, are clearly not good candidates for HME processing because of their high melting points and crystallinity, which would necessitate HME processing at temperatures well above those commonly used for the process and above the maximum tolerated temperature of many commonly used excipients.

An embodiment of the invention provides a hot-melt extruded composition that may include approximately 20%—80% weight of a plant-derived phenolic material; approximately 20%—85% weight of one or more edible or bioerodible excipients; approximately 0%—40% weight of a surface-active material; approximately 0%—40% weight of an oral absorption enhancer; and approximately 0%—10% weight of one or more pharmaceutical or food-grade additives. As a result, the plant-derived phenolic material has not degraded significantly in a hot-melt extruded composition that was prepared by heating the composition to a temperature below the melting point of the plant-derived phenolic material [12].

Methods for making and utilizing a hot-melt extruded composition incorporating phenolic plant material are an object of the invention.

11.2.4 Process for producing an antioxidant extract from the bearberry plant

This invention pertains to the use of plant extracts as antioxidants and natural food preservatives, and more specifically to bearberry extracts and procedures for manufacturing them. Ronald Bruce Pegg, Branka Barl, and Ryszard Amarowicz received the patent in 2003.

Flavor degradation, potential hazardous compounds, discoloration of pigments, and loss of nutritional content are consequences of lipid oxidation in food. Because of this, the oxidative breakdown of cooked beef lipids is particularly dangerous (e.g., autoxidation). Singlet oxygen, UV light, heat, meat ions, and pigments all function as catalysts in these processes. It appears that autoxidation is also influenced by the level of unsaturation in the lipids.

Antioxidants are molecules that, when present in low amounts in foods or the body, considerably delay or prevent oxidation. They help reduce autoxidation, rancidity, color loss, and nutritional loss in foods prior to heat processing. They do so by binding metal ion catalysts, reducing primary oxidation products to nonradical chemicals, breaking chains to prevent ongoing hydrogen abstraction from substrates, and forming a complex with the lipid molecule. Butylated hydroxyanisole (BHA), butylated hydroxytoluene (BHT), propyl gallate, and tert-butylhydroquinone are the most regularly utilized food-grade synthetic antioxidants.

Natural antioxidants are becoming more popular as a replacement for synthetic ones because of the possible carcinogenicity of BHA and BHT. Particular attention has been paid to the creation and application of antioxidants from edible plant species as a research focus. Several herbs and spices, such as rosemary, sage, oregano, thyme, clove, ginger, and marjoram, have been studied for their antioxidant properties in food. Researchers have shown that the active components found in spices and herbs, or extracts made from them, are usually phenolic acids, flavonoids, or tannins. An issue with some plant-based antioxidant preparations is that they might have a flavoring effect on the foods to which they are added. Although it can be beneficial in some situations, it is more often than not a negative trait. In powder and liquid form, Duralox and rosemary extract are plant-derived antioxidants that are commercially available preservatives.

Antioxidants, both synthetic and from natural sources, are utilized to maintain the nutritional value of a wide range of foods. Typically, antioxidants are added to meals when they can be easily incorporated. Antioxidant-rich sodium nitrite, for example, is a vital ingredient in curing meat products. Brine pickle is injected into whole muscle products as a brine pickle or added to meat batters directly. Spices and herbs, which include natural antioxidants, are also added to other meat formulations, such as fresh or cooked uncured sausages and salamis, or injected into hams as a pickle.

Antioxidants derived from natural or synthetic sources, such as BHT, cannot be used in meals that have been heated. This is due to the antioxidants' heat lability, which means that regular cooking temperatures degrade or eliminate their antioxidative potency.

Alternatively, a food preservative containing a bearberry plant extract is included in the new innovation. Additionally, the preservative in the invention is derived from the bearberry plant and is included in the food in one form or another. Muscle food might be included in the meal. The extracted preservative may also be used to preserve pork meat [13].

11.2.5 Use of bamboo leaf flavone in preparing cosmetics and food additives

Total flavonoid of the bamboo leaf can be used as an antiaging component in cosmetic formulations. Antiaging properties are a primary goal of this development. It has been shown that a flavonoid derived from bamboo leaves is efficient against free radicals, oxidative damage to skin cells, and radiation damage to the skin cells, microbes, and bacteria while lowering melanin development and skin aging without irritating or reacting to the skin or mucosa. The aroma of bamboo may be added to cosmetics in a unique way. It may be used in a variety of cosmetic formulations, including skin nourishment products, sunscreen, antiwrinkle and skin-whitening products, face cleansers, bath lotion, and more. In 2004, Ying Zhang Xiaoqin Wu and Boyi Lu were given this patent.

Cosmetics for daily use are the focus of the innovation. The use of antiaging skin-care components in cosmetics to bamboo leaf total flavones is the subject of innovation. Flavonoids found in bamboo leaf total flavones are a natural antiaging skin-care ingredient that can help reduce the appearance of fine lines and wrinkles. This ingredient can be found in a wide range of personal care products.

Cosmetics are a highly sought-after commodity, and their consumption tends to reflect the zeitgeist of the time in which they are purchased. Consumers are becoming increasingly wary of using cosmetics containing chemical substances as medical science continues to advance. This naturalization of raw materials has sparked a global boom in the development of natural resources in recent years. Slowing down the aging process has become an increasingly popular research issue as a result of rising living standards brought on by economic growth. Everyone aspires to have attractive, healthy, and youthful-looking skin. Besides protecting the skin, it is important to help minimize skin aging. This has led to an increase in the number of antiaging cosmetics on the market today.

Maintaining one's health and well-being is impossible without the proper care of one's skin. The body's first line of defense is its direct interaction with the outside world, and it is particularly vulnerable to environmental variables.

Stress, pollution, sunshine, and UV radiation all contribute to the formation of wrinkles on the skin, in addition to aging factors.

As we age, our skin begins to lose its suppleness and develop wrinkles and other pigmentation issues, such as melasma and age spots. There are two basic components to the aging of our skin. Free radical damage to the skin is thought to be a significant element in the aging process of the skin, according to the idea of aging free radicals. Malondialdehyde (MDA) is produced when the body's overabundance of reactive oxygen free radicals interacts with unsaturated fatty acids. The brown pigment is generated on the skin when MDA interacts with proteins on the cell membrane. This pigment then precipitates and takes on a variety of colors. The skin's collagen and elastin fibers can cross-link and denature under the influence of free radicals, resulting in brittleness and a loss of elasticity. Elastic fibers are prone to rupturing and forming wrinkles when the skin is dehydrated. Slower renewal metabolism and decreased proliferation and division of dermal fibroblasts are additional contributing factors to skin aging. The skin of the aged is noticeably thinner, and the number of skin keratinocytes and fibroblasts is markedly decreased. To combat the effects of aging, several skin-care treatments are designed to encourage the growth of new skin cells. Reduced skin free radical generation combined with increased superoxide dismutase (SOD) activity and a proliferative impact on skin cells may help speed up skin tissue regeneration and improve collagen formation, as well as protect skin hydration and slow down the aging process.

For successful skin care, the skin-care industry agrees on two points: (1) wet skin-care products should be used at a young age, and (2) skin must be protected from UV radiation. Despite the fact that fine wrinkles on the skin have been minimized, with current technology, some progress has been achieved, but the best strategy to prevent wrinkles from appearing is to delay and minimize their emergence. According to Chanel's Mausner, as the population ages and the environment deteriorates, people's skin will age and become more severe, necessitating the usage of long-lasting, highly efficient conditioning and preventive skin-care products. Cosmeceuticals, according to Elizabeth Arden, are the current trend in the skin-care market.

Flavonoids are found throughout the plant kingdom. More than 2000 species have been found so far, the majority of which are glycosides, with a few in their free form. They have a wide range of physiologic and biologic impacts. They have excellent UV and visible light absorption and are exceptionally stable in the visible and ultraviolet areas due to their conjugate structure. Antibacterial, antiphotosensitivity, antioxidation, detoxifying, and whitening properties are also found in naturally produced flavonoids. They have the ability to eliminate free radicals from the skin, prevent free radical damage to cells, stimulate skin metabolism, enhance skin suppleness, and postpone skin aging.

The current invention aims to supply bamboo leaf total flavonoids and antiaging skin-care ingredients produced from bamboo leaves. An application of bamboo leaf total flavones in cosmetics is given in the first aspect of the present invention. The bamboo leaf total flavones are applied in cosmetics as an antiaging skin-care element. A cosmetic product containing 0.001 to 10 weight% (more preferably 0.005 to 1 weight%) of bamboo leaf total flavones is provided in a second aspect of the present invention [14].

11.2.6 Production of catechin from natural sources using membrane-based technology

The goal of this invention is to develop a membrane-based technique for purifying and concentrating flavonoid chemicals such as flavones, flavanones, flavanols, flavonols, isoflavones, and flavon-3-ols from natural sources.

In the plant kingdom, flavonoids are secondary metabolites that are found in abundance. It has been shown that flavonoids have antioxidant and antiinflammatory properties as well as stimulating detoxification enzyme activity and inhibiting transcription factor activation as well as inducing apoptosis in the cell cycle, as well as regulating cell invasion and angiogenesis and interfering with receptor binding. Flavonoid components have become prominent in the pharmaceutical business as additives due to their medical benefits. Leafy green tea, citrus peels, berries, ginkgo biloba, parsley, pulses, tea, sea buckthorn, and onions are all excellent sources of flavonoids. Bamboo leaves, grapes, apples, and countless other natural sources also contain minor amounts of them. *Camellia sinensis* is employed here as a source for this experimental study.

Catechin chemicals have been extracted by a number of studies. The procedure of treating black tea-containing tea cream components in instant hot water and then treating the concentrated extract with catechins is covered by patent US4680193A. EP1767097A2 is a patent for a method of extracting epigallocatechin gallate from green tea. The tea extract was made by heating green tea extract to between 25 and 60°C before passing it through a nanofiltration membrane.

Catechins and polyphenols, two physiologically active chemicals, are extracted using a technique described in patent WO1999008693. The extracted compound is then used in food processing or pharmaceutical manufacturing. The extraction of polyphenols from the leaves of *C. Sinensis* has been done using microwave-aided extraction, although the procedure has no effect on the quality of the products that are produced. Chloroform, acetone, acetonitrile, and ethyl acetate have been used in several studies to extract catechins from the leaves of *C. Sinensis*, which is very undesired. A two-step extraction technique for the green *C. Sinensis* EGC and EGCG enhanced fraction was also described. Catechins from *C. Sinensis* may be extracted using lignocellulose as an adsorbent; however, this has only been reported by a few studies. The extraction of catechins has been reported to use a variety of methods. However, these methods fall short of delivering an effective extraction process. It is necessary to devise a new approach to overcoming the obstacles that now stand in the way of these procedures.

Concentrated aqueous catechins combination may be produced from plant sources and used in pharmaceutical-grade supplements as described in this study. There is a method of extracting catechins that does not require the use of chemical solvents and instead relies on water. Several benefits, including decreased energy consumption, product quality control using a suitable membrane, separation at moderate working temperatures, etc., make this process the most recommended.

This innovation involves a unique and eco-friendly method for extracting catechin from catechin-rich sources using membrane technology. The process involves using membrane cells for cross-flow or batch processing and collecting the membrane cell's catechin-rich permeate for various application [15].

11.2.7 Ginger extract and its preparing method and application

Zingiberaceae, which includes ginger, are perennial herbs with plump, fragrant rhizomes and a pungent, aromatic scent. Ginger is an essential spice, an important part of traditional Chinese medicine, and a versatile plant that may be utilized for medicinal purposes as well as culinary ones. Ginger has antioxidation properties, can eliminate free radicals, and protects the human body from being harmed by free radicals, according to studies. The invention pertains to the field of biomedicine, and more specifically, it relates to a ginger extract, as well as to a method of preparing it and its use in medicine.

The fresh rhizome of Rhizoma Zingiberis Recens (*Zingiber officinale*) is used in Chinese medicine to help digestion and treat stomach discomfort, diarrhea, and general malaise, among other symptoms. This use of Rhizoma Zingiberis Recens has been documented since the year 2000, and it has since surpassed previous records.

Rhizoma Zingiberis Recens' modern pharmacologic research suggests that it has antioxidative, antimicrobial, antiinflammatory, cholesterol-lowering, antiatherogenic, immune-boosting, antiemetic, antiallergic, and antikinetosis properties, as well as hypoglycemic and antiallergic properties, and there is an ethanol extract of Rhizoma Zingiberis Recens. Rhizoma Zingiberis Recens is used in the treatment of rheumatalgia, lumbago, and skelalgia, anemofrigid-damp arthralgia, scapulohumeral periarthritis, malaria, and acute bacillary dysentery, rheumatism, rheumatoid arthritis, lumbar anesthesia, and epidural anesthesia.

Rhizoma Zingiberis Recens has been shown to have functions such as increasing human body metabolism, antiinflammatory and analgesic properties, as well as regulating the function of the male prostate and treatment of prostatic disorders and sexual function barrier. As a result, Rhizoma Zingiberis Recens is frequently utilized in the treatment of male health problems. Rhizoma Zingiberis Recens comprises the pharmacologic research of the reproductive system: the water extract of Rhizoma Zingiberis Recens brings out mouse sperm deformity to cyclophosphamide to have a significant inhibitory effect. The prescription ethanol extraction of Rhizoma Zingiberis Recens and Rhizoma Curcumae Longue compatibility can effectively reduce the quality of rat prostate. The Rhizoma Zingiberis Recens extract of suitable dosage has certain stabilization.

One of the challenges in the field of free radical scavenging is how to generate a pure natural product capable of scavenging free radicals. Ginger extract and its manufacturing technique and use are primarily addressed by this invention (Patent No: CN106924707B). The ginger extract may be utilized to make a free radical—scavenging natural ginger extract. The invention proposes a method for preparing a ginger extract, which includes drying the Rhizoma Zingiberis Recens, and crushing to 70—90 mesh to produce Rhizoma Zingiberis Recens dry powder to address the technical issues. A further method involves the addition of crushed cellulase, pectinase, and cetyl trimethyl ammonium bromide (CTAB) to distilled water and uniformly mixing, wherein the material—liquid ratio of ginger dry powder to the distilled water is 1 g:50—60 mL, and the mass ratio of ginger dry powder to the crushed substances is 1 g:6—10 mg. The method is accomplished by placing the mixed liquid in the water bath at 55—65°C for 20—40 min, stirring, and freeze-drying; adding petroleum ether to the mixture; and drying at a low temperature [16].

11.2.8 Method for producing vanillin and syringaldehyde by catalytic oxidation of alkali lignin of sugarcane residue

A process for preparing lilacaldehyde and vanillin with alkali lignin of cane dregs includes such steps as use of acid to precipitate alkali lignin of cane dregs in waste pulp liquid, filtering, alkaline catalytic oxidization to generate low-molecular products, including lilacaldehyde and vanillin, extracting with organic solvent and then with sodium hydrogen sulfite, distillation, aldehyde-ammonia complexing, recrystallization, sublimation, and separation, and it features use of Fe_2O_3.CuO or Cu type of natural mordenite and Fe_2O_3 as an efficient catalyst to increase output rate and reduce alkali consumption.

The invention is about making syringaldehyde and vanillin from alkali lignin in pulp waste liquid bagasse with the help of a catalyst. Besides organic synthesis, the production method is an important way to get vanillin from natural plant lignin. Vanillin can be extracted from the lignin oxidation products of coniferous wood, and syringaldehyde and vanillin can be extracted from the lignin oxidation products of deciduous wood.

It is claimed in this invention that pulp waste liquid bagasse alkali lignin may be used to make syringaldehyde and vanillin. To begin, acid is used to precipitate the bagasse alkali lignin in the pulp waste liquid. The bagasse alkali lignin is then filtered, and alkaline catalytic oxidation is performed to generate low-molecular products such as syringaldehyde and vanillin. Finally, syringaldehyde compounds are extracted.

Catalytic oxidation of bagasse alkali lignin for the preparation of syringaldehyde and vanillin is provided by the following steps: alkaline lignin extraction from pulp waste liquid, acidification of the bagasse pulp waste liquid to pH 3.5–4.0 with 10% hydrochloric acid, and 50 min of heat preservation at 48–52°C to obtain bagasse alkaline lignin wet filter cake that may either be used for alkaline oxidation or dried to below 60% temperature for lignin extraction, depending on the final product's desired properties. The final step involves catalytic oxidation of bagasse alkali lignin to produce syringaldehyde and vanillin. In an autoclave, the oxidation reaction takes place. With sulfuric acid, it was evaporating the oxidation product extraction solution to dryness, dissolving with n-butanol, extracting syringaldehyde and vanillin with saturated sodium bisulfite water, evaporating to dryness, dissolving methanol, adding ammonia water, standing, filtering, precipitating syringaldehyde ammonia complex, and acidifying the extractive solution with sulfuric acid to pH 2–3.

Using an effective catalyst, the invention provides a process for producing syringaldehyde and vanillin from lignin that is high in yield, low in alkali consumption, and suited for recycling bagasse alkaline pulping waste liquid [17].

11.2.9 Processes for extracting carotenoids and for preparing feed materials

This invention develops a method of carotenoid extraction from various biomass, including the yeast *Phaffia Rhodozyma.* The extraction of carotenoids from these biomasses is accomplished by heating the carotenoid source at an elevated temperature with a solvent mixture that includes water, a hydrophobic carotenoid solvent such as vegetable oil, and a water-soluble co-solvent such as ethanol. Easy integration into the diet, improved bioavailability, and stability against oxidation are only a few of the advantages.

In 2004, Michael Kagan and Sergei Braun were awarded this patent. A method and apparatus for extracting carotenoids from naturally occurring or specially grown biomass, such as biomass rich in carotenoid pigments, is disclosed herein. There are several economic uses for these carotenoids, including pigments and antioxidants for both human and animal use. Because they regularly consume micro-crustacea containing the red pigment astaxanthin, salmonids raised in the wild develop a pink hue. Artificially added astaxanthin is used to provide the desirable pink coloring of salmonid meat when they are raised in captivity. Astaxanthin is needed in the quantity of 60 mg per kilogram of fish feed to obtain this shade of blue. It is also used to enhance the color of farmed fish such as sea bream and shrimp, as well as in aquaculture. Salmonid coloration has been achieved using both synthetic and natural astaxanthin. To keep costs down, synthetic formulations have mostly replaced natural sources. Astaxanthin-rich biomass such as yeast *P. rhodozyma*, algae *Haematococcus pluvalis*, and crustacean products have been directly included into the salmonid diet in natural-source formulations. Even though astaxanthin may be directly incorporated, it is not cost-effective compared with the synthetic product since the fish's digestive system does not have the capacity for extracting astaxanthin from biomass cells; in other words, this source has a poor bioavailability for astaxanthin. The natural sources of lycopene and carotene, two other economically significant carotenoids, are likewise more expensive at the moment than their synthetic counterparts. Astaxanthin and other carotenoids are economically important, and several strategies have been developed to optimize the production of carotenoid-rich biomasses and improve carotenoid extraction from them.

Using the current invention, a method for extracting a carotenoid from a carotenoid source, which includes heating the carotenoid source, a multiphase solvent combination comprising water, a hydrophobic carotenoid solvent, and a water-soluble co-solvent, is presented. It is possible that the carotenoid source contains water, either as a supplement or as a naturally occurring component. Multiphase mixtures often have two distinct phases, one aqueous and the other nonaqueous or oily; however, this is not always the case. During the treatment, the biomass is best agitated, for example swirled. The extraction is carried out over a length of time that is at least 30 min, but preferably between 30 min and 3 h. Hydrophobic solvents, such as edible oils, methyl acetates, ethyl acetates, butyl acetates, alkanes with carbon numbers 5 or higher, and chloroforms, are preferred because they combine hydrophobic qualities with acceptable solvent abilities for carotenoid pigments. Carotenoid is preferably chosen to have at least some limited capacity to dissolve the co-solvent, while the co-ability solvent's to transfer carotenoid dissolved in it to the solvent is determined by the co-partition solvent's coefficient. Alcohol, ketone, or ether can be used as a co-solvent. A monoalkyl ester of ethylene glycol (Cellosolve) or 1,3-dioxane or 1,4-dioxane is preferred as the water-soluble co-solvent, as are methanol, ethanol, n-propanol, and iso-propanol. A carotenoid solution in edible oil may be created directly by utilizing the edible oil as the solvent; however, in some instances, it is beneficial to use a hydrophobic solvent and then combine the hydrophobic solvent with edible oil and evaporate it from there. Preferably, the hydrophobic solvent evaporated during the extraction procedure will be re-used. Carotenoid solutions in edible oils can be prepared by combining carotenoid solution in a water-immiscible solvent with the oil and then evaporating the solvent from the combination, according to another aspect of this invention. Carotenoid extraction is carried out as previously described to produce a solution of carotenoid in edible oil, which is then added to feed components for the production of feed material, according to the invention [18].

11.2.10 Aromatic carbon-coated iron-aluminum nanocomposite and its green synthetic process

A green synthetic approach for synthesizing coated iron-aluminum nanocomposite was developed in this invention. Specifically, the focus of this research is to develop a procedure for the synthesis of the nanocomposite made by using the clove extract for diverse applications [19,20].

In the family of Myrtaceae, clove (*Syzgium aromaticum*) is regarded as an aromatic flower bud with therapeutic properties. In Asian, African, and Middle Eastern cuisine, it is an essential ingredient. Due to its strong antioxidant content, clove has been used for a variety of medical purposes. The ability to act as a better antioxidant agent is greatly enhanced by foods high in polyphenolic chemicals, particularly flavonoids. Flavonoids are polyphenolic substances that may be found in a variety of medicinal plants, fruits, vegetables, and drinks. Due to the presence of numerous hydroxyl groups at certain locations, such compounds have a greater antioxidant and anticancer activity, as well as a C2—C3 double bond. Among flavonoids' beneficial effects include their antihepatotoxic, osteoporotic, allergenic, and antiinflammatory capabilities. As a result, these chemicals are regarded as powerful regulators of cell cycle progression and might be studied further in the hopes of preventing carcinogenesis. Additionally, clove contains flavonoid glycosides (like rutin), which implies flavonoids bound to sugar. Using enzymes or acidic conditions, free flavonoid aglycones can be produced by hydrolysis of glycosidic bonds. Flavonoids including gallic acid (phenol), quercetin (flavonol), rutin (glycoside coupled flavonol), and catechin (flavan-3-ol) were studied in this work for the manufacture of clove extract.

Nanoparticles like Au and Ag have been synthesized via green synthesis for a long time because of their broad use in the biomedical area. It is easy and affordable to synthesize stable nanoparticles using plant extracts as a green synthesis source. The fluorescence and phosphorescence activity of quercetin and rutin has been the subject of several studies. Fluorescence intensity was shown to be affected by rutin and quercetin when they were combined with bovine serum albumin and hemoglobin. Several studies have shown that the fluorescence activity of these flavonols directly affects the detection of different proteins and DNA. Green nanocomposites, including fluorescence-based flavonols coating on their surface, have never been used before to construct nanocomposite-based metal sensors. Metal-metal nanocomposites comprising graphene oxide and activated carbon have been developed to date with the goal of delivering carbon-containing groups and functional groups via surface modifications for improved adsorption. So Purkait and coworkers synthesized and characterized a new green iron-aluminum nanocomposite and tested its ability to remove fluoride from a water supply.

Green synthetic method development for coated iron-aluminum nanocomposite synthesis is a major goal of the innovation. Additionally, a green synthesis procedure for photoluminescent, aromatic carbon-coated iron-aluminum nanocomposite is the goal of the invention. Methods for making photoluminescent, aromatic carbon-coated iron-aluminum nanocomposite using clove extract under microwave irradiation are the particular object of this invention. An additional goal is to create a cost-effective method of producing photoluminescent, aromatic carbon-coated iron-aluminum nanocomposite that is environmentally friendly.

The clove extract is obtained by stirring finely powdered dried cloves into boiling water at 80°C using a magnetic stirrer. It is necessary to keep the clove extract ratio greater than that of the aqueous metal-metal salt solution to ensure effective metal reduction and, therefore, easier synthesis of nanocomposites.

Metal chloride and aluminum chloride are both 0.1 M solutions. The pH is maintained at 6.9 ± 0.5 with 200 rpm of stirring. For 15 min, 600 Watts of microwave radiation is used to irradiate the area. Using a hot plate set to 70°C, the mixture was stirred for an additional 10–15 min. For a further 30–40 min, the mixture was maintained at room temperature. The sp2 hybridized carbon groups (C=C and C=O) and −OH groups with lone pair of electrons over the iron-aluminum nanocomposite coating are used to make a photoluminescent, aromatic carbon-coated iron-aluminum nanocomposite.

11.2.11 Compositions of catechin flavonoids mixture

Methods for separating a catechin combination using membrane separation technology are the subject of this invention. Secondary metabolites known as catechins are found throughout the plant kingdom. Catechin may be found in the green leaves of *C. sinensis*, which are a good source. Other natural sources also include them in lower amounts. This experiment was carried out using *C. sinensis* as a source.

Oxidative characteristics, stimulation of detoxifying enzyme activity, inhibition of transcription factor activation, suppression of cell-signaling pathways, induction of apoptosis, cell cycle control, and prevention of cell invasion and angiogenesis are all ascribed to catechins' health benefits. Catechin components have become prominent in the pharmaceutical business because of their therapeutic properties. Tumor cell elimination without hurting the normal cells of the same tumor carrier is still a difficult task despite substantial developments in medical technology for detection and therapy, making cancer a potentially lethal menace to the global population. During cancer chemotherapy, a number of commonly prescribed and effective medications have adverse side effects, including liver damage, oxidative stress, and immune system suppression in the patient with the tumor. As a result, successful cancer therapy needs specific targeting and minimal toxicity for normal host tissues, which catechins meet. Carbohydrate metabolism is disrupted when blood sugar levels rise over the typical range. There is strong epidemiologic evidence that dietary flavonoids may protect against diabetes; however, this has yet to be proven in humans. Polyphenols from *C. sinensis* have been shown in animal studies to reduce blood glucose levels. Because the insulin receptor, the insulin receptor substrate, the hosphoinositide 3-kinase enzyme, and the mitogen-activated protein kinase enzyme are all tyrosine-phosphorylated, the tea components in tea imitate insulin. Phosphoinositide 3-kinase regulates gene expression of phosphoenolpyruvate carboxykinase and gluconeogenic enzymes as well as protein tyrosine phosphorylation. Polyphenols' antioxidant qualities have also been shown to lessen the risk of illnesses caused by free radicals. Thus, catechins from *C. sinensis* can be termed antidiabetic in animals without causing any harm to them.

The pathophysiology of cardiovascular disease is assumed to have a significant oxidative component, especially in terms of lipid oxidation, and dietary antioxidants, such as catechins from *C. sinensis*, have been reported to provide preventive advantages. Sufficient antioxidant consumption, according to one explanation for atherogenesis, would limit low-density lipoprotein (LDL) oxidation and hence minimize the development of coronary heart disease.

Free-radical-induced oxidative stress affects renal illness, which is linked to a variety of disorders. In a renal epithelial cell line, catechins significantly reduced oxidative stress caused by free radicals and reduced cell damage. By decreasing the generation of oxidative uremic toxins and enhancing the renal blood circulation state, catechins alleviated excessive oxidation stress and renal hypertension. Catechins were used to enhance renal function by preventing mesangial cell growth. Catechins were discovered to be useful in reducing discomfort associated with renal illness.

Senescence is an aging process that occurs after the age of maturity, characterized by physiologic dysfunctions and a loss of homeostasis. Senescence/aging is assumed to be influenced by oxidative stress as a significant component. Tea catechins have been shown to have therapeutic effects on the aging brain and to extend the human lifetime by avoiding premature mortality. Sufficient daily consumption of catechins may be an efficient way to delay aging.

Tooth decay, gum disease, and tooth loss afflict more people than any other type of illness in the world combined. Oral bacteria may raise the risk of cardiovascular disease, stroke, and lung illness. Catechins have been included in toothpaste and mouthwashes as an auxiliary to mechanical plaque management because of their ability to operate as a way of plaque control. Caries and gingivitis can be prevented by these chemicals in a number of ways, including reducing existing plaque, preventing new plaque formation, inhibiting the expression of cariogenic determinants, suppressing specific cariogenic bacterial species, or inhibiting the metabolism of plaque bacteria.

The goal of the invention is to create formulations that include a catechin combination created using membrane-based technology, as described in Indian patent application number 240/KOL/2010. This technique of formulating has a catechin combination mixed with inert elements such as starch, sucrose, and other inert components that, when combined with catechin, do not produce any reaction products. At various quantities, components such as starch, sucrose, glucose, sorbitol, ethanol, flavor, and color were used in the formulation trials. The formulation's detailed components are listed in Table 11.1.

Moreover, researchers have successfully devised a technique for extracting plant-derived concentrated aqueous catechins mixtures. Catechins were extracted from the permeate of plant products that had been filtered via a polymeric membrane (MWCO 400 and 500 Da). An effective amount of 30%–80% (w/w) catechin component combination and 5%–50% (w/w)

Table 11.1 Composition of five different formulations of tablet preparation.

Sl. no.	Material	A% (wt/wt)	B% (wt/wt)	C% (wt/wt)	D% (wt/wt)	E% (wt/wt)
1	Catechin component mixture	40	55	30	40	80
2	Starch as a filler	50	7	20	5	15
3	Sucrose	3	32	25	5	–
4	Glucose	1.5	5.5	11.5	45	–
5	Sorbitol	2	2	5	2	–
6	Ethanol	3.498	5.498	5.498	3.498	–
7	Flavor	0.001	0.001	0.001	0.001	–
8	Color	0.001	0.001	0.001	0.001	–

Reproduced with permission for Dhadge et al. [15].

starch as a filler, together with or without the inert materials as additives, was derived from the decaffeinated and concentrated permeate. On the contrary, the more crystalline formulations D and E lacked molding characteristics because of their inferior molding qualities [15].

11.3 Summary

Plant seeds have long been utilized as sources of oil for a variety of applications, including nutritional, medicinal, and industrial. They are a by-product of industrial fruit processing and can be obtained straight from the process. To recover bioactive components from plant material, it is necessary to follow certain methods throughout the preextraction and extraction processes. In small-scale research, extraction methods such as hydrodistillation, Soxhlet extraction, and microwave-assisted extraction have traditionally been utilized. These solvents' extracting capacity (organic or inorganic) is entirely dependent on the polarity element of the target compounds, which determines which solvents are used and how effective they are. Various extraction methods have been developed in recent decades to overcome the limitations of classic extraction methods. In addition, phytochemical extraction for a variety of innovative uses is discussed. We have briefly discussed 11 distinct patents relevant to bioactive chemical extraction and application in this chapter. The summary of each invention along with the detailed background study for the patents are presented to provide a brief overview of the patent filing process.

The first patent in this chapter discussed the creation of a BDS SFE technology. A 0.01%–80% blend of a xanthone-rich mangosteen pericarp (rind) extract in unique combinations for pharmacologic, aesthetic, medicinal, or dermatological formulations that give considerable health benefits is the subject of the second patent. The utilization of hot-melt extraction from phytochemical isolation was highlighted in the third one. A technique for manufacturing an antioxidant extract from the bearberry plant was detailed in the fourth patent. Similary. The fifth highlighted how bamboo leaf flavone might be used to make cosmetics and food additives. The sixth one describes the production of catechin from natural sources utilizing membrane-based technology. This chapter also discusses a technique for manufacturing vanillin and syringaldehyde by catalytic oxidation of alkali lignin from sugarcane waste, as well as an aromatic carbon-coated iron-aluminum nanocomposite made from clove extract. Finally, a patent is described that details the formulation of catechin flavonoid mixed tablet formulations.

References

[1] R.F. da Silva, et al., Sustainable extraction bioactive compounds procedures in medicinal plants based on the principles of green analytical chemistry: a review, Microchemical Journal 175 (2022) 107184.
[2] T.N. Baite, B. Mandal, M.K. Purkait, Ultrasound assisted extraction of gallic acid from Ficus auriculata leaves using green solvent, Food and Bioproducts Processing 128 (2021) 1–11.
[3] P. Duarah, D. Haldar, M.K. Purkait, Technological advancement in the synthesis and applications of lignin-based nanoparticles derived from agro-industrial waste residues: a review, International Journal of Biological Macromolecules 163 (2020) 1828–1843.
[4] D. Haldar, M.K. Purkait, Micro and nanocrystalline cellulose derivatives of lignocellulosic biomass: a review on synthesis, applications and advancements, Carbohydrate Polymers 250 (2020) 116937.
[5] M.M. Aji, et al., Biopolymer (gum Arabic) incorporation in waste polyvinylchloride membrane for the enhancement of hydrophilicity and natural organic matter removal in water, Journal of Water Process Engineering 38 (2020) 101569.
[6] H.I. Mohamed, et al., Chapter 18 - date palm (*Phoenix dactylifera* L.) secondary metabolites: bioactivity and pharmaceutical potential, in: R.A. Bhat, K.R. Hakeem, M.A. Dervash (Eds.), Phytomedicine, Academic Press, 2021, pp. 483–531.
[7] A.K. Jha, N. Sit, Extraction of bioactive compounds from plant materials using combination of various novel methods: a review, Trends in Food Science and Technology 119 (2022) 579–591.
[8] N.M. Daud, et al., Valorisation of plant seed as natural bioactive compounds by various extraction methods: a review, Trends in Food Science and Technology 119 (2022) 201–214.
[9] S. Scott, The Importance of Patents for Scientists, Nature Precedings (2008), 1–1. https://doi.org/10.1038/npre.2008.197.
[10] C.A.H. Brian Whittle, I.R. Flockhart, D.V. Downs, P. Gibson, G. William Wheatley, Extraction of Pharmaceutically Active Components from Plant Materials, U.S. Patent, United state, 2008.
[11] A. Moffett, P. Shah, Pharmaceutical and Therapeutic Compositions Derived from Garcinia Mangostana L Plant, Google Patents, 2006.
[12] G. Dorairaju, A.E. Listro, D.R. Worthen, Hot-melt Extruded Compositions Containing Plant-Derived Phenolic Materials and Processes for the Preparation Thereof, Google Patents, 2012.
[13] B.B. Ronald Bruce Pegg, Ryszard Amarowicz, Process for Producing an Antioxidant Extract from the Bearberry Plant, Worldwide, 2000.
[14] X.W. Ying Zhang, B. Lu, Use of Total Flavonoid of Bamboo Leaf in Cosmetic Compositions as Anti-Aging Factor, in Google Patent 2004: Worldwide
[15] V.L. Dhadge, M. Changmai, M.K. Purkait, Purification of catechins from Camellia sinensis using membrane cell, Food and Bioproducts Processing 117 (2019) 203–212.
[16] G.W.L.H.T.C. ltd, Ginger extract and preparation method and application thereof, in: Google Patent C.N.I.P. Administration, 2020 (China).
[17] G.C.C. Ltd, Method for Producing Vanillin and Syringaldehyde by Catalytic Oxidation of Alkali Lignin of Sugercane Residue, in Google Patent, 2001. China.
[18] M. Kagan, S. Braun, Processes for Extracting Carotenoids and for Preparing Feed Materials, Google Patents, 2004.
[19] P. Mondal, M.K. Purkait, Green synthesized iron nanoparticles supported on pH responsive polymeric membrane for nitrobenzene reduction and fluoride rejection study: optimization approach, Journal of Cleaner Production 170 (2018) 1111–1123.
[20] P. Mondal, M.K. Purkait, Preparation and characterization of novel green synthesized iron–aluminum nanocomposite and studying its efficiency in fluoride removal, Chemosphere 235 (2019) 391–402.

Index

Note: 'Page numbers followed by "*f*" indicate figures and "*t*" indicate tables.'

A

Abelmoschus manihot, 203–204
Abutilon indicum, 204–205
Alkaloids, 8–13, 9f
  classification of, 9f
  heterocyclic alkaloids, 8–12, 10f
  nonheterocyclic alkaloids, 12–13
  properties of, 13
Aromatic carbon-coated iron-aluminum nanocomposite, 258–260
Artificial intelligence (AI), 122
  drug design and discovery, 125–127
  plant tissue culture, 123–125
  secondary metabolites from plants, 122–123
Asthma, treatment for, 201
Azadirachta indica, 178–181

B

Bamboo leaf flavone, 251–253
Bearberry plant, antioxidant extract from, 249–251
Bioaccessibility, 19–20
Bioactive compounds for pharmaceutical applications
  high-pressure Soxhlet extraction, 58
  limitations, 69–71, 70t
  microwave-assisted soxhlet extraction, 59
    decoction, 64
    direct steam distillation, 68–69
    hydrodistillation, 65–69
    infusion, 62–64
    maceration, 59–62
    modified maceration process, 61–62, 62f–63f
    percolation, 64–65
    water and steam distillation, 68
    water distillation, 67–68
  solubility, 55
  Soxhlet extraction, 56–59, 62f
  ultrasound-assisted soxhlet extraction, 58–59
Bioactive phytochemical compounds
  active pharmaceutical ingredients (API), 101–102
  alkaloids, 8–13, 9f
  bioaccessibility, 19–20
  bioavailability, 19–20
  encapsulation strategies for
    electrospinning, 151–153, 151f
    electrospraying, 148–151, 149f, 151f
    extrusion, 153–159
    freeze-drying, 144–148, 145f
    layer-by-layer disposition, 159–161
    natural resources, 141
    spray drying, 142–144, 143f
  future perspectives, 161–162
  green chemistry, 104t–105t
  International Council for Harmonization (ICH), 102
  others, 18–19
  pigments, 16–18
  polyphenols, 3–8, 5f–6f, 6t
  Registration, Evaluation, Authorization, and Restriction of Chemicals (REACH), 102
  steroids, 13–15
  terpenes, 15–16
  volatile organic compounds (VOCs), 102
Bioactive phytochemicals, high-throughput screening techniques for, 44–50
  assay development and optimization, 49
  high-throughput screening platforms, 45–49, 46f
  primary and secondary screening, 50
Bioavailability, 19–20

C

Cancer, 202–203
Catalytic oxidation, vanillin and syringaldehyde by, 256–257
Catechin, 253–254
  flavonoids mixture, 260–263, 262t
Centrifugal extrusion, 156–158
Computational methods, bioactive phytochemicals
  Artificial intelligence (AI), 122
    drug design and discovery, 125–127
    plant tissue culture, 123–125
    secondary metabolites from plants, 122–123
  genetic algorithms (GAs), 119–120
  machine learning (ML), 120–121
  molecular docking, 127–132, 129t–130t
    diseases treatment, 131–132
    drug design, 128–131, 135–136
    molecular dynamics simulation, diseases and drug design, 132–136, 133f
    simulation adaptation, 134–135
  protein database (PDB), 121
  root-mean-square deviation (RMSD), 121–122
Copper nanoparticles, 224–225
Cosmetics, 251–253
Curcuma longa, 187–188
Curcumin, 212

D

Deep eutectic solvent preparation, 112–114
  pharmaceutical industries, solvent-free reactions in, 114–115
Diabetes control, 201

E

Electrospinning, 151–153, 151f
Electrospraying, 148–151, 149f, 151f
Electrostatic extrusion, 158–159
Encapsulation strategies
  electrospinning, 151–153, 151f
  electrospraying, 148–151, 149f, 151f
  extrusion, 153–159
  freeze-drying, 144–148, 145f
  layer-by-layer disposition, 159–161
  natural resources, 141
  spray drying, 142–144, 143f
Enzyme-assisted extraction, 89–91
Eutectic solvents, 112–114, 113t
Extracting carotenoids, 257–258
Extrusion, 153–159
  centrifugal extrusion, 156–158
  electrostatic extrusion, 158–159
  hot-melt extrusion, 154–156
  melt injection extrusion process, 156

F

Ferulic acid, 210–212, 211f
Flash extraction, 93–94
Fluorous solvents, 107–109
Food additives, 251–253
Fracture healing, 169f
Freeze-drying, 144–148, 145f

G

Garcinia mangostana L., 246–248
Genetic algorithms (GAs), 119–120
Ginger extract, 254–255
Gold nanoparticles, 223–224
Green synthetic process, 258–260

H

Herb-derived bioactive phytochemicals
  Azadirachta indica, 178–181
  Curcuma longa, 187–188
  fracture healing, 169f
  icariin, 172–173
  immunity boosters, herbal plants as, 177–188
  Ocimum tenuiflorum, 184–185
  orthopedic diseases using herbal extracts, 168–176
  Phyllanthus emblica, 181–182
  Picrorhiza kurroa, 182–184
  Piper nigrum, 185–186
  tetrandrine, 173–175
  tropical delivery applications, herbal nanoformulation in, 188–190
  ursolic acid, 175–176
  Withania somnifera, 185

Zingiber officinale, 186–187
Heterocyclic alkaloids, 8–12, 10f
High-grade herbal product, 75
High-throughput screening platforms, 45–49, 46f
Hot-melt extruded compositions containing plant-derived phenolic materials, 248–249
Hot-melt extrusion, 154–156

I

Icariin, 172–173
Immunity boosters, herbal plants as, 177–188
Infrared-assisted extraction, 91–93
Ionic liquids, 109–112

L

Layer-by-layer disposition, 159–161

M

Machine learning (ML), 120–121
Medicinal efficacy of phytochemicals
curcumin, 212
ferulic acid, 210–212, 211f
myricetin, 213
quercetin, 209–210, 210f
Melt injection extrusion process, 156
Membrane-assisted extraction process, 94–95
Membrane-based technology, 253–254
Metallic nanoparticles
antibacterial, 229–232
anticancer, 233–234
antioxidant, 234
antiviral, 232–233
other applications, 234–235
Metallic nanoparticles biosynthesis, 220–226
Microwave-assisted extraction, 76–78
Microwave-assisted soxhlet extraction, 59
decoction, 64
direct steam distillation, 68–69
hydrodistillation, 65–69
infusion, 62–64
maceration, 59–62
modified maceration process, 61–62, 62f–63f
percolation, 64–65
water and steam distillation, 68
water distillation, 67–68
Molecular docking, 127–132, 129t–130t
diseases treatment, 131–132
drug design, 128–131, 135–136
molecular dynamics simulation, diseases and drug design, 132–136, 133f
simulation adaptation, 134–135
Mucuna pruriens, 207–208
Myricetin, 213

N

Natural products, 47–48
bioactive compound extraction from, 76–95
enzyme-assisted extraction, 89–91
flash extraction, 93–94
future perspectives, 95
infrared-assisted extraction, 91–93
membrane-assisted extraction process, 94–95
microwave-assisted extraction, 76–78
pressurized liquid extraction, 81–85
subcritical water extraction, 87–89
supercritical carbon dioxide extraction, 85–87
ultrasound-assisted extraction, 78–81, 79f
Natural resources, 141
Neoteric solvents for extraction
bioactive phytochemicals
active pharmaceutical ingredients (API), 101–102
green chemistry, 104t–105t
International Council for Harmonization (ICH), 102
Registration, Evaluation, Authorization, and Restriction of Chemicals (REACH), 102
volatile organic compounds (VOCs), 102
deep eutectic solvent preparation, 112–114

Neoteric solvents for extraction (*Continued*)
pharmaceutical industries, solvent-free reactions in, 114–115
synthetic solvents, 103–114
eutectic solvents, 112–114, 113t
fluorous solvents, 107–109
ionic liquids, 109–112
supercritical fluids, 103–107, 106t
Nigella sativa, 198–203, 199f
Abelmoschus manihot, 203–204
Abutilon indicum, 204–205
asthma, treatment for, 201
cancer, 202–203
common effects, 203
diabetes control, 201
Mucuna pruriens, 207–208
Senna auriculatus, 208–209
Solanum surattense, 206–207
Thespesia populnea, 205–206
Nonheterocyclic alkaloids, 12–13
Novel extraction technologies, 75–76
Nuclear magnetic resonance (NMR), 48

O

Ocimum tenuiflorum, 184–185
Orthopedic diseases using herbal extracts, 168–176

P

Patents on naturally derived pharmaceuticals
aromatic carbon-coated iron-aluminum nanocomposite, 258–260
bamboo leaf flavone, 251–253
bearberry plant, antioxidant extract from, 249–251
catalytic oxidation, vanillin and syringaldehyde by, 256–257
catechin, 253–254
flavonoids mixture, 260–263, 262t
cosmetics and food additives, 251–253
extracting carotenoids, 257–258
Garcinia mangostana L., 246–248
ginger extract, 254–255
green synthetic process, 258–260
hot-melt extruded compositions containing plant-derived phenolic materials, 248–249
membrane-based technology, 253–254
plant materials, extraction of pharmaceutically active components from, 245–246
sugarcane residue, alkali lignin of, 256–257
PH, 226–228
Pharmaceutically active compound
bioactive phytochemicals, high-throughput screening techniques for, 44–50
assay development and optimization, 49
high-throughput screening platforms, 45–49, 46f
primary and secondary screening, 50
extracted from flower and seed, 35–40, 36t–38t
extracted from leaves, 31–35, 32t–33t
extracted from stem bark, 40, 41t
extracted from the root, 42–43
other parts of the plant, 43–44
Phyllanthus emblica, 181–182
Picrorhiza kurroa, 182–184
Pigments, 16–18
Piper nigrum, 185–186
Plant-based bioactive molecules
bioaccessibility, 19–20
bioactive phytochemical compounds, 3–19
alkaloids, 8–13, 9f
bioaccessibility, 19–20
bioavailability, 19–20
others, 18–19
pigments, 16–18
polyphenols, 3–8, 5f–6f, 6t
steroids, 13–15
terpenes, 15–16
bioavailability, 19–20
future perspectives, 22–23
naturally occurring, commercialization of, 21–22
Plant-derived metal nanoparticles in pharmaceuticals

copper nanoparticles, 224–225
future perspectives, 235–237
gold nanoparticles, 223–224
limitations, 235–237
metallic nanoparticles
antibacterial, 229–232
anticancer, 233–234
antioxidant, 234
antiviral, 232–233
other applications, 234–235
metallic nanoparticles biosynthesis, 220–226
other metallic nanoparticles, 225–226
pH, 226–228
plant extract concentration, 229
reaction time, 228–229
silver nanoparticles, 222–223
temperature, 228
Plant extract concentration, 229
Plant materials, extraction of pharmaceutically active components from, 245–246
Polyphenols, 3–8, 5f–6f, 6t
properties of, 7–8
Pressurized liquid extraction, 81–85
Protein database (PDB), 121

Q

Quercetin, 209–210, 210f

R

Reaction time, 228–229
Root-mean-square deviation (RMSD), 121–122

S

Senna auriculatus, 208–209
Silver nanoparticles, 222–223
Solanum surattense, 206–207
Solid-phase extraction (SPE), 47–48
Solubility, 55
Soxhlet extraction, 56–59, 62f
Spray drying, 142–144, 143f
Steroids, 13–15
Subcritical water extraction, 87–89
Sugarcane residue, alkali lignin of, 256–257
Supercritical carbon dioxide extraction, 85–87
Supercritical fluids, 103–107, 106t
Synthetic solvents, 103–114
eutectic solvents, 112–114, 113t
fluorous solvents, 107–109
ionic liquids, 109–112
supercritical fluids, 103–107, 106t

T

Temperature, 228
Terpenes, 15–16
Tetrandrine, 173–175
Thespesia populnea, 205–206
Tropical delivery applications, herbal nanoformulation in, 188–190

U

Ultrasound-assisted extraction, 58–59, 78–81, 79f
Ursolic acid, 175–176

W

Withania somnifera, 185

Z

Zingiber officinale, 186–187

FSC
www.fsc.org
MIX
Papier | Fördert gute Waldnutzung
FSC® C083411

Kolibri 360 GmbH
Ferdinand-Jühlke-Straße 7
99095 Erfurt, Deutschland
produktsicherheit@kolibri360.de